Respiratory Disease Series: Diagnostic Tools and Disease Managements

Series Editors:

Hiroyuki Nakamura
Ibaraki Medical Center
Tokyo Medical University
Ibaraki, Japan

Kazutetsu Aoshiba
Ibaraki Medical Center
Tokyo Medical University
Ibaraki, Japan

This book series cover a variety of topics in respiratory diseases, with each volume providing an overview of the current state of knowledge, recent discoveries and future prospects for each disease. In each chapter the editors pose critical questions, which are often unresolved clinical issues. These are then discussed by the authors, providing insights and suggestions as to which developments need to be addressed. The series offers new information, which will inspire innovative ideas to further develop respiratory medicine.This collection of monographs is aimed at benefiting patients across the globe suffering from respiratory disease.
Edited by established authorities in the field and written by pioneering experts, this book series will be valuable to those researchers and physicians working in respiratory medicine. The series is aimed at a broad readership, and the books will also be a valuable resource for radiologists, emergency medicine physicians, pathologists, pharmacologists and basic research scientists.

More information about this series at http://www.springer.com/series/15152

Takeshi Kaneko
Editor

Clinical Relevance of Genetic Factors in Pulmonary Diseases

Springer

Editor
Takeshi Kaneko
Yokohama City University
Yokohama, Kanagawa, Japan

ISSN 2509-5552 ISSN 2509-5560 (electronic)
Respiratory Disease Series: Diagnostic Tools and Disease Managements
ISBN 978-981-10-8143-9 ISBN 978-981-10-8144-6 (eBook)
https://doi.org/10.1007/978-981-10-8144-6

Library of Congress Control Number: 2018948729

Printed on acid-free paper

This Springer imprint is published by the registered company Springer Nature Singapore Pte Ltd.
The registered company address is: 152 Beach Road, #21-01/04 Gateway East, Singapore 189721, Singapore

Preface

Cystic fibrosis, a monogenic hereditary disease that manifests in the lungs, is well known in Western countries and mainly affects Caucasians of Northern European descent, but is rarely seen in Asian populations. However, polygenic hereditary diseases of the lungs are commonly seen across all ethnicities, since most pulmonary diseases are thought to result from interactions between multiple genetic and environmental factors.

For example, chronic obstructive lung disease (COPD) is a common pulmonary disease and cigarette smoking is the main environmental risk factor for developing the disease. Since only approximately 15% of smokers develop COPD, genetic factors are considered to be important for the development of the disease. In fact, more than 100 genes that affect susceptibility to non-hereditary COPD have been reported to date, and each identified gene can explain only a small part of the etiology of COPD. In COPD, genetic factors only become important when environmental factors exist. In contrast, in bronchial asthma, genetic factors are more important than environmental factors. Consequently, bronchial asthma has a very high heritability rate, reportedly as high as 70%. Many genes have been identified that are possibly involved in the susceptibility, activity, and severity of bronchial asthma. These two diseases demonstrate how the contribution of genetic factors varies widely depending on the disease. In this book, we discuss the contribution of genetic factors to common pulmonary diseases that are encountered in daily practice.

The Human Genome Project was finished in 2003 and provided a complete and accurate sequence of the 3 billion DNA base pairs that make up the human genome. We are currently in an era of rapidly expanding knowledge about genetic medicine. It has become possible to determine the genetic contributions to common pulmonary diseases. Understanding the functions of genetic factors in each disease can contribute significantly to various fields of medicine and enable us to identify genotypes or phenotypes of each disease. Based on this information, new therapeutic strategies are being developed, leading to precision medicine. By translating genomic information into clinical practice, we can expect to minimize adverse events and obtain the maximum treatment effect.

Striking progress has been made recently in the treatment of various cancers, including lung cancer. Recent findings of oncogenic driver mutations resulted in a major paradigm shift in the management of non-small cell lung cancer (NSCLC). Treatment for this disease now focuses on a genetic biomarker-based strategy to develop personalized treatment with molecularly targeted agents. Indeed, the prognosis of NSCLC patients given treatments that are personalized based on their identified oncogenic driver mutations has dramatically improved, and their quality of life is significantly better.

To the best of my knowledge, there is currently no textbook that focuses on the roles that genetic factors play in pulmonary diseases. I am convinced that this book is very unique, not only in its discussion of gene abnormality in pulmonary diseases but also in its focus on applying cutting-edge discoveries in genetic medicine to daily clinical practice.

I hope that this book will improve our understanding of pulmonary diseases and lead to more appropriate treatment.

Yokohama, Japan Takeshi Kaneko

Contents

Part I
Introduction

Chapter 1
Clinical Development of Genomic Medicine in Pulmonary Diseases: Are Genetic Factors Enough to Determine the Phenotype and Inheritance of Pulmonary Diseases?

Mari Hikichi, Shuichiro Maruoka, and Shu Hashimoto

Abstract Many pulmonary disease genotypes have been identified in genome-wide association studies using microarray technology. These genetic variants are relatively common but generally explain little about the heritability of disease, a phenomenon known as "missing heritability." This suggests that a genomic approach alone might not be enough to determine the phenotype and heritability of pulmonary diseases. Since the airway is continuously exposed to various environmental factors, the gene–environment interaction is extremely important in the pathogenesis of pulmonary diseases. However, the mechanisms by which environmental factors contribute to the heritability and pathological development of pulmonary diseases remain unknown. Recently, it has been reported that not only the genome but also the epigenome and microbiome are involved in the determination of disease susceptibility and phenotype. Recent advances in analytical techniques have yielded enormous quantities of diverse types of individual biological information, including genomic, epigenomic, transcriptomic, proteomic, metabolomic, and microbiomic data. Using this vast array of biometric information, new pulmonary disease phenotypes will be identified and could be used to develop personalized medicines for patients with pulmonary diseases in the future. This review provides an overview of the current knowledge of the genomic medicine for better understanding of the heritability of pulmonary disease.

Keywords Epigenome · Genomic medicine · Gene–environment interaction
Microbiome · Personalized medicine

M. Hikichi · S. Maruoka (✉) · S. Hashimoto
Division of Respiratory Medicine, Department of Internal Medicine, Nihon University School of Medicine, Tokyo, Japan
e-mail: maruoka.shuichiro@nihon-u.ac.jp

T. Kaneko (ed.), *Clinical Relevance of Genetic Factors in Pulmonary Diseases*, Respiratory Disease Series: Diagnostic Tools and Disease Managements, https://doi.org/10.1007/978-981-10-8144-6_1

1.1 Introduction

Since the airway is in contact with the external environment, it is exposed to various environmental factors (e.g., tobacco, air pollutants, and allergens). Therefore, the etiologies of many respiratory diseases are affected by environmental factors. However, interactions between genetic and environmental factors represent a very important factor in the onset of respiratory diseases; in particular, differences in individual responsiveness to environmental factor exposure result from differences in genetic factors.

This chapter will provide an overview of the history of genomic medicine and outline the current situation and issues of genomic medicine in the context of respiratory disease, the influences of environmental factors on genetic factors (i.e., epigenetic and microbiome control mechanisms), and the applications to personalized medicine.

1.2 History of Genomic Medicine

From the viewpoint of genetic factors, respiratory diseases can be roughly divided into monogenic diseases (e.g., α-1 antitrypsin deficiency) and polygenic diseases (e.g., asthma, chronic obstructive pulmonary disease, and interstitial pneumonia). A monogenic disease is defined as a cellular-level functional abnormality caused by a single genetic variant (mutation). Genetically, such diseases often show very strong inheritance patterns. On the other hand, polygenic diseases, which involve multiple sets of genes, are common in the field of respiratory medicine. Advances in genomic medicine (genomics) according to genetic analyses, which allowed for the elucidation of not only respiratory diseases but also other pathological conditions, represent a major epoch in the history of medicine.

The genome is defined as the complete set of genetic information and its base sequences of DNA (genes) and chromosomes in the organism. This genomic information is thought to underlie the pathogenesis of diseases. Accordingly, studies have mainly focused on monogenic diseases, and genomic medicine has developed with advances in analytical techniques.

In the 1980s, the development of DNA polymorphic markers made it successful to conduct linkage analyses and thus determine the chromosomal loci of genetic diseases in both affected and unaffected family members. Disease genes were identified by positional cloning [1], in which candidate genes identified by linkage analysis were comprehensively analyzed to identify disease-specific mutations. In the 2000s, DNA microarray technology was implemented in practical applications. A microarray is an assay in which thousands to tens of thousands of DNA probes are affixed to a board at a high density. Such assays have enabled comprehensive gene expression analyses. Using this technology, mRNA extracted from a specimen is labeled with a fluorescent tag and hybridized to a DNA probe on a substrate.

Subsequently, the fluorescence intensity is measured with a scanner to quantify the expression level of a target gene. Since its introduction, innovations in microarray technology have progressed and reduced the costs of this assay each year. Currently, microarray is considered an established target gene screening tool in both basic and clinical research settings [2]. Microarray techniques have been used to conduct various comprehensive analyses, which have led to the subsequent identification of disease susceptibility genes for various respiratory diseases.

In 2003, the Human Genome Project identified all human genes [3]. Subsequently, the International HapMap Project was initiated on the basis of the identified human genes with the aim of analyzing patterns of genetic similarity and dissimilarity among races. These analyses revealed the existence of individual differences in human genomic information or "diversity." Furthermore, certain similarities in genomic diversity, or polymorphism, were identified. Tools have been developed to analyze genomic information not only for monogenic diseases but also for common diseases. A high-density microarray was developed to implement information about the tens to hundreds of millions of single-nucleotide polymorphisms (SNPs) distributed throughout the human genome; these SNPs were derived from the aforementioned Human Genome Project and International HapMap Project. Genome-wide association studies (GWASs) are possible because of this array. Accordingly, large-scale genotyping became possible, and the identification of "disease susceptibility genes" began in earnest.

1.3 Issues and Future Prospects of Genomic Medicine (Fig. 1.1)

One characteristic of GWAS-based disease susceptibility gene identification is that previously unreported genes can be identified with high levels of reproducibility within the same race. However, it has some issues that a SNP present at a high frequency in the disease population may itself have only weak effects, and many of the identified SNPs are mapped to nonprotein-coding regions, such as introns or intergenic regions. This theory is based on the "common disease-common variants hypothesis," and many of the identified "disease susceptibility genes" have a relatively small degree of influence (i.e., effect size) on disease onset, as well as low heritability (missing heritability) [4–6]. In other words, rare variants with large effect sizes and unknown polymorphisms might be undetectable by GWASs. From a technical point of view, next-generation sequencing (NGS), which is based on the massively parallel sequencing of DNA fragments, has facilitated analyses of rare variants that are less frequent but have greater influences on disease onset [7, 8]. Since 2008, international projects have used NGS to comprehensively analyze rare genetic polymorphisms that are difficult to detect through GWASs (The 1000 Genomes Project: 1kGP [9, 10]). Given the cost performance, it is efficient to analyze entire exons that contain very important protein-coding DNA sequences, which

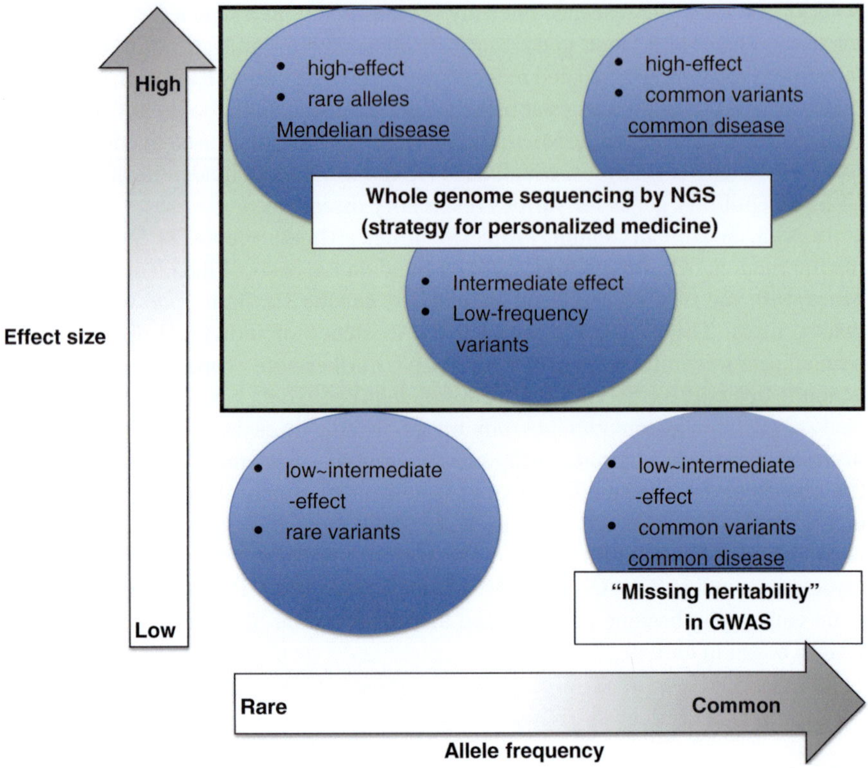

Fig. 1.1 Missing heritability in GWAS

correspond to only approximately 1% of the entire genome (exosome analysis). Exon arrays based on microarray technology are also commercially available and enable comprehensive analyses at a relatively low cost. Comprehensive respiratory disease analyses intended to complement the missing heritability of GWAS [11, 12] have been reported, and this technique could potentially become a mainstream analytical method in clinical genomic medicine research in the future.

1.4 Genomic Medicine and Environmental Factors

Advances in genomic medicine predict the arrival of an era in which individual genetic variations can accurately determine the "constitution prone to a specific disease." However, identical twin studies have shown that even subjects with identical genetic factors will not necessarily develop identical diseases, suggesting that the genetic code is not the only determinant of susceptibility to disease. Therefore, interactions with environmental factors are important [13, 14]. The lung, in particular, is the most susceptible organ to the influences of external environmental factors, such as dust, pollutants, and microorganisms, because it comes in contact with the outside world. In fact, many respiratory diseases are clearly induced and exacerbated by environmental factors.

Chronic obstructive pulmonary disease (COPD) is a condition in which irreversible airflow obstruction is caused by the chronic inhalation of and exposure to harmful substances such as tobacco smoke. However, not all smokers will develop COPD, leading to the suggestion that both environmental factors and disease susceptibility genes are necessary for pathogenesis. An α-1 antitrypsin deficiency is a monogenic disease causing familial COPD and has been linked to a mutation on the *SERPINA1* gene. Despite the strong influence of this single genetic abnormality on disease onset, the severity of respiratory effects may vary within the same family. Therefore, secondary stimuli, such as smoking, may determine these differences in severity [15].

Therefore, interactions between genetic factors (i.e., presence of disease susceptibility genes and differences in individual reactivity) and environmental factors (i.e., gene–environmental interaction) are very important in the pathogenesis of respiratory diseases. This is a factor associated with missing heritability.

1.5 Gene–Environmental Interaction via Epigenetics

Accordingly, is there a molecular mechanism by which environmental factors act on genetic factors, induce disease onset, and acquire heredity over generations? The genetic elements that cause differences among individuals of the same species have been identified as SNPs or DNA sequence mutations. However, although differences in the phenotypic traits of identical twins with identical DNA base sequences have been attributed to environmental factors, the molecular pathological mechanism was unknown. The field of "epigenetics" is expected to explain the mechanism.

In an organism, existing mechanisms can regulate gene expression to determine the phenotype of an individual without changing the DNA sequence. These mechanisms include DNA methylation, histone modification, and noncoding RNA (ncRNA). The academic study of these mechanisms is called "epigenetics," and the collected information is called the "epigenome." Cellular differentiation and embryogenesis are regulated by epigenetic modifications. Such modifications are susceptible to various environmental factors and can determine the phenotype of a disease. Furthermore, the epigenome, which determines the disease phenotype, is conserved across generations. Accordingly, epigenetics has attracted attention as a potential mechanistic link underlying gene–environmental interactions [9].

Historically, the word epigenetics was created by the British embryologist Waddington and colleagues to represent "a mechanism by which a genotype determines a phenotype during development" [16]. Riggs et al. later redefined this term as "a mitotically preserved change in the function of a gene other than the change in DNA sequence." In 1987, Holliday et al. identified the importance of

DNA methylation [17], which led to the discovery of histone protein modification, chromatin structure transformation, and ncRNA [18]. In a fertilized egg, gene expression within cells can be switched on or off. During development and differentiation, epigenetic changes determine which genes are expressed or not expressed, leading to unique cellular phenotypes. This epigenetic information is stored and transmitted to cells in the next generation, thus allowing subgroups of cells to maintain their unique phenotypes despite retaining the same DNA sequence.

As described above, as the epigenome differs considerably from the genome within each cell type, large-scale international epigenome projects such as the ENCODE project (Encyclopedia of DNA Elements) have been established to analyze epigenomic characteristics [19].

1.5.1 DNA Methylation

DNA methylation is a phenomenon observed in many biological organisms, from fungi to mammals. In vertebrates, DNA contains regions wherein cytosine (C) is followed by guanine (G) in a repeated sequence or CpG sites. DNA methyltransferase can add a methyl group to the 5-position carbon of a CpG site. In mammalian DNA, more than 80% CpG sites are methylated. Many of the CpG islands are located in the promoter region upstream of the gene, where they regulate gene expression. The DNA methylation pattern depends on conditions such as organs and environmental exposure. Different diseases may occur, depending on the organ in which the abnormal DNA accumulates, as well as the timing.

Smoking is an environmental factor associated with various respiratory diseases, with a particular influence on the pathogenesis of COPD. In addition, exposure to tobacco smoke may increase the risk of asthma development by approximately 20% [20]. Furthermore, studies of pregnant mothers suggest that internal exposure to tobacco smoking induces epigenetic changes in their offspring [21, 22]. Other reports suggest that during pregnancy, exposure to polycyclic aromatic compounds present in diesel exhaust particles induces DNA methylation at the promoter sites of genes encoding interferon gamma and acyl-coenzyme A synthetase long-chain family member 3 (*ACSL3*) in umbilical cord blood leukocytes, which may affect a child's risk of asthma development [23, 24]. Psychosocial stress also affects the epigenetic changes involved in the development of asthma. An evaluation of DNA derived from the peripheral blood cells of abused children (ages 6–14 years) in Puerto Rico revealed that promoter region methylation and a SNP (rs 2267735) in the *ADCYAP1R1* gene, which has been linked to post-traumatic stress disorder, correlate with the onset of asthma. This finding demonstrates the involvement of childhood stress in asthma pathogenesis via DNA methylation [25].

Some epigenomic analyses have adopted the methods used in GWASs and are therefore known as epigenome-wide association studies (EWASs) [26]. Yang et al. collected peripheral blood-derived DNA from a population of 97 asthmatic and

97 healthy children (aged 6–12 years) that included poor urban residents and conducted a comprehensive EWAS. The authors observed the hypomethylation of asthma-related genes, such as the gene encoding *IL-13*, in asthmatic children relative to healthy children [27]. Liang et al. also comprehensively analyzed the association of serum IgE concentration and DNA methylation in an EWAS. These authors identified sets of genes that linked low DNA methylation with high IgE concentrations in peripheral blood eosinophil-derived DNA from asthmatic patients [28]. An EWAS-based analysis has been also conducted for idiopathic pulmonary fibrosis (IPF) [29]. In addition, MeDIP-seq and MethylCap-seq, which respectively sequence DNA fragments containing methylated cytosine collected by immunoprecipitation with anti-methylated cytosine antibody (MeDIP) or by affinity enrichment with methylated cytosine-binding protein (MethylCap), are used as NGS-based genome-wide analysis methods. Whole-genome bisulfite sequencing, which is based on bisulfite conversion, was also developed [30]. In the future, advances in technology are expected to increase the ease and decrease the expenses associated with collecting epigenomic information.

1.5.2 Histone Modification

DNA strands wrap around histone proteins to form nucleosomes. Changes in chromatin structure these nucleosomes form can significantly affect the efficiencies of gene transcription, replication, and repair. The 20–30 amino acids that comprise the histone N-terminus have weak three-dimensional structures and are called histone tails. These tails can be chemically modified through methylation, acetylation, and phosphorylation to regulate gene expression. The enzyme histone acetyltransferase (HAT) acetylates histones, whereas histone deacetylase (HDAC) deacetylates histones to terminate transcription. HAT acetylates the histone tail to neutralize the charge between DNA and the histone, which relaxes binding and promotes transcription. HDAC can terminate transcription by tightening the wrapping of DNA around histones via deacetylation.

Thus, HAT and HDAC balance each other to regulate gene expression.

Compared with healthy subjects, the inflamed airways of asthmatic patients show enhanced HAT activity and attenuated HDAC activity [31]. Furthermore, decreased HDAC2 activity is observed in the respiratory tracts of COPD patients, particularly those who smoke. Moreover, enhanced IL-8 expression consequent to widespread histone 4 acetylation in the *IL8* promoter region has been observed and correlated with COPD severity [32]. In addition, theophylline, a therapeutic agent used to treat COPD, may improve respiratory function by enhancing HDAC activity [33].

ChIP-seq, which combines chromatin immunoprecipitation (ChIP) and NGS, is used for genome-wide analyses of histone modification and chromatin-binding proteins.

1.5.3 ncRNA

The generic term ncRNA is used to distinguish nonprotein-encoding RNAs from protein-encoding mRNAs. Recent transcriptome analyses (i.e., comprehensive transcript analyses) have included not only protein-encoding mRNAs but also ncRNAs with various gene expression regulatory functions, and the expression levels of these RNAs were found to correlate with cell phenotype [34, 35]. MicroRNAs (miRNAs) are a type of ncRNA for which the precursors are encoded in specific miRNA genomic regions. Following transportation from the nucleus to the cytoplasm and cleavage into 21–22-base miRNA fragments by Dicer, a miRNA binds to the 3′-untranslated region of an mRNA to suppress translation and promote mRNA degradation.

miRNA expression profiles can now be comprehensively quantified using microarrays. These microarray analyses have identified a set of miRNAs involved in the pathogenesis and severity of asthma, COPD, and IPF [36].

miRNAs have potential as biomarkers and therapeutic targets, leading to interest in further research and development with the aim of identifying future clinical applications.

1.6 Gene–Environmental Interaction via Microbiomics

Living organisms harbor many microbiological organisms, such as intestinal bacteria, which play a role in mucosal immunity maintenance and defenses against infection. Technological advances such as next-generation sequencers and 16S rRNA gene sequencing have enabled comprehensive analyses of bacterial genetic information (metagenomic analysis). The recent observation of a group of bacteria that is previously difficult to identify has attracted attention as a novel type of biological information related to disease onset. The microbiotal genome is called the microbiome.

The microbiome is specific to each individual, with low levels of similarity between a parent and child or among siblings. Therefore, this “second genome” represents a research area (microbiomics) that is comparable to the genome and epigenome and could be applied to personalized medicinal approaches. The microbiome is reportedly affected by various environmental factors, can influence immune regulation, and is related to various conditions such as allergic and autoimmune diseases, malignant tumors, and obesity [37].

Until recently, the lung was considered aseptic; however, studies conducted using the latest bacterial detection technology have revealed the existence of a lung microbiota. Within the respiratory field, numerous related papers have been published, and the potential elucidation of pathology and treatment is being debated [38].

Compared with healthy subjects, the respiratory tract microbiota in asthmatics reportedly differs with respect to bacterial species diversity and patterns [39]. Some reports have identified bacteria species involved in the pathology and severity of airway hyperresponsiveness [40, 41]. Similarly, decreases in microbiotal diversity are thought to influence both the acute exacerbation and severity of COPD [42–44] and IPF [45]. Thus, an inappropriate microbiotal composition (dysbiosis) may affect the pathogenesis of respiratory diseases [44].

Both human genomic information and coexisting bacterial (microbiotal) genomic information of bacteria (microbiome) might affect disease onset. The microbiome, therefore, is an important genetic factor that should be considered with respect to respiratory disease onset mechanisms.

Infancy is the most important period for microbiotal establishment. Both antibiotic usage and the environment affect the types of microbiota that engraft during infancy. This microbiota could potentially induce the development of respiratory disease later in life [46–48]. Therefore, early intervention for microbiome adjustment during infancy has been recognized as important for preventing the onset of respiratory diseases.

1.7 Genomic Medicine and Personalized Medicine (Fig. 1.2)

A new asthma phenotype classification (endotype), using biomarkers reflective of molecular pathology and clinical information, has been proposed [49]. Medical care is shifting from conventional medical care designed for "average patients" to personalized medicine based on individual biometric information [50].

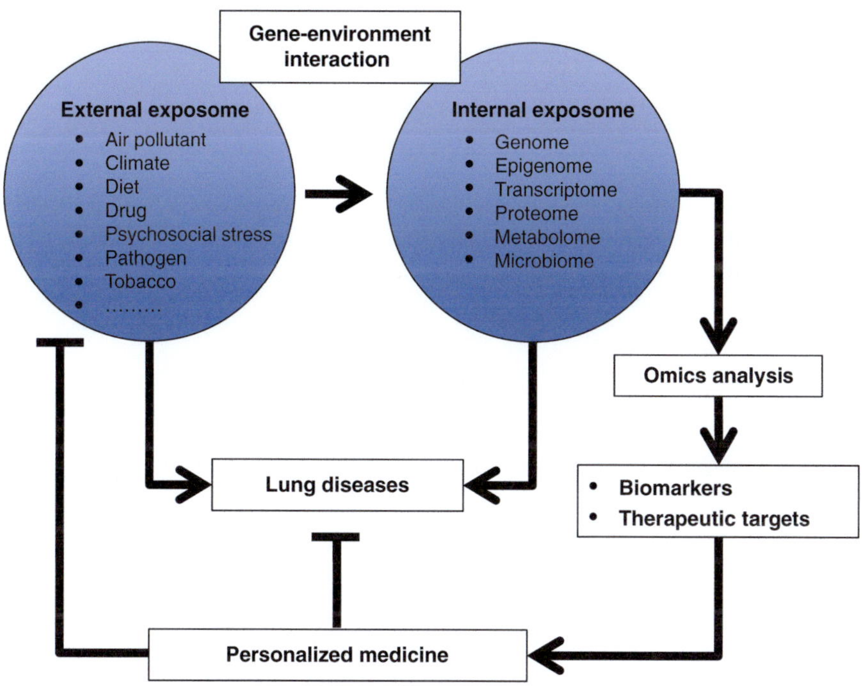

Fig. 1.2 Personalized medicine based on the omics data profiling

The recent advances in analytical techniques have yielded enormous quantities of various types of individual biological information. Integrated omics (-omics = -ome + -ics) analyses have been conducted to incorporate information about the genome, epigenome, transcriptome (i.e., genomic DNA transcripts), proteome (i.e., proteins), metabolome (metabolites), and in vivo microbiome (microbiotal genetic information). Furthermore, the concept of an exposome, which considers pathological conditions from the viewpoint of exposure to environmental factors, has been proposed in addition to the above types of biological information [51].

Personalized medicine is expected to provide very effective treatments; however, there remains the possibility of increased medical costs. Precision medicine is a type of personalized medicine that considers cost-effectiveness and obtains individual biological information from a specific disease-related group to create appropriate treatment methods and disease prevention. In the State of the Union address given by US President Obama on January 20, 2015, the "Precision Medicine Initiative" was announced and gained worldwide attention. Active work with respiratory diseases mainly involves the selection of molecular targeted therapeutic agents and the avoidance of side effects based on genetic analyses of lung cancer [52]. Pharmacogenomic research evaluates the relationship between genes and drug responses. Pharmacogenomic information can allow predictions of susceptibility and side effects to therapeutic agents [53]. Accordingly, pharmacogenomics is thought to play an important role in drug treatment and drug discovery research in the context of personalized medicine not only for lung cancer but also for other respiratory diseases.

1.8 Conclusion

Continuous advances in microarray technology and NGS have facilitated the analyses of genetic predispositions with improved convenience and cost-effectiveness. The enormous amounts of individual biometric information have led us to expect that in the future, individualized preemptive medicine will prevent the onset of respiratory diseases via early intervention.

References

1. Collins FS. Positional cloning: let's not call it reverse anymore. Nat Genet. 1992;1:3–6.
2. Campbell JD, Spira A, Lenburg ME. Applying gene expression microarrays to pulmonary disease. Respirology. 2011;16:407–18.
3. International Human Genome Sequencing C. Finishing the euchromatic sequence of the human genome. Nature. 2004;431:931–45.
4. McCarthy MI, Abecasis GR, Cardon LR, et al. Genome-wide association studies for complex traits: consensus, uncertainty and challenges. Nat Rev Genet. 2008;9:356–69.

5. Manolio TA, Collins FS, Cox NJ, et al. Finding the missing heritability of complex diseases. Nature. 2009;461:747–53.
6. Maher B. Personal genomes: the case of the missing heritability. Nature. 2008;456:18–21.
7. Yang IV, Schwartz DA. The next generation of complex lung genetic studies. Am J Respir Crit Care Med. 2012;186:1087–94.
8. Radder JE, Zhang Y, Gregory AD, et al. Extreme trait whole genome sequencing identifies PTPRO as a novel candidate gene in emphysema with severe airflow obstruction. Am J Respir Crit Care Med. 2017;196(2):159.
9. Seibold MA, Schwartz DA. The lung: the natural boundary between nature and nurture. Annu Rev Physiol. 2011;73:457–78.
10. Genomes Project C, Abecasis GR, Altshuler D, et al. A map of human genome variation from population-scale sequencing. Nature. 2010;467:1061–73.
11. Petrovski S, Todd JL, Durheim MT, et al. An exome sequencing study to assess the role of rare genetic variation in pulmonary fibrosis. Am J Respir Crit Care Med. 2017;196(1):82.
12. Jamal-Hanjani M, Wilson GA, McGranahan N, et al. Tracking the evolution of non-small-cell lung cancer. N Engl J Med. 2017;376(22):2109.
13. Fraga MF, Ballestar E, Paz MF, et al. Epigenetic differences arise during the lifetime of monozygotic twins. Proc Natl Acad Sci U S A. 2005;102:10604–9.
14. Thomsen SF, Duffy DL, Kyvik KO, Backer V. Genetic influence on the age at onset of asthma: a twin study. J Allergy Clin Immunol. 2010;126:626–30.
15. DeMeo DL, Campbell EJ, Brantly ML, et al. Heritability of lung function in severe alpha-1 antitrypsin deficiency. Hum Hered. 2009;67:38–45.
16. Sirlin JL, Waddington CH. Cell sites of protein synthesis in the early chick embryo, as indicated by autoradiographs. Exp Cell Res. 1956;11:197–205.
17. Holliday R. The inheritance of epigenetic defects. Science. 1987;238:163–70.
18. Goldberg AD, Allis CD, Bernstein E. Epigenetics: a landscape takes shape. Cell. 2007;128:635–8.
19. Consortium EP. An integrated encyclopedia of DNA elements in the human genome. Nature. 2012;489:57–74.
20. Cook DG, Strachan DP. Health effects of passive smoking. 3. Parental smoking and prevalence of respiratory symptoms and asthma in school age children. Thorax. 1997;52:1081–94.
21. Joubert BR, Haberg SE, Nilsen RM, et al. 450K epigenome-wide scan identifies differential DNA methylation in newborns related to maternal smoking during pregnancy. Environ Health Perspect. 2012;120:1425–31.
22. Breton CV, Byun HM, Wenten M, Pan F, Yang A, Gilliland FD. Prenatal tobacco smoke exposure affects global and gene-specific DNA methylation. Am J Respir Crit Care Med. 2009;180:462–7.
23. Tang WY, Levin L, Talaska G, et al. Maternal exposure to polycyclic aromatic hydrocarbons and 5′-CpG methylation of interferon-gamma in cord white blood cells. Environ Health Perspect. 2012;120:1195–200.
24. Perera F, Tang WY, Herbstman J, et al. Relation of DNA methylation of 5′-CpG island of ACSL3 to transplacental exposure to airborne polycyclic aromatic hydrocarbons and childhood asthma. PLoS One. 2009;4:e4488.
25. Chen W, Boutaoui N, Brehm JM, et al. ADCYAP1R1 and asthma in Puerto Rican children. Am J Respir Crit Care Med. 2013;187:584–8.
26. Michels KB, Binder AM, Dedeurwaerder S, et al. Recommendations for the design and analysis of epigenome-wide association studies. Nat Methods. 2013;10:949–55.
27. Yang IV, Pedersen BS, Liu A, et al. DNA methylation and childhood asthma in the inner city. J Allergy Clin Immunol. 2015;136:69–80.
28. Liang L, Willis-Owen SA, Laprise C, et al. An epigenome-wide association study of total serum immunoglobulin E concentration. Nature. 2015;520:670–4.
29. Yang IV, Pedersen BS, Rabinovich E, et al. Relationship of DNA methylation and gene expression in idiopathic pulmonary fibrosis. Am J Respir Crit Care Med. 2014;190:1263–72.

30. Rakyan VK, Down TA, Balding DJ, Beck S. Epigenome-wide association studies for common human diseases. Nat Rev Genet. 2011;12:529–41.
31. Ito K, Caramori G, Lim S, et al. Expression and activity of histone deacetylases in human asthmatic airways. Am J Respir Crit Care Med. 2002;166:392–6.
32. Ito K, Ito M, Elliott WM, et al. Decreased histone deacetylase activity in chronic obstructive pulmonary disease. N Engl J Med. 2005;352:1967–76.
33. Ito K, Lim S, Caramori G, et al. A molecular mechanism of action of theophylline: induction of histone deacetylase activity to decrease inflammatory gene expression. Proc Natl Acad Sci U S A. 2002;99:8921–6.
34. Carninci P, Kasukawa T, Katayama S, et al. The transcriptional landscape of the mammalian genome. Science. 2005;309:1559–63.
35. Birney E, Stamatoyannopoulos JA, Dutta A, et al. Identification and analysis of functional elements in 1% of the human genome by the ENCODE pilot project. Nature. 2007;447:799–816.
36. Comer BS, Ba M, Singer CA, Gerthoffer WT. Epigenetic targets for novel therapies of lung diseases. Pharmacol Ther. 2015;147:91–110.
37. Blaser MJ, Falkow S. What are the consequences of the disappearing human microbiota? Nat Rev Microbiol. 2009;7:887–94.
38. Dickson RP, Martinez FJ, Huffnagle GB. The role of the microbiome in exacerbations of chronic lung diseases. Lancet. 2014;384:691–702.
39. Hilty M, Burke C, Pedro H, et al. Disordered microbial communities in asthmatic airways. PLoS One. 2010;5:e8578.
40. Huang YJ, Nelson CE, Brodie EL, et al. Airway microbiota and bronchial hyperresponsiveness in patients with suboptimally controlled asthma. J Allergy Clin Immunol. 2011;127:372–81. e371–373.
41. Huang YJ, Nariya S, Harris JM, et al. The airway microbiome in patients with severe asthma: associations with disease features and severity. J Allergy Clin Immunol. 2015;136:874–84.
42. Sze MA, Dimitriu PA, Suzuki M, et al. Host response to the lung microbiome in chronic obstructive pulmonary disease. Am J Respir Crit Care Med. 2015;192:438–45.
43. Molyneaux PL, Mallia P, Cox MJ, et al. Outgrowth of the bacterial airway microbiome after rhinovirus exacerbation of chronic obstructive pulmonary disease. Am J Respir Crit Care Med. 2013;188:1224–31.
44. Faner R, Sibila O, Agusti A, et al. The microbiome in respiratory medicine: current challenges and future perspectives. Eur Respir J. 2017;49(4)
45. Han MK, Zhou Y, Murray S, et al. Lung microbiome and disease progression in idiopathic pulmonary fibrosis: an analysis of the COMET study. Lancet Respir Med. 2014;2:548–56.
46. Teo SM, Mok D, Pham K, et al. The infant nasopharyngeal microbiome impacts severity of lower respiratory infection and risk of asthma development. Cell Host Microbe. 2015;17:704–15.
47. Biesbroek G, Tsivtsivadze E, Sanders EA, et al. Early respiratory microbiota composition determines bacterial succession patterns and respiratory health in children. Am J Respir Crit Care Med. 2014;190:1283–92.
48. Duijts L, Jaddoe VW, Hofman A, Moll HA. Prolonged and exclusive breastfeeding reduces the risk of infectious diseases in infancy. Pediatrics. 2010;126:e18–25.
49. Lotvall J, Akdis CA, Bacharier LB, et al. Asthma endotypes: a new approach to classification of disease entities within the asthma syndrome. J Allergy Clin Immunol. 2011;127:355–60.
50. Agusti A, Anto JM, Auffray C, et al. Personalized respiratory medicine: exploring the horizon, addressing the issues. Summary of a BRN-AJRCCM workshop held in Barcelona on June 12, 2014. Am J Respir Crit Care Med. 2015;191:391–401.
51. Siroux V, Agier L, Slama R. The exposome concept: a challenge and a potential driver for environmental health research. Eur Respir Rev. 2016;25:124–9.
52. Hirsch FR, Scagliotti GV, Mulshine JL, et al. Lung cancer: current therapies and new targeted treatments. Lancet. 2017;389:299–311.
53. Wang L, McLeod HL, Weinshilboum RM. Genomics and drug response. N Engl J Med. 2011;364:1144–53.

Chapter 2
Approaches to Understanding the Genetic Basis of Complex Diseases: Overview—What Is the Rationale for the Genome-Wide Approach to Understand Complex Diseases, Its Application and Limitations

Mayumi Tamari and Tomomitsu Hirota

Abstract Pulmonary diseases are complex disorders caused by a number of environmental and genetic factors. Recent advances in technologies and study designs have revealed the genetic components of common diseases. Genetic mapping is an unbiased method to comprehensively identify genes and biological pathways involved in diseases or traits. Genome-wide association studies (GWASs) have convincingly identified disease-associated loci. Most of the associated variants identified by GWASs are located in noncoding regions, and the functional link between those disease-associated variants and clinical phenotypes remains unclear. Recent progress in next-generation sequencing (NGS) technologies has improved the functional annotation of the human genome and highlighted the importance of noncoding regions. Epigenetic studies, transcriptome analyses, and characterization of *cis*-regulatory regions have revealed a wide variety of molecular phenotypes: RNA expression and stability, transcription factor binding, DNA methylation, histone modifications, and protein levels in various cell types and tissues. Recent

M. Tamari (✉)
Core Research Facilities for Basic Science (Molecular Genetics), Research Center for Medical Science, The Jikei University School of Medicine, Tokyo, Japan

Laboratory for Respiratory and Allergic Diseases, Center for Integrative Medical Sciences, Institute of Physical and Chemical Research (RIKEN), Yokohama, Kanagawa, Japan
e-mail: mayumitamari@jikei.ac.jp

T. Hirota
Core Research Facilities for Basic Science (Molecular Genetics), Research Center for Medical Science, The Jikei University School of Medicine, Tokyo, Japan

T. Kaneko (ed.), *Clinical Relevance of Genetic Factors in Pulmonary Diseases*, Respiratory Disease Series: Diagnostic Tools and Disease Managements, https://doi.org/10.1007/978-981-10-8144-6_2

genome editing technology and pluripotent stem cells are also helpful to assess the functional effects of genetic risk variants in disease-relevant cell types. Interdisciplinary research to elucidate the relationships between risk variants and molecular phenotypes in the pathologically relevant cell types is necessary to identify the targets of the risk loci and improve our mechanistic understanding of diseases.

Keywords Genome-wide association study · Genetic variants · Noncoding region Disease-relevant cell types

2.1 Introduction

A number of technologies and study designs have identified genetic components of common diseases. The Human Genome Project is an international project that was launched in 1990 to determine the consensus sequence of the human genome [1]. The human nuclear DNA contains around three billion base pairs, and the draft sequence of the human genome was reported in 2001 [2]. Genetic variants are differences of DNA sequences among individuals. These include single nucleotide polymorphisms (SNPs), insertion/deletions (indels), inversions, block substitutions, and copy number variants (CNVs). Among them, SNPs are the most frequent genetic variants (95%) [3]. The HapMap and 1000 Genomes Project have reported approximately 40,000,000 variants in the human genome. Human genetics is the scientific study of inherited human variations, and genetic mapping is a hypothesis-free method to identify the localization of genes that influence the phenotypes on the bases of correlations with genetic variations [4]. Genome-wide association study (GWAS) is an unbiased method that is used to comprehensively identify the genetic components of human diseases and phenotypes [5]. To date, GWASs have identified a number of disease susceptibility loci for common diseases. The great majority of disease-associated variants (>80%) defined by GWASs are located in intronic or intergenic regions [6], though the functional links between those risk variants and diseases remain to be investigated. Recent technological progress has made possible accurate, cost-effective, and high-throughput sequencing, which has contributed to improving our knowledge of the complexity and diversity of genomes in phenotypes and diseases [7]. Next-generation sequencing (NGS) is applied not only for genetic mapping but also for epigenomics and transcriptomics. Epigenetic modifications of the human genome such as DNA methylation and histone modification have been characterized, and large-scale reference epigenome databases are publicly available (http://www.roadmapepigenomics.org). RNA sequencing (RNA-Seq) data are also openly available on several websites such as GTEx Portal (http://www.gtexportal.org/home/) and Ensemble (http://www.ensembl.org/info/website/tutorials/expression.html). Intensive studies annotating the genomic regions have facilitated the discovery of functional targets in the associated loci [8].

2.2 Genome-Wide Association Studies (GWASs)

2.2.1 GWAS Method

Biologic insights identified by GWASs improve our knowledge of the pathophysiology of respiratory diseases. GWASs assess the majority of common genetic variations, mainly SNPs, rapidly and cost-effectively, and try to identify genetic variants that are statistically associated with a disease or trait [5]. The results of published GWASs are summarized in GWAS Catalog (http://www.ebi.ac.uk/gwas/). Phenotypes of pulmonary diseases investigated by GWASs are shown in Table 2.1.

Table 2.1 Phenotypes of pulmonary diseases investigated by GWAS

Phenotypes	Subphenotypes
Bronchial asthma	
	Asthma (SNP × SNP interaction)
	Aspirin-exacerbated respiratory disease in asthmatics
	Post-bronchodilator lung function in asthma (FEV1, FEV1/FVC)
	Response to inhaled corticosteroid treatment in asthma (change in FEV1)
	Bronchial hyperresponsiveness in asthma
	Atopic march
	IgE levels in asthmatics
	Asthma and hay fever
	Pulmonary function in asthmatics
Chronic obstructive pulmonary disease	
	Pulmonary emphysema
	Emphysema distribution in smoking
	Smoking cessation in chronic obstructive pulmonary disease
Interstitial lung disease	
	Idiopathic pulmonary fibrosis
Pulmonary function	
	Pulmonary function decline
	Airflow obstruction
Tumors of the lung	
	Lung adenocarcinoma
	EGFR mutation-positive lung adenocarcinoma
	Squamous cell carcinoma
	Response to platinum-based chemotherapy in non-small cell lung cancer
	Platinum-induced hepatotoxicity in non-small cell lung cancer

(continued)

Table 2.1 (continued)

Phenotypes	Subphenotypes
	Platinum-induced myelosuppression in non-small cell lung cancer
	Malignant pleural mesothelioma
Others	
	Cystic fibrosis severity
	Primary spontaneous pneumothorax
	Sarcoidosis
	Tuberculosis
	Acute lung injury
	Bronchopulmonary dysplasia
	Obstructive sleep apnea
	Cough in response to angiotensin-converting enzyme inhibitor drugs

Those results are summarized in GWAS Catalog (https://www.ebi.ac.uk/gwas/)

2.2.1.1 Microarrays for GWASs

Two platforms of genotyping arrays (products from Illumina and Affymetrix) have been used in most GWASs [9]. Although conventional GWAS arrays were created to tag common variants in European populations, multiethnic genotyping arrays have been developed for genetic association studies across diverse populations. Imputation is a statistical method that is used to infer untyped genotypes by using a reference panel of individuals extensively genotyped [10]. Meta-analysis that combines multiple GWAS results can increase the power to detect an effect. Imputation is useful for meta-analysis to merge data from GWASs using different platforms. Small sample sizes may lead to insufficient statistical power and type II errors. Imputation provides a high-resolution overview of association results with increased statistical power to identify susceptibility loci.

2.2.1.2 Data Quality Issues

After genotyping, several quality control procedures for samples and markers are necessary to minimize potential errors and biases in GWAS results. For sample quality, relatedness, sex inconsistencies, and population substructures are assessed. To find sample identity problems caused by blunders in sample handling, clinical and self-reported data such as sex and familial relationships are reconciled with genetic data. Population stratification can cause type I and type II statistical errors. To assess evidence of population stratification, principal component analysis (PCA) of the genotype data from the samples and on European, African, and East Asian (Japanese and Han Chinese) individuals derived from public databases is performed. The smartpca program is often used to calculate the principal components of genetic data and to remove outliers prior to GWAS [11]. Sample genotyping call rates are also used to remove insufficient samples. For marker quality, markers with low genotyping call rates or minor allele frequencies <0.01 and markers that are not within Hardy-Weinberg equilibrium are usually excluded from the analysis as poor-quality variants. If the associations of variants are assessed by other methods such as TaqMan assay and Invader assay in a replication study, the concordance rates of genotyping results between the GWAS array and other methods should be shown.

2.2.1.3 Statistical Analysis for GWAS

The significance of the association with each genetic variant in the GWAS and validation study is statistically assessed using techniques such as the one-degree-of-freedom Cochran-Armitage trend test. Data from the GWAS and a validation study are combined by the Mantel-Haenszel method. An association result with a large number of data points is usually shown as a Manhattan plot (Fig. 2.1). The $-\log_{10} P$ values of genetic variants in the GWAS are plotted against their respective chromosomal positions. The odds ratio and 95% confidence interval (CI) are calculated from a 2 × 2 allele frequency table. Meta-analysis of Transethnic Association studies (MANTRA) has been developed to conduct transethnic meta-analysis of GWASs [12]. The Breslow-Day test is used to examine heterogeneity across the studies. The thresholds of statistical significance are adjusted for multiple testing, and the genome-wide significance level of $P < 5.0 \times 10^{-8}$ is the most commonly used threshold.

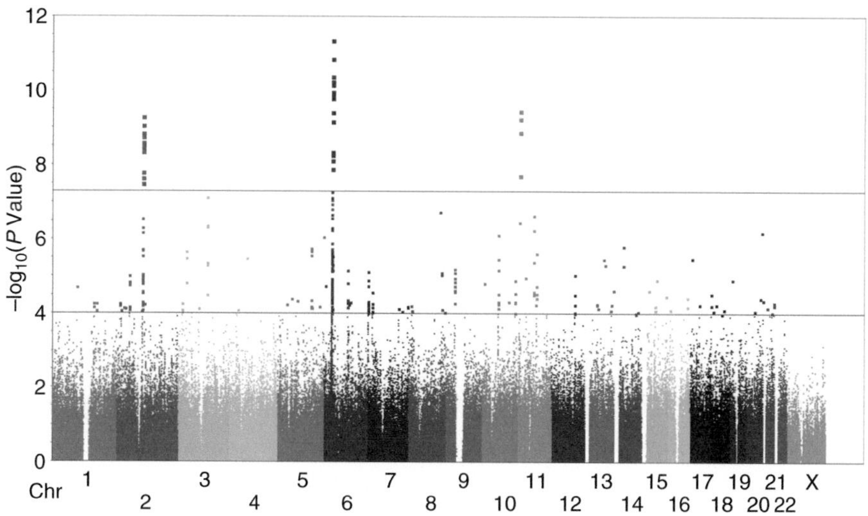

Fig. 2.1 Manhattan plot showing the $-\log_{10} P$ values in the GWAS plotted against their respective positions on autosomes and the X chromosome. The red line indicates the genome-wide significance threshold ($P = 5 \times 10^{-8}$)

2.2.2 *Transethnic Analysis of GWASs*

Most earlier GWASs were conducted in European populations to minimize population stratification effects. Recently, a number of GWASs have been performed in populations with ethnically diverse genetic ancestries. Transethnic studies across worldwide populations enable us to conduct a large-scale replication studies and to increase statistical power [13]. Although population-stratification-related confounding causes false positives in GWASs, shared signals across multiple distant ancestral populations are helpful to identify functional and causal variants and can prioritize loci for further replication and sequencing studies. Methods for meta-analysis assume one of two theoretical models, the fixed effects and random effects models [13]. Fixed effects models assume that an association observed in one cohort will have a similar effect size in other cohorts. Random effects models assume that effect sizes are highly variable but that they usually follow the normal distribution. MANTRA software is a powerful tool for detecting overlapping associations and fine mapping of risk variants and has been used to conduct transethnic meta-analysis of GWASs [13].

2.2.2.1 Population-Specific Loci

Allele frequencies of genetic variants, linkage disequilibrium, and haplotype structures are often different between ethnic populations. Population-specific risk variants are often observed in inflammatory diseases. It has been considered that the evolution of the human genome and populations probably influences the genetic components of common diseases, and infectious diseases are a major selective pressure. A recent study has reported that the susceptibility loci for inflammatory disease are enriched with genetic signatures for positive natural selection [14]. The study implied that the recurrent epidemics of the bubonic plague in European populations might function as putative selective events [14]. Another study has reported that a risk allele of celiac disease, allele *SH2B3* rs3184504A, shows stronger activation of the pathway of NOD2 recognition [15]. Celiac disease is a common inflammatory disease and affects 1–2% of the Western population. SH2B3 plays a role in protective immunity against bacterial infection. The study suggests a selective sweep for *SH2B3*, which arose at some time between 1200 and 1700 years ago [15].

2.2.3 *Missing Heritability*

Heritability is defined as the portion of phenotype variability in the population that can be explained by the genotype. Earlier GWASs identified a number of genomic regions associated with common diseases; however, their odds ratios were small

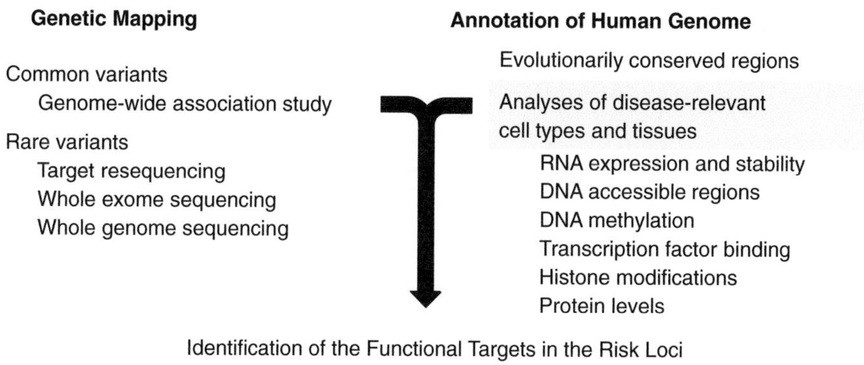

Fig. 2.2 Methodologies to investigate functional link between disease-associated variants and clinical phenotypes

(often <1.3) [16]. Those genetic susceptibility variants can explain very little of the heritability of common diseases (often <10%), and this gap is called "missing heritability." Furthermore, the majority of loci are not in linkage disequilibrium with coding exons. A variety of factors have been considered to explain missing heritability: contributions of untested genetic variations such as rare variants or copy number variation, epistatic effects, myriad common variants of small effects, synthetic association with common variants, gene–environment interactions, lack of statistical power, population stratification, parent-of-origin effects, and epigenomic effects [17]. Sequence-based analyses of common diseases to investigate rare disease-associated variants have been undertaken (Fig. 2.2).

2.2.4 *Phenome-Wide Association Studies (PheWASs)*

Multiple phenotypes are sometimes associated with the same gene or variant, and these are called cross-phenotype associations [18]. Electronic health records and epidemiologic research provide a large amount of detailed phenotypic data. The Electronic Medical Records and Genomics (eMERGE) network is a consortium of US medical research institutions that was founded in order to perform a GWAS using electronic health records. A phenome is the set of all phenotypes, and one PheWAS tested a set of genetic variants for associations with an assemblage of human diseases and traits [18]. The direction of inference in a PheWAS from the genetic variant to the outcome is different from that in a GWAS. The PheWAS can comprehensively investigate the impacts of genetic variants with established functions on clinical phenotypes and the influences of environmental exposures and life stages. These studies may contribute to the identification of novel targets for the prevention of various conditions.

2.3 Sequencing Analysis for Common Diseases

2.3.1 Next-Generation Sequencing

Next-generation sequencing (NGS) using miniaturization technology can determine the precise order of nucleotides in multiple regions of the genome rapidly and inexpensively [19]. Those fragments derived from NGS platforms are pieced together by mapping to the human reference genome. NGS technologies have been used in a wide variety of genomic studies and include de novo genome sequencing, DNA resequencing, transcriptome sequencing, and genomic location analyses. Sequencing depth is the average number of times that a given nucleotide is represented in a collection of random raw sequences. The issue of sequencing depth is discussed in a recent review [20].

2.3.2 Rare-Variant Association Analyses

Conventional arrays used in earlier GWASs did not contain a number of rare variants, and earlier GWASs focused on common variants with minor allele frequencies of 5% or more. Therefore, the contributions of rare variants to susceptibility to common diseases have not been fully investigated. It has been suggested that some of the modest associations identified by GWASs may be pointers to rare variants with much larger effects [7]. Advances in sequencing technologies and reductions in cost have made it possible to evaluate the contribution of rare variants to the risks for diseases [21]. International approaches to characterize rare variants and to increase understanding of the mechanisms of disease have been conducted [3]. One study assessed the genomes of 1092 subjects from a total of 14 populations by using a combination of low-coverage whole-genome and whole-exome sequencing and found that rare variants show geographic differentiation [3]. Therefore it is important to consider ethnicity in rare-variant association analyses. Furthermore, increasing sample size is necessary to achieve sufficient statistical power and to detect rare events in genome-wide scans.

2.3.2.1 Deep Resequencing Around Candidate Regions

Synthetic association is a phenomenon in which “the disease class causing an observed association may consist of multiple low-frequency variants across large regions of the genome” [22]. Fine mapping of candidate loci using resequencing techniques has become economically feasible. Recent studies of targeted region sequencing have reported rare coding variants with strong effects on Crohn disease and hypertriglyceridemia [21]. However, a number of association studies for rare variants have revealed that most variants show only modest to small effects on the variability of phenotypes [23]. Increasing sample sizes and transethnic analyses have been utilized to obtain sufficient power. The top signal observed across different ethnic populations can be helpful to prioritize regions for resequencing. At present, genotyping with arrays is still considered to be useful to assess genetic variants with minor allele frequencies >1% compared with resequencing analyses.

2.3.2.2 Targeted Resequencing Analysis in Asthma

A recent study explored rare variants in asthma susceptibility by resequencing candidate genes [24]. The study examined a total of nine genes that had the strongest signatures of purifying selection among 53 candidate genes for asthma susceptibility: *ADRB2*, *AGT*, *CFTR*, *CHIA*, *DPP10*, *IKBKAP*, *IL12RB1*, *PLA2G7*, and *TGFB1*. The exons and flanking noncoding genomic regions were sequenced using 450 patients (108 Euro-Americans and 342 African-Americans) with asthma and 515 controls (248 Euro-Americans and 267 African-Americans). Rare variants in four genes (*AGT*, *DPP10*, *IKBKAP*, and *IL12RB1*) were associated with asthma in the African-American populations, and those in *IL12RB1* were associated with asthma in Euro-American populations. Most of the rare variants in those genes were population specific. Associations between asthma and nonsynonymous rare variants in the *DPP10* and *IL12RB1* gene were identified in the African-American and Euro-American populations, respectively. Overall, rare noncoding rare variants in flanking regions of the exons predominantly contributed to asthma susceptibility [24].

2.3.3 Whole-Exome Sequencing (WES) and Whole-Genome Sequencing (WGS)

Whole-genome sequencing (WGS), whole-exome sequencing (WES), targeted sequencing of candidate genes, and exome arrays, respectively, are methodologies for rare variant assessment (Fig. 2.3). With the decreasing cost of NGS, WES, and WGS, it has become possible to catalogue genetic variants in noncoding regions. WES is clinically used to search for genetic mutations and access the ~2% of the human genome focusing on protein-coding exons [25]. Polyphen2 (http://genetics.bwh.harvard.edu/pph2/) and SIFT (http://sift.bii.a-star.edu.sg/) can predict the possible impact of an amino acid substitution on the function and structure of a protein. WGS can investigate all types of genetic variants, single nucleotide variants, copy number variants, and structural variants (Fig. 2.3). WES and WGS have been widely used to find unknown causes of diseases such as Mendelian diseases. However, very large sample sizes are necessary for those studies of common diseases to identify low-frequency risk alleles with sufficient statistical power.

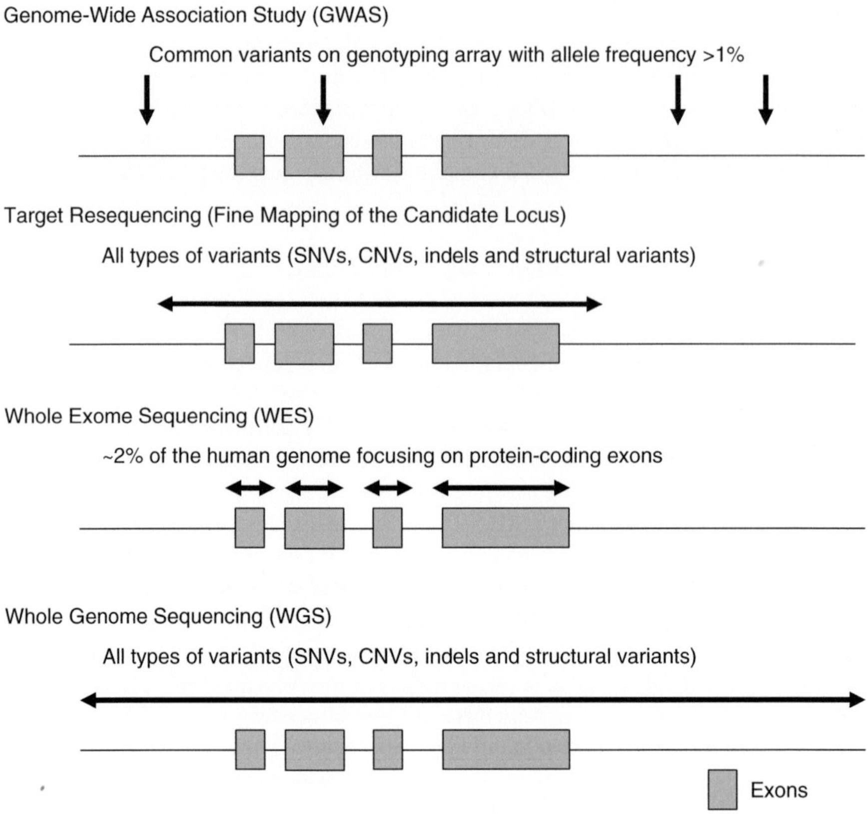

Fig. 2.3 Targets of genetic mapping analyses. SNVs, single nucleotide variants; CNVs, copy number variations; indels, insertions and deletions

2.4 Structure and Function of the Human Genome

2.4.1 Cis-regulatory Regions

The majority of GWAS-identified associations are localized in noncoding regions of the genome. It is necessary to improve our understanding of the structure and function of the human genome to determine the roles of genetic risk variants of diseases. It has been suggested that disease-related genetic variants are enriched in regulatory regions, which are active in cell types involved in disease pathogenesis [26]. Methodologies to investigate functional links between disease-associated variants and clinical phenotypes are summarized in Fig. 2.2.

2.4.1.1 Features of Cis-regulatory Region DNA

Genomic regions that determine where and when genes are transcribed are termed *cis*-regulatory regions. The regions consist of *cis*-regulatory elements. Transcription factor binding sites (TFBSs), usually ~15 bp in length, are core elements of *cis*-regulatory regions [25]. Identification of functional *cis*-regulatory regions is crucial to assess the impacts of genetic variants on gene expression and to understand the functions of the noncoding regions. The *cis*-regulatory regions have several features: open chromatin, chromatin confirmation, nucleosome, histone modification, TFBSs, DNA methylation, conservation, and GC content [25]. Chromatin consists of DNA and proteins that make up chromosomes. The nucleosome is an organizational unit of chromatin that consists of a DNA segment and a histone octamer. Nucleosomes are depleted in many promoter and enhancer regions. DNaseI-hypersensitive sites are considered to be active regions that have regulatory functions such as enhancers, silencers, promoters, and insulators. Open chromatin regions, which are accessible for transcription factors and other proteins, are identified by DNaseI hypersensitivity assay. The nucleotide composition of the genome such as the GC content can highlight CpG islands. The presence of CpG islands is a hallmark of promoters. A recent study reported influences of CpG islands and GC content on nucleosome depletion of promoters [27].

2.4.1.2 Analysis of Chromatin Conformation

Chromatin loop formation enables enhancers and promoters to interact physically to regulate expression. This formation can be analyzed by chromatin conformation assay, which investigates genomic regions interacting closely in a three-dimensional architecture. Chromosome conformation capture techniques are powerful tools to investigate chromatin interactions in the three-dimensional space of the nucleus [28]. After cross-linking of chromatin, shearing and ligation steps fuse DNA fragments from two distant genomic regions. High-throughput sequencing of those fragments provides information on distant targets of regulatory elements [28].

2.4.1.3 Analysis of Transcription Factors and Histone Modifications

Specific antibodies can assess histone modifications and transcription factor bindings. Chromatin immunoprecipitation-sequencing (ChIP-seq) is a widely used method for genome-wide assessment of transcription factor and DNA interactions [29]. Histone N-terminal tails are posttranslationally modified and affect the chromatin structure. The Roadmap Epigenomics Consortium has reported analysis of 111 reference human epigenomes and contains histone modification profiles as well

Table 2.2 Association between genomic regions and histone modification marks

Promoter regions	H3K4me3
Enhancer regions	H3K4me1
Transcribed regions	H3K36me3
Polycomb regions	H3K27me3
Heterochromatin regions	H3K9me3
Increased activation of enhancer and promoter regions	H3K27ac, H3K9ac

as information on the accessibility and methylation of DNA and RNA expression [30]. Associations between histone marks and functional regions assessed in that study are shown in Table 2.2. Asthma is a Th2 cell-mediated chronic airway inflammatory disease. A recent study mapped the genome-wide of histone modification profiles of helper T cells using asthmatic and healthy subjects [31]. The study identified disease-specific enhancers that gained the H3K4me2 mark during Th2 cell development [31]. Interestingly those Th2 cell-specific enhancer regions are highly enriched for susceptible variants of asthma [31].

2.4.1.4 Analysis of Conserved Regions

It has been considered that conserved sequences among species are likely to be functional regions. Comparative genomics across mammalian or vertebrate genomes has improved our knowledge of noncoding elements. Conserved regions suggest their functional roles are influenced by natural selection [25, 28]. There are 500 ultraconserved elements in the human genome in which ≥200 bases are perfectly conserved among human, mouse, and rat [1]. Most of those elements are highly enriched in tissue-specific active enhancers in embryonic development [1].

2.4.1.5 DNA Methylation

DNA methylation is a heritable epigenetic mechanism that consists of the addition of a methyl (-CH3) group to a cytosine nucleotide. DNA methylation in a promoter region can modify the function of the gene and typically acts to repress gene transcription. Perturbations of DNA methylation patterns are frequently observed in human diseases [32]. Recent technologies enable us to assess genome-wide DNA methylation profiles.

2.4.1.6 Epigenome-Wide Association Study (EWAS)

IgE plays an important role in atopic immune responses. An epigenome-wide association study of total serum IgE concentrations was reported in 2015 [33]. In that study, whole-blood DNA methylation levels at genome-wide CpG sites were investigated using Illumina HumanMethylation27 arrays. This array was developed for investigation of individual CpG sites within proximal promoter regions of 14,475 genes. The study found associations between IgE levels and low methylation at 36 loci in a meta-analysis with a false discovery rate $<10^{-4}$. Annotated genes such as *IL5RA*, *PGR2*, *PGR3*, and *GATA1* located in those loci encode characteristic molecules of eosinophils [33]. The most significant association was identified at cg01998785, adjacent to *LPCAT2*, which encodes lysophosphatidylcholine acetyltransferase 2. LPCAT2 plays a role in the production of platelet-activating factor (PAF) in inflammatory cells. Novel therapeutically tractable pathways involving IgE production were suggested in that study [33].

2.4.1.7 Databases of Regulatory Elements

GWAS susceptibility loci show tissue-specific enrichment at histone marks, DNase I hypersensitivity sites (DHS), and other regulatory elements, and studies of those genomic regions are useful to prioritize causal genetic variants to be investigated [34]. The aim of the Encyclopedia of DNA Elements (ENCODE) project is to clarify functional elements in the human genome comprehensively [35]. The project has reported that approximately 80% of the human genome is annotated as functional [35]. The NIH Roadmap Epigenomics Program, which builds on the ENCODE project, was launched in 2003 to improve our understanding of gene regulation, cellular differentiation, and human disease (http://www.roadmapepigenomics.org). The project has also annotated predicted regulatory elements such as enhancers in the human genome sequence. Enrichment analyses of GWAS-identified regions provide insights about the functional mechanisms of disease.

2.4.2 RNA

2.4.2.1 Features of RNA

It is considered that the human genome contains about 20,000 protein-coding genes (mRNAs) and a number of noncoding RNAs that are involved in gene expression via transcriptional or posttranscriptional modifications [36]. Understanding of the diversity and functions of those RNAs is necessary for the functional characterization of disease-susceptibility regions [36]. Small nuclear RNA (snRNA) processes pre-mRNA, and small nucleolar RNA (snoRNA) processes ribosomal RNA (rRNA), transfer RNA (tRNA), and snRNA. Antisense RNA (aRNA) and long noncoding RNA (lncRNA) are involved in gene regulation. MicroRNA (miRNA), a small noncoding RNA (small ncRNA), is involved in mRNA degradation and posttranscriptional inhibition. Small interfering RNA (siRNA) plays roles in posttranscriptional gene silencing through interference with the expression of specific genes with complementary sequences and degradation of mRNA after transcription. Piwi-interacting RNA (piRNA) interacts with Piwi proteins, and these RNA-protein complexes protect genomic integrity.

2.4.2.2 Expression Quantitative Trait Loci (eQTLs)

Regulatory elements are DNA regions including promoters, enhancers, and insulators that regulate expression of target genes. Genetic studies of gene expression play a key role in linking genetic variations to phenotypes. Expression quantitative trait loci (eQTLs) are genomic regions that contain one or more genetic variants that influence the expression level of a given gene [37]. eQTLs are useful to investigate the effects of genetic variants on gene expression [37]. However, most of those studies examined blood cells, lymphoblastoid cells, and accessible tissues such as fat or skin. The Genotype-Tissue Expression (GTEx) project was started to establish a database showing the relationships between genetic variants and gene expression in human tissues (http://www.gtexportal.org/) [38]. The project plans to assess the relationships between whole-genome sequence variations and RNA sequencing data for ≥50 tissues from almost a thousand postmortem donors [38]. Another study assessed the contribution of genetic variants to gene regulation from chromatin to proteins in detail [39]. Interestingly, about 65% of eQTLs show effects through chromatin, and about 35% of eQTLs are enriched in transcribed regions, and the study identified a total of 2893 splicing eQTLs [39]. The study suggested three primary regulatory mechanisms linking common variants to complex diseases: effects via chromatin, direct effects on expression, and direct effects on pre-mRNA splicing [39]. Furthermore, interactions between genetic factors and environmental factors are considered to contribute to disease risk. Response eQTLs (reQTLs), which are associated with differential expression after stimulation, which have been investigated include human dendritic cells stimulated with LPS, influenza and interferon-β [40], monocytes stimulated with interferon-γ, and LPS [41]. These resources will improve our understanding of the pathophysiology of immune-mediated diseases.

2.4.2.3 Enhancer RNAs

Enhancer RNAs (eRNAs) are noncoding RNAs transcribed from enhancers and act as functional enhancers [42]. Transcription factors bind enhancer elements and recruit cofactors and RNA polymerase II (RNAPII) to target genes to regulate gene expression. Transcription factors also interact with cofactors, protein complexes that do not have DNA-binding properties but modify the chromatin structure. Cofactors play an important role in DNA loop formation and maintenance, and cohesin stabilizes the DNA loop formed between enhancers and promoter elements [42]. eRNAs regulate the chromatin accessibility of promoters and RNAPII binding and facilitate the formation or stability of the loop formation of enhancers and promoter elements [42].

2.4.2.4 Long Noncoding RNA

Long noncoding RNAs (lncRNAs) are nonprotein-coding transcripts that are longer than 200 nucleotides. Cap analysis of gene expression (CAGE) data provides information on multiple transcription start sites with high precision [43]. A recent study generated a comprehensive atlas of human lncRNAs with high-confidence 5′ ends by using FANTOM5 CAGE data, and a total of 19,175 potentially functional lncRNAs were identified [43]. In the study, 1970 and 3166 lncRNAs were implicated in GWAS traits and eQTLs, respectively, and conserved lncRNAs were significantly enriched in those regions [43].

2.4.3 Functional Roles of Coding Regions

Nonsynonymous risk variants such as nonsense and missense variants can result in a change in protein structure and/or function. Synonymous risk variants are located in coding exons but do not alter the amino acid sequence. Recent studies have shown that synonymous variants can alter translation rates and influence protein folding [8]. Another study has reported that approximately 15% of human codons are dual-use codons that simultaneously specify both amino acids and transcription factor recognition sites [44]. Those findings imply that synonymous variants might have functional effects. Splicing is the editing of the precursor mRNA that removes introns and joins exons. Exonic splicing enhancers (ESEs) consisting of specific hexamer sequences and an AG sequence play a role in recruitment of the splicing complex to pre-mRNA. It has been reported that genetic risk variants, which disrupt ESE, lead to exon skipping that results in a shorter protein [45].

2.5 Functional Links between Risk Variants and Phenotypes

2.5.1 Prediction of Causal Disease Variants

Although GWASs have identified thousands of susceptibility loci for a diverse set of diseases, the causal variants and mechanisms remain unclear. A recent study developed a fine-mapping algorithm, probabilistic identification of causal SNPs (PICS), to predict candidate causal variants and integrated the genetic data with transcription and *cis*-regulatory element annotations for 21 autoimmune diseases [46]. The study investigated primary human immune cells, resting and stimulated CD4+ T cells, regulatory T cells, CD8+ T cells, B cells, and monocytes. It mapped a total of six histone modifications by ChIP-seq and conducted RNA-Seq and also incorporated data from the NIH Epigenomics Project and ENCODE. Interestingly, about 60% of causal variants have been mapped to immune cell enhancers and tend to be located near binding sites for master regulators of immune responses [46]. However, only 10–20% of those variants appear to alter transcription factor binding motifs directly [46]. Further studies are necessary to explain the influences of other noncoding risk variants in gene regulatory models. Chromatin loop formation and nonprotein-coding transcripts are especially interesting as targets for study.

2.5.2 *Trait Mapping Using Transcriptome Data*

The primary purpose of genetic mapping is not to predict disease risks but to improve knowledge of disease mechanisms [4]. Although we cannot identify the causal genes and mutations, understanding of disease pathways can suggest strategies for diagnosis, therapy, and prevention [4]. A gene-based association method using reference transcriptome data, PrediXcan, has been developed to find trait-associated genes [47]. GWASs compare five to ten million genotyped or imputed variants, and stringent Bonferroni correction has been widely used for multiple testing. Gene-based tests have a benefit with regard to the multiple testing burden, with approximately 20,000 tests conducted for 10,000 genes with high-quality prediction in most tissues. PrediXcan is focused on the regulation of gene expression and estimates the genetically determined component [47]. Whole-genome tissue-dependent prediction models are used with reference transcriptome datasets such as the GTEx Project and GEUVADIS (http://www.geuvadis.org) and estimate genetically regulated gene expression [47]. Another study using gene-based analysis of regulatory variants identified four putative novel asthma risk genes involved in nucleotide synthesis (*B4GSLT3* and *USMG5*) and signaling (*P2RY13* and *P2RY14*) [48]. The study identified associations between asthma and eQTL for those four genes. Interestingly, P2ry13 and P2ry14 are upregulated in airway epithelial cells, eosinophils, and neutrophils after allergen challenge in a mouse model [48].

2.5.3 *Multiomic Studies*

Although interindividual variability of immune responses is well recognized, recent studies have assessed only a few factors. To advance our knowledge of the variability of human immune responses more comprehensively, the Human Functional Genomics Project (HFGP) (http://www.humanfunctionalgenomics.org) was launched in 2013 [49]. The project integrates omic techniques with stringent phenotyping of immune responses in diseased and healthy subjects [49]. The HFGP database will contribute to the progress of functional genomic studies of human immune-mediated disorders. Another study performed high-resolution genome, epigenome, and transcriptome sequencing analyses of human immune cells (CD14+ monocytes, CD16+ neutrophils, and naïve CD4+ T cells) [50]. This multiomic study revealed genome-epigenome coordination in cell-specific contexts and functionally mapped disease mechanisms to autoimmune-related loci [50].

2.5.4 Functional Validation of Predictions by Using a Genome Editing System

The clustered regularly interspaced short palindromic repeats (CRISPR)/CRISPR-associated gene system (CAS) is a precise and efficient genome editing technology that can be used in living eukaryotic cells [51]. We can assess functional effects of genetic risk variants such as gene expression, transcription factor recruitment, and protein structure by using such model systems. Although most susceptible variants identified by GWASs are located in noncoding regions of the genome, a large proportion of them are not conserved across different species. Pluripotent stem cells such as induced pluripotent stem cells (iPSCs) can be differentiated into a wide variety of cell types and contribute to cell-based disease modeling [8]. Genome editing by using the CRISPR technology in appropriate cells will be a powerful tool for characterization of risk alleles in disease development.

2.6 Toward Clinical Application of Genetic Researches

GWASs have highlighted previously unexpected biological pathways and revealed the overlap between risk variants among different diseases by comparisons of GWAS results across diseases. Such findings are helpful to identify effective drug targets. GWAS findings are also valuable for biomarker identification and disease subclassification and useful to select treatments and drug dosages [16, 46].

2.6.1 Super-enhancers and Diseases

Super-enhancers, a subset of enhancers, play important roles in the definition of cell identity [52]. The definition of super-enhancers is useful to identify regulatory regions that control genes involved in cell-type specification. Disease susceptibility variants for immune-mediated disorders are especially enriched with T-cell super-enhancers compared with typical enhancers or super-enhancers in other cell types [53]. Interestingly, tofacitinib, which inhibits Janus kinase disproportionately, alters the structures of super-enhancers and the expression of risk genes of rheumatoid arthritis [53]. Further investigation of super-enhancers in disease-relevant cell types might be helpful for understanding pathophysiology and for the identification of new drug targets.

2.6.2 Drug Repositioning

Drug repositioning also called reprofiling is the application of known drugs for treatment of new diseases. Protein products of genes or pathways that are identified by GWASs can be assessed to determine whether they are targets for approved therapies or drugs in development. A recent study conducted a GWAS meta-analysis of rheumatoid arthritis using >100,000 individuals of European and Asian descent, and a total of 42 new risk loci at genome-wide significant levels were reported [54]. The study also identified 98 candidate genes at 101 susceptible loci that are existing drug targets, by using bioinformatics methods, and has implied the possibility of repositioning drugs approved for other uses [54]. ChEMBL (https://www.ebi.ac.uk/chembl/compound) is an open database for drug discovery that contains information on a large number of drug-like bioactive compounds. Another GWAS assessed a total of 48,943 subjects selected from extremes of the pulmonary function distribution and conducted a replication study using 95,375 subjects [55]. The study identified a total of 43 novel association signals for pulmonary function and was able to highlight drug targets such as genes in the inositol phosphate metabolism pathway and CHRM3 in the development of asthma and COPD by using the ChEMBL database [55]. GWAS and comprehensive genetic studies provide crucial information for drug discovery.

2.7 Conclusion

Genetic mapping methods such as GWAS, target resequencing, WES, and WGS have discovered genetic components of common human diseases. However, the associations explain only a small fraction of the phenotypic variance. Extensive phenotypic information from larger sample sizes and recording of environmental factors are crucial to improve our understanding of the genetic bases of common diseases. Functional links between disease-related variants and clinical phenotypes also remain to be clarified. Intensive studies on the epigenome, transcriptome sequencing analyses, and characterization of *cis*-regulatory regions in various cell types and tissues are currently in progress. Further interdisciplinary research including deep phenotyping and genotyping studies and functional studies of risk variants in disease-relevant cell types are necessary for the application of genetic knowledge to clinical practice.

References

1. Lander ES. Initial impact of the sequencing of the human genome. Nature. 2011;470:187–97.
2. Lander ES, Linton LM, Birren B, Nusbaum C, Zody MC, Baldwin J, et al. International Human Genome Sequencing Consortium. Initial sequencing and analysis of the human genome. Nature. 2001;409:860–921.
3. Abecasis GR, Auton A, Brooks LD, DePristo MA, Durbin RM, Handsaker RE, Kang HM, Marth GT, McVean GA. 1000 Genomes Project Consortium. An integrated map of genetic variation from 1,092 human genomes. Nature. 2012;491:56–65.
4. D A, Daly MJ, Lander ES. Genetic mapping in human disease. Science. 2008;322:881–8.
5. Manolio TA. Genomewide association studies and assessment of the risk of disease. N Engl J Med. 2010;363:166–76.
6. Hindorff LA, Sethupathy P, Junkins HA, Ramos EM, Mehta JP, Collins FS, Manolio TA. Potential etiologic and functional implications of genome-wide association loci for human diseases and traits. Proc Natl Acad Sci U S A. 2009;106:9362–7.
7. Cirulli ET, Goldstein DB. Uncovering the roles of rare variants in common disease through whole-genome sequencing. Nat Rev Genet. 2010;11:415–25.
8. Zhang X, Bailey SD, Lupien M. Laying a solid foundation for Manhattan—'setting the functional basis for the post-GWAS era'. Trends Genet. 2014;30:140–9.
9. Bush WS, Moore JH. Chapter 11: Genome-wide association studies. PLoS Comput Biol. 2012;8:e1002822.
10. Marchini J, Howie B. Genotype imputation for genome-wide association studies. Nat Rev Genet. 2010;11:499–511.
11. Price AL, Patterson NJ, Plenge RM, Weinblatt ME, Shadick NA, Reich D. Principal components analysis corrects for stratification in genome-wide association studies. Nat Genet. 2006;38:904–9.
12. Morris AP. Transethnic meta-analysis of genomewide association studies. Genet Epidemiol. 2011;35:809–22.
13. Li YR, Keating BJ. Trans-ethnic genome-wide association studies: advantages and challenges of mapping in diverse populations. Genome Med. 2014;6:91.
14. Raj T, Kuchroo M, Replogle JM, Raychaudhuri S, Stranger BE, De Jager PL. Common risk alleles for inflammatory diseases are targets of recent positive selection. Am J Hum Genet. 2013;92:517–29.
15. Zhernakova A, Elbers CC, Ferwerda B, Romanos J, Trynka G, Dubois PC, et al. Evolutionary and functional analysis of celiac risk loci reveals SH2B3 as a protective factor against bacterial infection. Am J Hum Genet. 2010;86:970–7.
16. Manolio TA. Bringing genome-wide association findings into clinical use. Nat Rev Genet. 2013;14:549–58.
17. Eichler EE, Flint J, Gibson G, Kong A, Leal SM, Moore JH, et al. Missing heritability and strategies for finding the underlying causes of complex disease. Nat Rev Genet. 2010;11:446–50.
18. Bush WS, Oetjens MT, Crawford DC. Unravelling the human genome-phenome relationship using phenome-wide association studies. Nat Rev Genet. 2016;17:129–45.
19. Goodwin S, McPherson JD, McCombie WR. Coming of age: ten years of next-generation sequencing technologies. Nat Rev Genet. 2016;17:333–51.
20. Sims D, Sudbery I, Ilott NE, Heger A, Ponting CP. Sequencing depth and coverage: key considerations in genomic analyses. Nat Rev Genet. 2014 Feb;15(2):121–32.
21. Lee S, Abecasis GR, Boehnke M, Lin X. Rare-variant association analysis: study designs and statistical tests. Am J Hum Genet. 2014;95:5–23.
22. Dickson SP, Wang K, Krantz I, Hakonarson H, Goldstein DB. Rare variants create synthetic genome-wide associations. PLoS Biol. 2010;8:e1000294.
23. Auer PL, Lettre G. Rare variant association studies: considerations, challenges and opportunities. Genome Med. 2015;7:16.

24. Torgerson DG, Capurso D, Mathias RA, Graves PE, Hernandez RD, Beaty TH, et al. Resequencing candidate genes implicates rare variants in asthma susceptibility. Am J Hum Genet. 2012;90:273–81.
25. Mathelier A, Shi W, Wasserman WW. Identification of altered cis-regulatory elements in human disease. Trends Genet. 2015;31:67–76.
26. Maurano MT, Humbert R, Rynes E, Thurman RE, Haugen E, Wang H, et al. Systematic localization of common disease-associated variation in regulatory DNA. Science. 2012;337:1190–5.
27. Fenouil R, Cauchy P, Koch F, Descostes N, Cabeza JZ, Innocenti C, et al. CpG islands and GC content dictate nucleosome depletion in a transcription-independent manner at mammalian promoters. Genome Res. 2012;22:2399–408.
28. Alexander RP, Fang G, Rozowsky J, Snyder M, Gerstein MB. Annotating non-coding regions of the genome. Nat Rev Genet. 2010;11:559–71.
29. Furey TS. ChIP-seq and beyond: new and improved methodologies to detect and characterize protein-DNA interactions. Nat Rev Genet. 2012;13:840–52.
30. Roadmap Epigenomics Consortium, Kundaje A, Meuleman W, Ernst J, Bilenky M, Yen A, Heravi-Moussavi A, et al. Integrative analysis of 111 reference human epigenomes. Nature. 2015;518:317–30.
31. Seumois G, Chavez L, Gerasimova A, Lienhard M, Omran N, Kalinke L, et al. Epigenomic analysis of primary human T cells reveals enhancers associated with TH2 memory cell differentiation and asthma susceptibility. Nat Immunol. 2014;15:777–88.
32. Schübeler D. Function and information content of DNA methylation. Nature. 2015;517:321–6.
33. Liang L, Willis-Owen SA, Laprise C, Wong KC, Davies GA, Hudson TJ, et al. An epigenome-wide association study of total serum immunoglobulin E concentration. Nature. 2015;520:670–4.
34. Price AL, Spencer CC, Donnelly P. Progress and promise in understanding the genetic basis of common diseases. Proc Biol Sci. 2015;282:20151684.
35. ENCODE Project Consortium. An integrated encyclopedia of DNA elements in the human genome. Nature. 2012;489:57–74.
36. Lee TI, Young RA. Transcriptional regulation and its misregulation in disease. Cell. 2013;152:1237–51.
37. Battle A, Montgomery SB. Determining causality and consequence of expression quantitative trait loci. Hum Genet. 2014;133:727–35.
38. Consortium GTE. The Genotype-Tissue Expression (GTEx) project. Nat Genet. 2013;45:580–5.
39. Li YI, van de Geijn B, Raj A, Knowles DA, Petti AA, Golan D, et al. RNA splicing is a primary link between genetic variation and disease. Science. 2016;352:600–4.
40. Lee MN, Ye C, Villani AC, Raj T, Li W, Eisenhaure TM, et al. Common genetic variants modulate pathogen-sensing responses in human dendritic cells. Science. 2014;343:1246980.
41. Fairfax BP, Humburg P, Makino S, Naranbhai V, Wong D, Lau E, et al. Innate immune activity conditions the effect of regulatory variants upon monocyte gene expression. Science. 2014;343:1246949.
42. Li W, Notani D, Rosenfeld MG. Enhancers as non-coding RNA transcription units: recent insights and future perspectives. Nat Rev Genet. 2016;17:207–23.
43. Hon CC, Ramilowski JA, Harshbarger J, Bertin N, Rackham OJ, Gough J, et al. An atlas of human long non-coding RNAs with accurate 5′ ends. Nature. 2017;543(7644):199.
44. Stergachis AB, Haugen E, Shafer A, Fu W, Vernot B, Reynolds A, et al. Exonic transcription factor binding directs codon choice and affects protein evolution. Science. 2013;342:1367–72.
45. Gregory AP, Dendrou CA, Attfield KE, Haghikia A, Xifara DK, Butter F, et al. TNF receptor 1 genetic risk mirrors outcome of anti-TNF therapy in multiple sclerosis. Nature. 2012;488:508–11.
46. Farh KK, Marson A, Zhu J, Kleinewietfeld M, Housley WJ, Beik S, et al. Genetic and epigenetic fine mapping of causal autoimmune disease variants. Nature. 2015;518:337–43.
47. Gamazon ER, Wheeler HE, Shah KP, Mozaffari SV, Aquino-Michaels K, Carroll RJ, et al. A gene-based association method for mapping traits using reference transcriptome data. Nat Genet. 2015;47:1091–8.

48. Ferreira MA, Jansen R, Willemsen G, Penninx B, Bain LM, Vicente CT, et al. Gene-based analysis of regulatory variants identifies 4 putative novel asthma risk genes related to nucleotide synthesis and signaling. J Allergy Clin Immunol. 2017;139(4):1148.
49. Netea MG, Joosten LA, Li Y, Kumar V, Oosting M, Smeekens S, et al. Understanding human immune function using the resources from the Human Functional Genomics Project. Nat Med. 2016;22:831–3.
50. Chen L, Ge B, Casale FP, Vasquez L, Kwan T, Garrido-Martín D, et al. Genetic drivers of epigenetic and transcriptional variation in human immune cells. Cell. 2016;167:1398–414.
51. Lander ES. The Heroes of CRISPR. Cell. 2016;164:18–28.
52. Hnisz D, Abraham BJ, Lee TI, Lau A, Saint-André V, Sigova AA, et al. Super-enhancers in the control of cell identity and disease. Cell. 2013;155:934–47.
53. Vahedi G, Kanno Y, Furumoto Y, Jiang K, Parker SC, Erdos MR, et al. Super-enhancers delineate disease-associated regulatory nodes in T cells. Nature. 2015;520:558–62.
54. Okada Y, Wu D, Trynka G, Raj T, Terao C, Ikari K, et al. Genetics of rheumatoid arthritis contributes to biology and drug discovery. Nature. 2014;506:376–81.
55. Wain LV, Shrine N, Artigas MS, Erzurumluoglu AM, Noyvert B, Bossini-Castillo L, et al. Genome-wide association analyses for lung function and chronic obstructive pulmonary disease identify new loci and potential druggable targets. Nat Genet. 2017;49:416–25.

Part II
Genetic Disorders in Pulmonary Disease

Chapter 3
Bronchial Asthma: Is Asthma Inherited?

Nobuyuki Hizawa

Abstract Asthma runs strongly in families and has a heritability rate of up to 70%. Genetic studies offer a structured means for understanding the causes of asthma and for identifying targets of treatment for the syndrome. As with studies of other common complex diseases, genetic studies of asthma have led to considerable advances in the understanding of this disease. Genome-wide association studies have greatly advanced the identification of the most important genes predisposing individuals to asthma. Several genes act in pathways that communicate the presence of epithelial damage to the adaptive immune system; identification of these genes has provided a new focus for the development of effective therapies. However, these loci explain only a small proportion of the heritability of the disease because the phenotypic heterogeneity of asthma greatly complicates genetic analysis. A specific phenotype is likely to be more closely related to a specific pathogenetic mechanism, and focusing on a particular phenotype may increase the power of genetic studies and consequently lead to a better understanding of an endotype defined by a distinct functional or pathobiological mechanism. Genetic predisposition to the dysregulation of particular pathways may further help to define subgroups of asthma. In the end, this approach may lead to diagnosis for patients based, in part, on their genetic makeup and to new therapeutic prospects. In addition, further work is necessary to understand the biological consequences of the known susceptibility variants; the most immediate challenge in this field is the systematic analysis of the precise functions of these genes in the pathogenesis of asthma. Detailed functional dissection of the roles of these genes in asthma will point the way to new therapies for the disease.

Keywords Asthma · Endotype · GWAS · TSLP · ORMDL3 · CDHR3 · HCG22

N. Hizawa
Department of Pulmonary Medicine, Faculty of Medicine, University of Tsukuba, Tsukuba, Japan
e-mail: nhizawa@md.tsukuba.ac.jp

T. Kaneko (ed.), *Clinical Relevance of Genetic Factors in Pulmonary Diseases*, Respiratory Disease Series: Diagnostic Tools and Disease Managements,
https://doi.org/10.1007/978-981-10-8144-6_3

3.1 Introduction

Asthma runs in families, and children of asthmatic parents are at increased risk of asthma. Studies of twins and of families of asthmatic individuals have shown that asthma occurs in a pattern consistent with heritable factors [1]; twin and family studies suggest that 60–70% of asthma is heritable [2]. In the past 30 years, researchers have tried to find the genes that account for this heritability. Initial efforts investigating candidate genes in a relatively small number of cases and controls produced at best varying results; however, a major breakthrough came with the introduction of the genome-wide association study (GWAS) [3]. The varied clinical patterns seen in asthma reflect individual genetic profiles combined with environmental exposures that initiate persistent bronchial inflammation and tissue injury and lead to pathophysiological abnormalities and airway wall remodeling [4]. The heterogeneity of asthma makes optimizing treatment a challenge, especially for patients that respond poorly to current therapies [5]. In recent years, the concept of the endotype has become increasingly important in the study of asthma. A phenotype is defined as a group of similar clinically observable characteristics that lacks a documented and direct etiologic relationship with a distinct pathophysiological mechanism. In contrast, the term endotype is used to describe "a subtype of a disease defined by a unique or distinctive functional or pathophysiological mechanism" [6]. Hypothetically, variation in environment influences on individual genotypes can lead to heterogeneous endotypes of asthma. Several clinical phenotypes can overlap in one patient, and the same clinical phenotype could result from different endotypes. Understandings of endotype will, therefore, lead to an improved understanding of disease heterogeneity and progression and contribute to the development of new targeted treatments. Consequently, future treatment options are likely to target individual endotypes that are each defined by a distinct pathophysiological mechanism such as type-2 inflammation, viral infection, bacterial colonization, dysregulated lung growth, and systemic inflammation.

3.2 Genome-Wide Association Studies

Over the past decade, GWASs have been used extensively to investigate the genetic bases of common complex diseases, including asthma [7, 8]. Before GWASs, many candidate-gene studies were done for asthma susceptibility [9, 10]; however, most of the positive associations were not replicated in GWAS because of differences in either phenotype definition or the populations studied (either in terms of ancestry or environmental exposures) or because of false positives and small sample sizes in the original candidate-gene studies.

GWASs use genotyping arrays with up to millions of probes for single-nucleotide polymorphism (SNP) markers located throughout the genome. This method provides an unbiased or hypothesis-independent means to identify the underlying genetic variants that contribute to a disease, its severity, and intermediate phenotypes, such as lung function and bronchial hyperresponsiveness in the case of asthma. The first completed GWAS for asthma involved 994 childhood-onset asthma patients and 1243 non-asthma controls; this study identified asthma-associated SNPs within chromosome 17q21 that span the *ORMDL3/GSDMB* genes [11]. These SNPs showed highly significant association with childhood asthma, and the associations with asthma were also replicated in two independent cohorts. The validity of the GWAS findings regarding *ORMDL3* was confirmed using eQTL; markers associated with asthma were also strongly associated ($p < 10^{-22}$) in cis with transcript levels of *ORMDL3* [12]. This association has been widely replicated in several European ancestry samples [13, 14], as well as in Asians [15] and Hispanics [16]. Larger case-control populations have identified additional loci consistently associated with asthma; these include *IL33* on chromosome 9p24, *HLA-DR/DQ* on 6p21, *IL1RL1/IL18R1* on 2q12, *TSLP* on 5q22, and *IL13* on 5q31 [17, 18]. In an expanded GWAS by the European-based GABRIEL Consortium (10,365 individuals with physician-diagnosed asthma and 16,110 unaffected individuals), 5 genes in addition to the *ORMDL3* locus were strongly associated with asthma [14], of which 2, *IL-33* and the chromosome 2 locus *IL1RL1/IL18R1*, were replicated in the EVE Consortium [19]. In an independent GWAS on eosinophil counts in Icelanders, the *IL33* and *IL1RL1* SNPs were similarly strongly associated with asthma, but with atopic asthma, not nonatopic asthma [18]. IL33 is a member of the IL-1 family that induces Th2 cytokines, and its receptor, ST2, exists as membrane and circulating soluble protein. IL-33 is produced by mast cells following IgE-mediated activation [20]. Greater IL33 expression has been observed in the airway smooth muscle cells [21] and airway epithelium of patients with asthma than in those of healthy individuals [22].

Although much progress has been made in recent years in identifying genes involved in the risk of developing asthma, alleles identified through GWAS account for a relatively small fraction of missing heritability [3]. Several explanations include overestimation of heritability of the complex traits and underestimation of the effects of alleles identified through GWAS. In addition, yet-to-be identified common as well as rare alleles might explain the missing heritability. Moreover, gene-gene and gene-environment interactions might explain another fraction of the heritability of asthma. Genotype effects for many regulatory variants may be context or environment specific, and these variants may fail to reach genome-wide thresholds of significance in typical GWAS. To explore a multi-genetic approach, an Australian GWAS [23] assessed the use of genetic loci identified by the European GABRIEL Consortium to predict disease status. Although the multi-SNP score generated from the ten most associated loci reported in the GABRIEL study was significantly associated with asthma in the Australian study population ($p = 8{\cdot}2 \times 10^{-15}$), the sensitivity and specificity of this multi-SNP score were low. This result has little clinical relevance, as the multi-SNP scores tested had very poor discriminative ability, with values for the area under the receiver operator characteristic curve (AUC) not exceeding 0.58. These findings highlight the need for even more complex genetic models and improved phenotyping for disease prediction. Another study aimed to construct a multi-locus profile of genetic predisposition to asthma—a genetic risk score—from a comprehensive case-control GWAS of asthma [14] and then to calculate this score in an unselected cohort followed from birth to midlife [24] with extensive asthma phenotyping across nine assessments spanning the ages of 9–38 years. The study then tested how GWAS-discovered genetic risks were related to the development, persistence, and biological characteristics of asthma in this cohort. Of the 880 cohort members included in the analysis, those at higher genetic risk developed asthma earlier in life than did those with lower genetic risk. Of the cohort members with childhood-onset asthma, those with higher genetic risk were more likely to develop life-course-persistent asthma than were those with a lower genetic risk. Participants with asthma at higher genetic risk more often had atopy, airway hyperresponsiveness, and incompletely reversible airflow obstruction than did those with a lower genetic risk. Those with higher genetic risk were also more likely to miss school or work and be admitted to hospital because of asthma. Genotypic information about asthma risk was independent of and additive to information derived from cohort members' family histories of asthma. These findings indicate that genetics plays a greater role in childhood-onset asthma. Genetic risk assessments might be able to predict which childhood-onset asthma cases remit and which become life-course-persistent, who might develop impaired lung function, and what the burden of asthma is in terms of missed school and work and hospital admissions, although these predictions are currently not sufficiently sensitive or specific to support point-of-care decision-making. Although the modest effect sizes of the common variants, both individually and in combination, and the small fraction of heritability that is explained by these variants preclude practical prediction, it is important to note that the primary goal of GWAS is not only prediction of individual risk but also discovery of biological pathways underlying polygenic diseases and traits [25].

3.3 The Role of Allergy in the Pathogenesis of Asthma

GWASs provide the potential for important insights into disease mechanisms through the identification of previously unrecognized biological pathways associated with disease pathogenesis. Many asthma genes, including those previously identified by positional cloning, are expressed within the respiratory epithelium; this finding highlights the importance of epithelial barriers in causing asthma [14]. Based on a previous GWAS of asthma in Spanish individuals, a gene set enrichment analysis identified the Wnt signaling pathway genes in asthma susceptibility, providing support for the central role of epithelia in asthma development [26]. In contrast, our study found an association between serum total IgE and the *HLA-C* gene within the class I region of the major histocompatibility complex (MHC) on chromosome 6 [27]; the gene was not associated with asthma. In fact, the genes controlling IgE levels have surprisingly little overlap with the genes mediating asthma susceptibility, suggesting that atopy is secondary to asthma, not a primary driver of the disease [14]. This contention is supported by the absence of a relationship between atopic sensitization and asthma in many populations [28]. Genetic studies of children with atopic dermatitis have shown that defects in barrier proteins such as FLG [29] and SPINK5 [30] commonly predispose individuals to the disease, indicating that increases in IgE levels may be secondary to barrier failure. The integrity of the airway epithelium in patients with asthma is often disrupted, with loss of epithelial cell-cell contacts [31]. Because structural epithelial barrier function is highly involved in the ability of the epithelium to regulate the immune system and many of the recently identified susceptibility genes for asthma are expressed in airway epithelium, changes at the airway epithelial barrier may also play a central role in sensitization to allergens and in the pathogenesis of allergic asthma.

3.4 Heterogeneity of Asthma

Genetic variants are often assumed to contribute equally to disease susceptibility. However, it is increasingly clear that asthma is not a single disease but a disorder with vast heterogeneity in pathogenesis, severity, and treatment response. A specific disease definition may be used that identifies a subgroup of asthma patients in whom specific-risk alleles might have stronger effects. There is evidence from existing data to support this concept. For example, the 17q locus *ORMDL3*/*GSDML* appears to have a pronounced effect on risk of childhood-onset asthma but very little effect on adult-onset asthma [13]. Another example of this approach was recently published by Bonnelyke et al., who studied Danish children with asthma and frequent exacerbations, for which they were hospitalized. With these childhood asthma cases involving severe exacerbations, the known asthma genes (i.e., *ORMDL3*, *IL33*, and *IL1RL1*) were identified, and they appeared to have larger effect sizes than in previous GWASs; additionally, a previously unrecognized asthma gene (*CDHR3*, cadherin-related protein 3) was identified [32].

The heterogeneity of asthma phenotypes may also be identified as clusters of measurements from different dimensions of the disease (e.g., the clinical features, physiology, immunology, pathology, hereditary components, environmental influences, and response to treatment). A large-scale cluster analysis was performed with 726 patients with asthma in the Severe Asthma Research Program (SARP) [33]. This study used 628 variables compressed into 34 weighted variables and identified 5 separate clusters. The strongest predictors were $FEV_1\%$ and age at onset. Another cluster analysis with a different cohort revealed similar findings [34]. Asthma can develop at any stage of life, and asthma phenotypes show age-related variations [35]; together, these findings suggest that adult-onset asthma may comprise some distinct subset of asthma phenotypes. The development of asthma in older adults is also influenced by smoking; compared with younger adults with asthma (18–34 years), older adults with asthma are more likely to report a history of smoking (54% vs. 34%) [36]. Using cluster analysis, we examined the existence of distinct phenotypes of late-onset asthma in Japanese patients with adult asthma [37].

We then associated genotypes at the *CCL5* and *ADRB2* genes with the clusters of asthma identified. In the airways of asthma, CCL5 has detrimental effects through the recruitment of immune cells that enhance inflammatory processes. We previously reported that the -28G gain-of-function allele in the *CCL5* promoter region is associated with late-onset asthma that develops at the age of 40 years or later [38]. We also studied a functionally relevant SNP on the *ADRB2* gene, Arg16Gly, because it is among the most extensively studied in relation to asthma [39]. Although this coding variant is not an important determinant of asthma per se, some data suggest that the Arg16 allele might influence the phenotype of asthma. In the Hutterites, the homozygosity of the Arg16 allele is associated with lower lung function in adults, suggesting that this allele may influence either lung growth or the rate of decline in lung function with age [40]. In the British 1958 cohort, again, the Arg16 allele had some influence on prognosis of wheezing in childhood, with persistent asthma or wheezing, or both, being common at 42 years of age in individuals carrying this variant [41]. The genetic effect of the Arg16 allele on lung function is also influenced by smoking; the Arg16 allele was associated with lower lung function in children, especially when there was a significant exposure to tobacco smoke [42]. Using 8 variables (age, sex, age at onset of the disease, smoking status, total serum IgE, %FEV1, FEV_1/FVC) and specific IgE responsiveness to common inhaled allergens, we conducted a two-step cluster analysis involving 880 Japanese patients with adult asthma and identified 6 phenotypes, as follows [37]: cluster A ($n = 155$), older age at onset, no airflow obstruction; cluster B ($n = 170$), childhood onset, normal-to-mild airflow obstruction; cluster C ($n = 119$), childhood onset, longest disease duration, moderate-to-severe airflow obstruction; cluster D ($n = 108$), older age at onset, severe airflow obstruction; cluster E ($n = 130$), middle age at onset, no airflow obstruction; and cluster F ($n = 198$), older age at onset, mild-to-moderate airflow obstruction. The *CCL5*-28C>G genotype was significantly associated with three of the clusters A, B, and D (OR 1.65, $p = 0.0021$; 1.67, 0.018; and 1.74, 0.011, respectively). The *ADRB2* Arg16Gly genotype was also associated with two of the clusters, B and D (OR 0.47, $p = 0.0004$; and 0.63 and 0.034, respectively). Our study identified meaningful adult asthma phenotypes linked to the functional *CCL5* and *ADRB2* genotypes.

3.5 Genes Responsible for Specific Endotypes

Clusters of phenotypes are likely to encompass specific endotypes—subgroups of these diseases, each with distinct molecular mechanisms. Therefore, in genetic studies, limiting the analysis to individuals with a specific phenotype of asthma may help define disease subtypes or endotypes, presenting great opportunities for better understanding of asthma pathogenesis and heterogeneity and, ultimately, for improving prevention and treatment of the disease. In fact, GWAS have yielded exciting results and revealed unexpected genes with variants that contribute to some distinct endotypes underlying the asthma syndrome, as described below.

3.5.1 Genes Responsible for Type-2 Allergic Inflammation

In Japan, a GWAS and a replication study that together comprised 7171 individuals with adult asthma and 27,912 controls have identified 5 loci associated with susceptibility to adult asthma [43]. These loci included the major histocompatibility complex and thymic stromal lymphopoietin (TSLP). TSLP is an epithelium-derived cytokine and has been identified as a master switch for type-2 allergic inflammation [44]. A human anti-TSLP monoclonal immunoglobulin G2-lambda that binds human TSLP and prevents receptor interaction, AMG 157 (ClinicalTrials.gov number, NCT01405963), has been shown to reduce allergen-induced bronchoconstriction and measures of airway inflammation [45].

Another GWAS was performed for pediatric asthma in Asian populations. By examining 6428 Asians, HLA-DPA1*0201/DPB1*0901 were found to be associated with pediatric asthma. Interestingly, the SNP rs987870 associated with pediatric asthma in this region confers protection against Th-1-type immune diseases, such as type 1 diabetes and rheumatoid arthritis, suggesting that this HLA class II region could determine Th1/Th2 dominance and could partially explain the inverse relationship between asthma and Th-1-type immune diseases [46].

A meta-analysis of three independent GWASs of Latinos and African Americans with asthma showed that multiple intronic variants in TYRO3 were associated with asthma [47]. TYRO3 is a member of the TAM (TYRO3, AXL, and MERTK) receptor tyrosine kinase (RTK) subgroup, and genetic ablation of a receptor tyrosine kinase encoded by Tyro3 in mice or the functional neutralization of its orthologue in human dendritic cells also resulted in enhanced type-2 immunity. These findings, together, indicated a critical role of TYRO3 in negatively regulating type-2 responses.

3.5.2 Genes Responsible for Increased Susceptibility to Viral Infection

Respiratory viral infection is a common feature of some major human airway diseases, including asthma. Exposure to respiratory viruses in early life is very common, and such exposure constitutes an independent risk factor for lung function abnormalities in adulthood, especially when the consequence of the childhood infection is severe acute lower respiratory tract infection (LRTI). Approximately 80–85% of asthma exacerbations in children, adolescents, and less frequently adults are associated with upper respiratory tract viral infections, and human rhinovirus (HRV) accounts for 60–70% of these virus-associated exacerbations. HRV-induced wheezing illnesses in early life are a significant risk factor for subsequent development of asthma, and growing evidence supports a role of recurrent HRV infections in the development and progression of several aspects of airway remodeling in asthma. The first GWAS for asthma identified a novel asthma-associated locus on chromosome 17q12-q21 that encompassed two genes, *ORMDL3* and *GSDMB* [11]. Variations at this locus are associated with an approximately twofold increased risk of recurrent wheezing, asthma, asthma exacerbations, and bronchial hyperresponsiveness from early infancy to school age but not with increased risk of eczema, rhinitis, or allergic sensitization [48]. Furthermore, the 17q21 locus is associated with asthma in children who have had RV wheezing illnesses and with expression of two genes at this locus, suggesting a role of 17q21 variants in the development of RV wheezing illnesses during early childhood as an underlying mechanism conferring susceptibility to early-onset asthma [49]. ORMDL3 is an endoplasmic reticulum (ER)-resident protein that appears to influence a stress response pathway known as the "unfolded protein response" (UPR) [50]. There is a striking association between elevated ORMDL3 expression and increased type I IFN production in response to RV, suggesting that higher ORMDL3 (the 17q21 risk genotype) response to RV with augmented ER stress could promote increased IFN responses or other pro-inflammatory consequences that predispose to the development of asthma [51].

Another GWAS of a specific asthma phenotype characterized by recurrent, severe exacerbations occurring between 2 and 6 years of age provided strong evidence for a newly recognized susceptibility gene, *CDHR3*, which encodes cadherin-related family member 3 and is highly expressed in the airway epithelium [32]. Compared with wild-type CDHR3, the CDHR3 (Cys529→Tyr, rs6967330) variant, which was linked to wheezing illnesses and hospitalizations for childhood asthma based on genetic analysis, exhibited approximately tenfold increase in RV-C binding and RV progeny yields when transfected into cells in vitro; these findings indicate that the CDHR3 variant that is associated with asthma susceptibility facilitates RV-C entry into host cells and that the variant could be a risk factor for RV-C wheezing illnesses [52].

In our sub-analysis of a large Japanese GWAS [43], to identify additional asthma-associated loci, only 240 asthma patients and 734 healthy controls, all recruited from a single geographical region, were included; additionally, only nonsmoking asthmatic patients or those with a limited smoking history of <10 pack years were included [53]. These inclusion criteria reduced the number of participants who had asthma-like symptoms due to environmental factors such as smoking and thereby increased our ability to identify asthma-specific genetic effects. Using this approach, evidence that *hyaluronan synthase 2* (*HAS2*) is associated with asthma emerged. This gene encodes a glucosaminoglycan that is present in the extracellular matrix and is strongly expressed in the lungs. Furthermore, an asthma-associated SNP was shown to affect regulation of *HAS2* mRNA expression. Hyaluronan plays an essential role in many physiological and pathological processes, including cell migration, morphogenesis, tissue regeneration, wound repair, and tumor cell growth and invasion. The airway inflammation associated with asthma involves the accumulation of a hyaluronan-rich matrix following viral infection; the degraded hyaluronan matrix is removed by the leukocytes/macrophages that enter the tissue. Notably, the degraded hyaluronan matrix acts as a "danger signal" responsible for initiating host responses to the inflammatory process and likely participates in determining the extent of the response to viral infections [54].

3.5.3 Genes Responsible for Bacterial Colonization in Airways

The lower airways are all colonized with airway microbiota, and the airway microbiomes in patients with asthma differ from those in healthy control subjects [55]. Although it is unknown whether the differences are the cause or consequence of the disease or treatments to the disease [56], it is likely that disease-related bacterial colonization impacts negatively on the clinical course by increasing the symptoms (chronic cough and expectoration), accelerating the rate of FEV_1 decline, promoting the occurrence of exacerbations, or some combination thereof [57, 58]. One-month-old neonates with bacterial colonization in the hypopharyngeal region (*Streptococcus pneumoniae*, *Haemophilus influenzae*, *Moraxella catarrhalis*, or a combination) have an increased risk for recurrent wheezing and asthma early in life, and this increased risk is independent of atopy [59]. These findings indicate that bacterial colonization has a role in some disease phenotypes, especially those phenotypes with neutrophilic inflammation. Importantly, these patients are consistently found to be largely refractory to ICS treatment and thus have fewer treatment options than other groups [60].

Previously, we reported that the genes encoding CCL5, tissue factor (TF), Clara cell secretory protein (CC16), or catalase (CAT) are associated with adult/late-onset asthma in a Japanese population [38, 61–63]. Assuming that differentiating asthma on the basis of age at disease onset increases the power of genetic studies and will enhance our understanding of asthma pathogenesis, we performed a GWAS focusing on late-onset asthma (age of onset ≥40 years) in a two-stage genetic association study of 4933 Japanese adults [64]. A meta-analysis combining data from three studies, two discovery and one replication, showed increased frequencies of the C alleles at both rs2523870 and rs2517548 in the late-onset asthma group (meta-$p = 3.77 \times 10^{-7}$ and 3.98×10^{-7}, respectively). These SNPs are close to each other; both are located between *HLA complex group 22* (*HCG22*) and *mucin 22* (*MUC22*) and are in tight linkage disequilibrium. SNP-gene associations for these two SNPs obtained by expression quantitative trait loci (eQTL) analysis indicated that *HCG22* mRNA expression in lymphoblastoid cell lines is strongly correlated with the number of C alleles, the asthma susceptibility alleles at either rs2523870 or rs2517548 ($p = 8.54 \times 10^{-87}$ or 3.23×10^{-84}, respectively). When we plotted the OR for association between rs2523870 and age-of-onset-specific subsets of asthma, the OR gradually increased as the age-of-onset cutoff increased up to the 50 years or older category (Fig. 3.1); this finding clearly indicates that the genetic contribution of rs2523870 increases as the age at onset of asthma increases.

Interestingly, *HCG22* was originally identified as a candidate gene for diffuse panbronchiolitis (DPB) in the MHC class I region of chromosome 6p21.3 [65]. DPB is an idiopathic inflammatory disease characterized by chronic neutrophilic bronchiolitis and rhinosinusitis that causes mucus hyper-secretion and airflow obstruction. The average age of onset of DPB is 40 years, and two-thirds of those affected are non-smokers. HCG22 has characteristics similar to those of mucin, with tandem repeats consisting of serine and threonine-rich peptides. *HCG22*, a

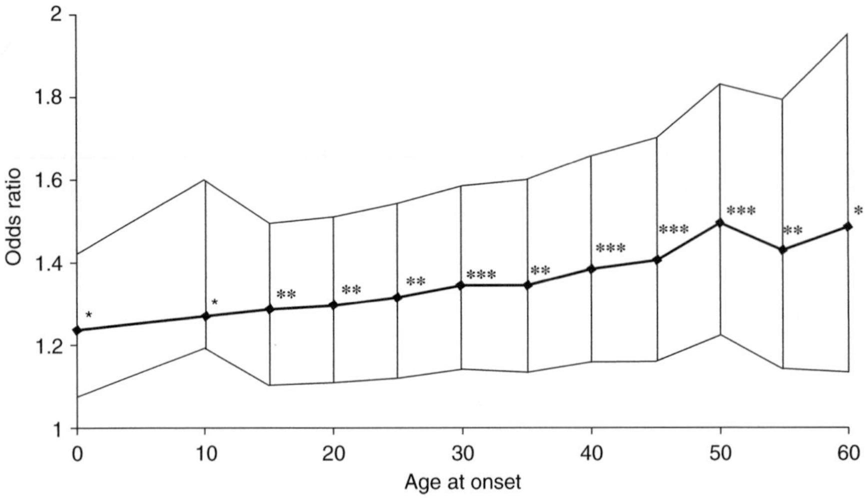

Fig. 3.1 Odds ratios for associations between *HCG22* and onset age-specific subsets of asthma. The OR gradually increases as the cutoff for the age-of-onset increases until the onset age reaches 50 years or later. ORs significantly >1 are highlighted (*$p < 0.005$, **$p < 0.001$, and ***$p < 0.0005$). Ref. [64]

novel mucin-like gene, forms a mucin-like gene cluster together with *MUC22*, *MUC21*, and *DPCR1*. Expression of *HCG22* is increased in lung tissues. When we investigated the genetic impact of rs2523870 on the development of DPB ($n = 108$) or COPD ($n = 307$) using 4044 healthy adults as controls, the C allele at rs2523870 (the risk allele for late-onset asthma) was also associated with DPB ($p = 3.06 \times 10^{-4}$; OR = 1.65) and with COPD ($p = 6.14 \times 10^{-3}$; OR = 1.28). The genetic associations found in patients with DPB or COPD and those with late-onset asthma along with the finding that both rs2523870 and rs2517548 are highly correlated with increased expression of *HCG22* strongly indicate that these SNPs confer increased risk of late-onset asthma and suggest that a common pathogenetic mechanism or a specific endotype underlies late-onset asthma, DPB, and COPD.

The HCG22 protein product is most closely related to peritrophin-A, which has a chitin-binding domain. Interestingly, another GWAS found that the chitinase 3-like 1 (*CHI3L1*) gene encoding YKL-40, another chitin-binding protein, was associated with asthma, bronchial hyperresponsiveness (BHR), and reduced lung function [66]. The *CHI3L1* variant was most strongly associated with elevated serum YKL-40 levels ($p = 1.1 \times 10^{-13}$) [64]. Subsequently, an intronic SNP in *CHI3L1* was shown to be associated with both circulating YKL-40 levels and asthma severity [67]. Neutrophils may be an important source of the increased levels of chitinases and chitinase-like proteins [68]. In fact, sputum YKL-40 levels strongly correlated with neutrophilic asthma [69].

Accumulation and activation of airway neutrophils are important in chronic airway diseases such as asthma, COPD, and DPB, and the activated neutrophils recruited to the airways play several key roles in mucus hyper-secretion. The genetic effects of *HCG22* and *CHI3L1* may, therefore, underlie some of the distinct asthma phenotypes characterized by impaired mucosal immunity and increased susceptibility to bacterial infection. With regard to the endotype characterized by bacterial colonization, recent insights into the airway microbiome suggest potential effects of aberrant airway microbiomes in patients with asthma on the pathobiology of the disease. Children living on farms are exposed to a wider range of microbes than are children not living on farms, and this exposure explains a substantial fraction of the inverse relation between asthma and growing up on a farm [70]. These findings indicate that the diversity of an environmental microbiome can influence lung health and disease. Detection of bacterial colonization may allow early intervention by exposing susceptible individuals to a wide range of microbes, which may help ameliorate or prevent chronic inflammatory lung diseases in later life. Long-term macrolide therapy is highly effective in the treatment of DPB [71]. In addition, macrolide antibiotics have been demonstrated to be efficacious in the treatment of severe neutrophilic asthma [72, 73]. Macrolides such as erythromycin, clarithromycin, and azithromycin not only have antimicrobial properties but also broad anti-inflammatory and immunomodulatory effects [74]. Nevertheless, chronic use of macrolides is associated with the occurrence of macrolide-resistant bacteria in the commensal flora of the pharynx of individual patients and also induces the risk of an increase in antibiotic resistance at the population level [75]. An electronic nose, which is a new noninvasive technology capable of distinguishing volatile organic compound (VOC) breath-prints in exhaled breath, can identify the presence of airway bacterial colonization in clinically stable patients with COPD [76]. Further research will determine the usefulness of breath-prints for diagnosing an endotype that may be particularly responsive to macrolide therapy.

3.5.4 Genes Responsible for Reduced Pulmonary Function

David Barker proposed an original hypothesis stating that fetal development is an important influence on the development of adult disease [77], and this hypothesis is relevant to asthma and COPD [78]. Adverse factors affecting lung development during fetal life and early childhood reduce the attainment of maximum lung function and accelerate declines in lung function during adulthood; therefore, these adverse factors predispose individuals to reduced lung function and increased respiratory morbidity, particularly asthma and COPD, throughout life [79, 80]. A GWAS performed in Japanese adults with asthma identified the most significant association at rs404860 in the major histocompatibility complex (MHC) region, which is near another SNP previously associated with lung function [43]. *TSLP* is a likely asthma-susceptibility locus, and we found that *TSLP* variants are associated with lower lung function in healthy individuals [81], which is consistent with the contention that genetic determinants of lung function influence susceptibility to asthma.

To date, GWASs on pulmonary function (e.g., predicted percentage of forced expiratory volume in 1 s [%FEV_1] and ratio of forced expiratory volume in 1 s to forced vital capacity [FEV_1/FVC]) have identified a number of risk loci in multiethnic populations [82–84]. Although our previous GWAS did not identify SNPs associated with pulmonary function at the level of genome-wide significance in a Japanese population, it does demonstrate that the heritability of pulmonary function can be explained by additive effects of multiple common SNPs, providing compelling evidence for a strong genetic influence on FEV_1/FVC [85]. Furthermore, our findings indicate that lung function genes identified in previous GWASs in non-Japanese populations account for 4.3–12.0% of the entire estimated heritability of FEV_1/FVC in a Japanese population. Therefore, we constructed a multi-SNP genetic risk score (GRS) for reduced FEV_1/FVC using genotype information for 16 genes associated with lower FEV_1/FVC in a GWAS of Japanese populations as well as in previous GWASs of non-Japanese populations [86]. The GRS, which combines the modest effects of multiple SNPs into a single variable, is calculated as the weighted sum of the number of high-risk alleles. Both reduced growth and accelerated lung function decline lead to lower lung function levels in adults, but the GRS calculated using the 16 SNPs was not associated with annual lung function decline in the healthy participants; therefore, we believe that these 16 SNPs (or gene pathways involving these 16 SNPs) may be involved in deregulated lung growth or development rather than in the accelerated decline of lung function. The "Development regulation of epithelial-to-mesenchymal transition (EMT)" pathway was annotated by the Gene Relationships Among Implicated Loci (GRAIL) program based on these 16 SNPs. Specifically, the EMT pathway contained three genes: *TGFB2*, *TNF*, and *NOTCH4*.

This GRS for lower FEV_1/FVC was consistently associated with the onset of asthma ($p = 9.6 \times 10^{-4}$) in two independent Japanese populations as well as with the onset of COPD ($p = 0.042$). The Cochran-Armitage trend test shows that the prevalence of asthma increases as GRS values increase ($p = 0.0059$) (Fig. 3.2). In contrast, the prevalence of atopic status does not change according to GRS values ($p = 0.46$), indicating that the association between the GRS and the presence of asthma is independent of atopic status. Clustering of asthma patients based on GRS values indicates that an increased GRS may be responsible for the development of a particular phenotype of asthma, a phenotype that is characterized by early onset, atopy, and more severe airflow obstruction. In a multinomial logistic regression analysis, the strongest association between GRS values and asthma was found in this particular cluster ($p = 3.6 \times 10^{-5}$). In fact, a similar cluster that is characterized by early-onset, atopic asthma with advanced airflow limitation has also been identified [87, 88]. Overall, these data highlight the potential application of genomics in developing novel strategies to precision medicine that may improve long-term respiratory outcomes for children with lower lung function. Such strategies may enable earlier identification of at-risk infants and of the specific pathways involved in disease pathogenesis in individual cases, which will allow for earlier and more specific interventions to achieve greater respiratory health after altered lung development in early childhood.

The progression from early life insults to pediatric disease and finally chronic obstructive airway disease in adulthood involves complex genetic, epigenetic, and

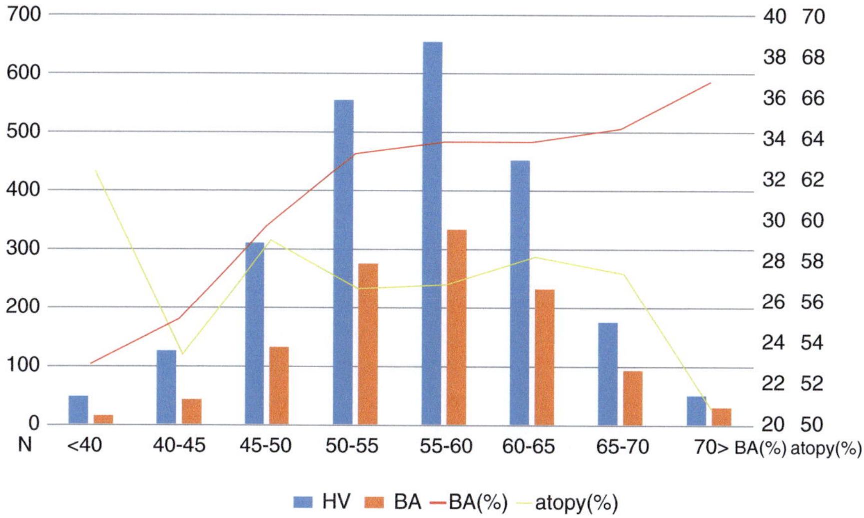

Fig. 3.2 Prevalence of asthma according to genetic risk score values for lower lung function. The horizontal axis shows the GRS ranges. The left vertical axis shows the number of healthy individuals and asthmatic patients for each GRS range. The right vertical axis shows the percentages of asthmatic patients and atopic individuals for each GRS range. The upper line shows the percentage of atopic individuals for each given GRS range. The lower line shows the percentage of asthmatic patients for each given GRS range. Atopy was defined as the presence of specific IgE antibody toward at least one common inhaled allergen. HV, healthy volunteer; BA, bronchial asthma. Ref. [86]

environmental interactions. In terms of the endotype characterized by impaired lung function, genetic variants that were identified in adults to be associated with lung function were not associated with neonatal lung function, but they were associated with the development of lung function measures during early childhood [89]. These findings suggest that a window of opportunity exists for interventions that target these genetic mechanisms. In fact, long-term improvements in air quality are associated with statistically and clinically significant positive effects on lung-function growth in children [90]. Measurement of lung function in early life, therefore, may help us in preventing reduced lung function and in maintaining respiratory health among children.

3.6 Conclusion

Asthma is a complex respiratory disorder, and susceptibility to the disease involves interplay between genetic and environmental factors. Unbiased genetic approaches, especially GWASs, have identified genetic factors important to the pathogenesis of asthma, but so far these factors account for only a small proportion of the heritability of asthma. There remains a need to determine the contribution of these polymorphisms to clinically relevant endpoints in asthma. A recent study of global gene expression in asthma revealed that expression of epithelial growth and repair and neuronal function genes were most strongly associated with severe asthma [91]. This suggested that epithelial integrity and related processes are of primary importance especially to the development of severe asthma, which is in line with current genetic findings. A concerted effort is, therefore, needed to sub-stratify asthma beyond the stratifications based on type-2 pathways and to use appropriate biomarkers that can identify patients likely to respond to specific and respective biologics. The application of modern technologies to the study of genomic alterations associated with viral infection, bacterial colonization, or lung growth may facilitate targeted development of new treatment options for patients with specific molecular abnormalities. These approaches will provide greater insight into the mechanisms altered in individuals carrying the relevant risk alleles, and such applications represent one component of personalized medicine.

References

1. Daniels SE, Bhattacharrya S, James A, et al. A genome-wide search for quantitative trait loci underlying asthma. Nature. 1996;383(6597):247–50.
2. Duffy DL, Martin NG, Battistutta D, Hopper JL, Mathews JD. Genetics of asthma and hay fever in Australian twins. Am Rev Respir Dis. 1990;142:1351–8.
3. Ober C, Yao TC. The genetics of asthma and allergic disease: a 21st century perspective. Immunol Rev. 2011;242:10–30.
4. Busse WW, Lemanske RF Jr. Asthma. N Engl J Med. 2001;344:350–62.
5. Carr TF, Bleecker E. Asthma heterogeneity and severity. World Allergy Organ J. 2016;9(1):41. eCollection 2016.
6. Wenzel S. Severe asthma: from characteristics to phenotypes to endotypes. Clin Exp Allergy. 2012;42:650–8.
7. Manolio TA. Genomewide association studies and assessment of the risk of disease. N Engl J Med. 2010;363:166–76.
8. McCarthy MI, Abecasis GR, Cardon LR, et al. Genome-wide association studies for complex traits: consensus, uncertainty and challenges. Nat Rev Genet. 2008;9:356–69.
9. Weiss ST, Raby BA, Rogers A. Asthma genetics and genomics 2009. Curr Opin Genet Dev. 2009;19:279–82.
10. Holloway JW, Yang IA, Holgate ST. Genetics of allergic disease. J Allergy Clin Immunol. 2010;125(suppl 2):S81–94.
11. Moffatt MF, Kabesch M, Liang L, et al. Genetic variants regulating ORMDL3 expression contribute to the risk of childhood asthma. Nature. 2007;448(7152):470–3.
12. Dixon AL, Liang L, Moffatt MF, et al. A genome-wide association study of global gene expression. Nat Genet. 2007;39:1202.
13. Bouzigon E, Corda E, Aschard H, et al. Effect of 17q21 variants and smoking exposure in early-onset asthma. N Engl J Med. 2008;359:1985.
14. Moffatt MF, Gut IG, Demenais F, et al. A large-scale, consortium-based genomewide association study of asthma. N Engl J Med. 2010;363:1211–21.
15. Hirota T, Harada M, Sakashita M, et al. Genetic polymorphism regulating ORM1-like 3 (Saccharomyces cerevisiae) expression is associated with childhood atopic asthma in a Japanese population. J Allergy Clin Immunol. 2008;121:769.

16. Wu H, Romieu I, Sienra-Monge JJ, et al. Genetic variation in ORM1-like 3 (ORMDL3) and gasdermin-like (GSDML) and childhood asthma. Allergy. 2009;64:629.
17. Torgerson DG, Ampleford EJ, Chiu GY, et al. Meta-analysis of genome-wide association studies of asthma in ethnically diverse North American populations. Nat Genet. 2011;43:887–92.
18. Gudbjartsson DF, Bjornsdottir US, Halapi E, et al. Sequence variants affecting eosinophil numbers associate with asthma and myocardial infarction. Nat Genet. 2009;41:342–7.
19. Myers RA, Himes BE, Gignoux CR, et al. Further replication studies of the EVE Consortium meta-analysis identifies 2 asthma risk loci in European Americans. J Allergy Clin Immunol. 2012;130:1294.
20. Hsu CL, Neilsen CV, Bryce PJ. IL-33 is produced by mast cells and regulates IgE-dependent inflammation. PLoS One. 2010;5:e11944.
21. Préfontaine D, Lajoie-Kadoch S, Foley S, et al. Increased expression of IL-33 in severe asthma: evidence of expression by airway smooth muscle cells. J Immunol. 2009;183:5094.
22. Préfontaine D, Nadigel J, Chouiali F, et al. Increased IL-33 expression by epithelial cells in bronchial asthma. J Allergy Clin Immunol. 2010;125:752.
23. Ferreira MA, Matheson MC, Duffy DL, et al, for the Australian Asthma Genetics Consortium. Identification of IL6R and chromosome 11q13.5 as risk loci for asthma. Lancet. 2011;378:1006–14.
24. Sears MR, Greene JM, Willan AR, et al. A longitudinal, population-based, cohort study of childhood asthma followed to adulthood. N Engl J Med. 2003;349:1414–22.
25. Hirschhorn JN. Genomewide association studies--illuminating biologic pathways. N Engl J Med. 2009;360(17):1699–701.
26. Barreto-Luis A, Corrales A, Acosta-Herrera M, et al. A pathway-based association study reveals variants from Wnt signaling genes contributing to asthma susceptibility. Clin Exp Allergy. 2017. https://doi.org/10.1111/cea.12883].
27. Yatagai Y, Sakamoto T, Masuko H, et al. Genome-wide association study for levels of total serum IgE identifies HLA-C in a Japanese population. PLoS One. 2013;8(12):e80941.
28. Weinmayr G, Weiland SK, Bjorksten B, et al. Atopic sensitization and the international variation of asthma symptom prevalence in children. Am J Respir Crit Care Med. 2007;176:565–74.
29. Palmer CN, Irvine AD, Terron-Kwiatkowski A, et al. Common loss-of-function variants of the epidermal barrier protein filaggrin are a major predisposing factor for atopic dermatitis. Nat Genet. 2006;38:441–6.
30. Walley AJ, Chavanas S, Moffatt MF, et al. Gene polymorphism in Netherton and common atopic disease. Nat Genet. 2001;29:175–8.
31. Holgate ST. Epithelium dysfunction in asthma. J Allergy Clin Immunol. 2007;120(6):1233–44.
32. Bønnelykke K, Sleiman P, Nielsen K, et al. A genome-wide association study identifies CDHR3 as a susceptibility locus for early childhood asthma with severe exacerbations. Nat Genet. 2014;46:51–5.
33. Moore WC, Meyers DA, Wenzel SE, et al. Identification of asthma phenotypes using cluster analysis in the Severe Asthma Research Program. Am J Respir Crit Care Med. 2010;181:315–23.
34. Haldar P, Pavord ID, Shaw DE, et al. Cluster analysis and clinical asthma phenotypes. Am J Respir Crit Care Med. 2008;178:218–24.
35. Wenzel SE. Asthma: defining of the persistent adult phenotypes. Lancet. 2006;368:804–13.
36. Diette GB, Krishnan JA, Dominici F, et al. Asthma in older patients: factors associated with hospitalization. Arch Intern Med. 2002;162:1123–32.
37. Kaneko Y, Masuko H, Sakamoto T, et al. Asthma phenotypes in Japanese adults - their associations with the CCL5 and ADRB2 genotypes. Allergol Int. 2013;62(1):113–21.
38. Hizawa N, Yamaguchi E, Konno S, et al. A functional polymorphism in the RANTES gene promoter is associated with the development of late-onset asthma. Am J Respir Crit Care Med. 2002;166:686–90.
39. Hizawa N. Beta-2 adrenergic receptor genetic polymorphisms and asthma. J Clin Pharm Ther. 2009;34(6):631–43.

40. Summerhill E, Leavitt SA, Gidley H, et al. beta(2)-adrenergic receptor Arg16/Arg16 genotype is associated with reduced lung function, but not with asthma, in the Hutterites. Am J Respir Crit Care Med. 2000;162(2 Pt 1):599–602.
41. Hall IP, Blakey JD, Al Balushi KA, et al. Beta2-adrenoceptor polymorphisms and asthma from childhood to middle age in the British 1958 birth cohort: a genetic association study. Lancet. 2006;368(9537):771–9.
42. Zhang G, Hayden CM, Khoo SK, et al. Beta2-Adrenoceptor polymorphisms and asthma phenotypes: interactions with passive smoking. Eur Respir J. 2007;30(1):48–55.
43. Hirota T, Takahashi A, Kubo M, et al. Genome-wide association study identifies three new susceptibility loci for adult asthma in the Japanese population. Nat Genet. 2011;43:893–6.
44. Licona-Limón P, Kim LK, Palm NW, Flavell RA. TH2, allergy and group 2 innate lymphoid cells. Nat Immunol. 2013;14(6):536–42.
45. Gauvreau GM, O'Byrne PM, Boulet LP, et al. Effects of an anti-TSLP antibody on allergen-induced asthmatic responses. N Engl J Med. 2014;370:2102.
46. Noguchi E, Sakamoto H, Hirota T, et al. Genome-wide association study identifies HLA-DP as a susceptibility gene for pediatric asthma in Asian populations. PLoS Genet. 2011;7(7):e1002170.
47. Chan PY, Carrera Silva EA, De Kouchkovsky D, et al. The TAM family receptor tyrosine kinase TYRO3 is a negative regulator of type 2 immunity. Science. 2016;352(6281):99–103.
48. Bisgaard H, Bønnelykke K, Sleiman PM, et al. Chromosome 17q21 gene variants are associated with asthma and exacerbations but not atopy in early childhood. Am J Respir Crit Care Med. 2009;179(3):179–85.
49. Çalışkan M, Bochkov YA, Kreiner-Møller E, et al. Rhinovirus wheezing illness and genetic risk of childhood-onset asthma. N Engl J Med. 2013;368:1398–407.
50. Cantero-Recasens G, Fandos C, Rubio-Moscardo F, Valverde MA, Vicente R, et al. The asthma-associated ORMDL3 gene product regulates endoplasmic reticulum-mediated calcium signaling and cellular stress. Hum Mol Genet. 2010;19:111–21.
51. Liu YP, Rajamanikham V, Baron M, et al. Association of ORMDL3 with rhinovirus-induced endoplasmic reticulum stress and type I Interferon responses in human leucocytes. Clin Exp Allergy. 2017;47(3):371–82.
52. Bochkov YA, Watters K, Ashraf S, et al. Cadherin-related family member 3, a childhood asthma susceptibility gene product, mediates rhinovirus C binding and replication. Proc Natl Acad Sci U S A. 2015;112(17):5485–90.
53. Yatagai Y, Sakamoto T, Yamada H, et al. Genomewide association study identifies HAS2 as a novel susceptibility gene for adult asthma in a Japanese population. Clin Exp Allergy. 2014;44(11):1327–34.
54. Scheibner KA, Lutz MA, Boodoo S, Fenton MJ, Powell JD, Horton MR. Hyaluronan fragments act as an endogenous danger signal by engaging TLR2. J Immunol. 2006;177:1272–81.
55. Hilty M, Burke C, Pedro H, et al. Disordered microbial communities in asthmatic airways. PLoS One. 2010;5:e8578.
56. Sethi S, Maloney J, Grove L, et al. Airway inflammation and bronchial bacterial colonization in chronic obstructive pulmonary disease. Am J Respir Crit Care Med. 2006;173:991–8.
57. Desai H, Eschberger K, Wrona C, et al. Bacterial colonization increases daily symptoms in patients with chronic obstructive pulmonary disease. Ann Am Thorac Soc. 2014;11:303–9.
58. Zhang Q, Illing R, Hui CK, Downey K, et al. Bacteria in sputum of stable severe asthma and increased airway wall thickness. Respir Res. 2012;13:35.
59. Bisgaard H, Hermansen MN, Buchvald F, et al. Childhood asthma after bacterial colonization of the airway in neonates. N Engl J Med. 2007;357:1487–95.
60. Green RH, Brightling CE, Woltmann G, Parker D, Wardlaw AJ, Pavord ID. Analysis of induced sputum in adults with asthma: identification of subgroup with isolated sputum neutrophilia and poor response to inhaled corticosteroids. Thorax. 2002;57:875–9.
61. Isada A, Konno S, Hizawa N, et al. A functional polymorphism (-603A --> G) in the tissue factor gene promoter is associated with adult-onset asthma. J Hum Genet. 2010;55:167–74.

62. Taniguchi N, Konno S, Hattori T, et al. The CC16 A38G polymorphism is associated with asymptomatic airway hyper-responsiveness and development of late-onset asthma. Ann Allergy Asthma Immunol. 2013;111:376–81.
63. Taniguchi N, Konno S, Isada A, et al. Association of the CAT-262C>T polymorphism with asthma in smokers and the nonemphysematous phenotype of chronic obstructive pulmonary disease. Ann Allergy Asthma Immunol. 2014;113:31–6.
64. Yatagai Y, Hirota T, Sakamoto T, et al. Variants near the HLA complex group 22 gene confer increased susceptibility to late-onset asthma in Japanese populations. J Allergy Clin Immunol. 2016;138(1):281. pii: S0091-6749(16)00024-5.
65. Hijikata M, Matsushita I, Tanaka G, et al. Molecular cloning of two novel mucin-like genes in the disease-susceptibility locus for diffuse panbronchiolitis. Hum Genet. 2011;129:117–28.
66. Ober C, Tan Z, Sun Y, et al. Effect of variation in CHI3L1 on serum YKL-40 level, risk of asthma, and lung function. N Engl J Med. 2008;358:1682.
67. Gomez JL, Crisafi GM, Holm CT, et al. Genetic variation in chitinase 3-like 1 (CHI3L1) contributes to asthma severity and airway expression of YKL-40. J Allergy Clin Immunol. 2015;136:51.
68. Żurawska-Płaksej E, Ługowska A, Hetmańczyk K, et al. Neutrophils as a source of chitinases and chitinase-like proteins in type 2 diabetes. PLoS One. 2015;10(10):e0141730.
69. Hinks TSC, Brown T, Lau LCK, et al. Multidimensional endotyping in patients with severe asthma reveals inflammatory heterogeneity in matrix metalloproteinases and chitinase 3–like protein 1. J Allergy Clin Immunol. 2016 Jul;138(1):61–75.
70. Ege MJ, Mayer M, Normand AC, et al. Exposure to environmental microorganisms and childhood asthma. N Engl J Med. 2011;364(8):701–9.
71. Nagai H, Shishido H, Yoneda R, Yamaguchi E, Tamura A, Kurashima A. Long-term low-dose administration of erythromycin to patients with diffuse panbronchiolitis. Respiration. 1991;58(3-4):145–9.
72. Brusselle GG, VanderStichele C, Jordens P, et al. Azithromycin for prevention of exacerbations in severe asthma (AZISAST): a multicentre randomised double-blind placebo-controlled trial. Thorax. 2013;68:322–9.
73. Simpson JL, Powell H, Boyle MJ, Scott RJ, Gibson PG. Clarithromycin targets neutrophilic airway inflammation in refractory asthma. Am J Respir Crit Care Med. 2008;177(2):148–55.
74. Spagnolo P, Fabbri LM, Bush A. Long-term macrolide treatment for chronic respiratory disease. Eur Respir J. 2013;42(1):239–51.
75. Serisier D. Risks of population antimicrobial resistance associated with chronic macrolide use for inflammatory airway diseases. Lancet Respir Med. 2013;1:262–74.
76. Sibila O, Garcia-Bellmunt L, Giner J, et al. Identification of airway bacterial colonization by an electronic nose in Chronic Obstructive Pulmonary Disease. Respir Med. 2014;108(11):1608–14.
77. Barker DJ, Winter PD, Osmond C, et al. Weight in infancy and death from ischemic heart disease. Lancet. 1989;2:577–80.
78. Sharma S, Chhabra D, Kho AT, Hayden LP, Tantisira KG, Weiss ST. The genomic origins of asthma. Thorax. 2014;69(5):481–7.
79. Haland G, Carlsen KC, Sandvik L, et al. Reduced lung function at birth and the risk of asthma at 10 years of age. N Engl J Med. 2006;355:1682–9.
80. Stocks J, Hislop A, Sonnappa S. Early lung development: lifelong effect on respiratory health and disease. Lancet Respir Med. 2013;1(9):728–42.
81. Masuko H, Sakamoto T, Kaneko Y, et al. Lower FEV1 in non-COPD, nonasthmatic subjects: association with smoking, annual decline in FEV1, total IgE levels, and TSLP genotypes. Int J Chron Obstruct Pulmon Dis. 2011;6:181–9.
82. Hancock DB, Eijgelsheim M, Wilk JB, et al. Meta-analyses of genome-wide association studies identify multiple loci associated with pulmonary function. Nat Genet. 2010;42(1):45–52.
83. Repapi E, Sayers I, Wain LV, et al. Genome-wide association study identifies five loci associated with lung function. Nat Genet. 2010;42(1):36–44.

84. Soler AM, Loth DW, Wain LV, et al. Genome-wide association and large-scale follow up identifies 16 new loci influencing lung function. Nat Genet. 2011;43(11):1082–90.
85. Yamada H, Yatagai Y, Masuko H, et al. Heritability of pulmonary function estimated from genome-wide SNPs in healthy Japanese adults. Respir Investig. 2015;53(2):60–7.
86. Yamada H, Masuko H, Yatagai Y, et al. Role of lung function genes in the development of asthma. PLoS One. 2016;11(1):e0145832.
87. Fitzpatrick AM, Teague WG, Meyers DA, et al. Heterogeneity of severe asthma in childhood: confirmation by cluster analysis of children in the National Institutes of Health/National Heart, Lung, and Blood Institute Severe Asthma Research Program. J Allergy Clin Immunol. 2011;127(2):382–9.
88. Lodrup Carlsen KC, Mowinckel P, Hovland V, Haland G, Riiser A, Carlsen KH. Lung function trajectories from birth through puberty reflect asthma phenotypes with allergic comorbidity. J Allergy Clin Immunol. 2014;134(4):917–23.
89. Kreiner-Møller E, Bisgaard H, Bønnelykke K. Prenatal and postnatal genetic influence on lung function development. J Allergy Clin Immunol. 2014;134(5):1036–42.
90. Gauderman WJ, Urman R, Avol E, et al. Association of improved air quality with lung development in children. N Engl J Med. 2015;372(10):905–13.
91. Modena BD, Bleecker ER, Busse WW, et al. Gene expression correlated to severe asthma characteristics reveals heterogeneous mechanisms of severe disease. Am J Respir Crit Care Med. 2017;195(11):1449. https://doi.org/10.1164/rccm.201607-1407OC.

Chapter 4
COPD: Hereditary (A1-AT) and Non-hereditary—What Are the Roles of Genetic Factors in the Pathogenesis of COPD?

Nobuyuki Horita

Abstract Although smoking is a considerable risk factor for COPD development, genetic susceptibility is believed to play a key role in the development of COPD. This is because approximately 15% of the smoking population eventually suffer from this disease, while the others sustain normal lungs despite their smoking habit. A well-known causal gene of COPD is the serine protease inhibitor A1 (SERPINA1) gene, which causes hereditary severe α1-antitrypsin (A1-AT) deficiency. After SERPINA1 was identified as causal gene for A1-AT deficiency leading to COPD, many other genes that alter the risk of non-hereditary COPD were identified. Especially, the recent development of the genome-wide association study (GWAS) is a powerful tool to identify hypothesis-free genes. Even though recent studies have revealed more than 100 genes that affect the risk of non-hereditary COPD, the impact of each gene is not very strong, and they usually change the risk of COPD with a risk ratio of between 0.7 and 1.5. Thus, identified genes can explain only a small part of the etiology of COPD. In this chapter, we will review the roles of genetic factors in the pathogenesis of hereditary and non-hereditary COPD.

Keywords Chronic obstructive pulmonary disease · Gene · Meta-analysis Genome-wide association study

4.1 Introduction

Chronic obstructive pulmonary disease (COPD) is a systematic inflammatory disease which is mainly diagnosed by smoking history, pulmonary obstruction, and clinical symptoms. The main symptoms include cough, sputum, and shortness of

N. Horita
Department of Pulmonology, Yokohama City University Graduate School of Medicine, Yokohama, Japan

T. Kaneko (ed.), *Clinical Relevance of Genetic Factors in Pulmonary Diseases*, Respiratory Disease Series: Diagnostic Tools and Disease Managements,
https://doi.org/10.1007/978-981-10-8144-6_4

breath on exertion. It is the third leading cause of death in the world, with more than three million people dying from COPD a year [1–3]. Although smoking is a considerable risk factor for COPD development, genetic susceptibility is believed to play a key role in the development of COPD. This is because approximately 15% of the smoking population eventually suffer from this disease, while the others sustain normal lungs despite their smoking habit. A well-known causal gene of COPD is the serine protease inhibitor A1 (SERPINA1) gene, which causes hereditary severe α1-antitrypsin (A1-AT) deficiency [4]. A1-AT is clinically characterized by liver disease and early-onset emphysematous change. Although large amount of A1-AT is produced in the liver, its main function is to protect the lung from proteolytic damage from neutrophils. A serum level of A1-AT below 11 μmol/L increases the risk for COPD. For years, SERPINA1 was the only genetic factor whose relationship with COPD was revealed. Given that SERPINA1 gene polymorphism increases the COPD, it could have been hypothesized that other genes can be related to CODP risk. In this chapter, we will review the genetic aspect of COPD.

4.2 COPD Is a Multifactorial Genetic Disease

The Mendelian inheritance model provides a simple rule that explains genomic contribution to a disease development. A family tree with three or four generations is usually sufficient to identify a Mendelian-inherited disease, though few cases might be affected because of new gene mutations. However, most hereditary disease and hereditary traits of human do not simply follow this Mendelian model. COPD is believed to be a multifactorial disease caused by complex etiologies such as many genes, epigenetic factors, and environmental factors. It is far more difficult to reveal the causal genes of a multifactorial disease than to reveal those of a Mendelian-inherited disease. Traditional methods to identify the causal genes of a multifactorial disease are a family tree study, a twin study, an adaptive study, sibling analysis, case-control studies, linkage analysis, and association studies. The recent development of the genome-wide association study (GWAS) is a powerful tool to identify hypothesis-free genes [5]. Even though recent studies have revealed more than 100 genes that affect the risk of COPD, the impact of each gene is not very strong, and they usually change the risk of COPD with a risk ratio of between 0.7 and 1.5. In addition, a large number of genes that were reported to be associated with COPD development were not reconfirmed in replication studies. Thus, identified genes can explain only a small part of the etiology of COPD [6, 7] (Table 4.1).

Gene structure is often complicated. Some genes have components across many chromosomes. Certain lines of deoxyribonucleic acid are shared by two or more genes. Therefore, one single nucleotide polymorphism (SNP) can alter the structure of two or more genes. On the other hand, there can be many SNPs in a gene.

Table 4.1 List of possible COPD causal genes

A disintegrin and metalloprotease domain 33 (ADAM33)
Adrenergic receptor beta 2 (ADRB2)
Alpha-2-macroglobulin (A2M)
Angiotensin I converting enzyme 1 (ACE1)
Aquaporin 5 (AQP5)
Arachidonate 5-lipoxygenase-activating protein (ALOX5AP)
ATP-binding cassette, subfamily C, member 1 (ABCC1)
B-cell leukemia/lymphoma 2 (BCL2)
Bradykinin receptor B2 (BDKRB2)
Caspase 10, apoptosis-related cysteine peptidase (CASP10)
Catalase (CAT)
Cathepsin S (CTSS)
CD14 molecule (CD14)
CD40 molecule (CD40)
CD63 molecule (CD63)
CD86 molecule (CD86)
Cell division cycle 6 homolog (CDC6)
Chemokine ligand 5 (CCL5)
Chemokine receptor 2 (CCR2)
Chitinase 3-like 1 (CHI3L1)
Chloride channel accessory 1 (CLCA1)
Cholinergic receptor, nicotinic, alpha 3 (CHRNA3)
Cholinergic receptor, nicotinic, alpha 5 (CHRNA5)
Classical class 11 subregion of the MHC (HLA)
Collagen, type IV, alpha 3 (COL4A3)
Colony stimulating factor 2 (CSF2)
Colony stimulating factor 3 (CSF3)
C-reactive protein (CRP)
Cyclin-dependent kinase inhibitor 1A (CDKN1A)
Cystic fibrosis transmembrane conductance regulator (CFTR)
Cytochrome b-245, alpha polypeptide (CYBA)
Cytochrome P450, family 1, subfamily A, polypeptide 1 (CYP1A1)
Cytochrome P450, family 1, subfamily A, polypeptide 2 (CYP1A2)
Cytochrome P450, family 2, subfamily E, polypeptide 1 (CYP2E1)
Cytochrome P450, family 2, subfamily F, polypeptide 1 (CYP2F1)
Cytochrome P450, family 3, subfamily A, polypeptide 5 (CYP3A5)
Cytotoxic T-lymphocyte-associated protein 4 (CTLA4)
Defensin, beta 1 (DEFB1)
Defensin, beta 4A (DEFB4A)
Elastin (ELN)
Endothelin 1 (EDN1)

(continued)

Table 4.1 (continued)

Endothelin receptor type B (EDNRB)
Epoxide hydrolase 1 (xenobiotic) (EPHX1)
Estrogen receptor 1 (ESR1)
Family with sequence similarity 13, member A (FAM13A)
Fibroblast growth factor 10 (FGF10)
Glutamate-cysteine ligase, catalytic subunit (GCLC)
Glutamate-cysteine ligase, modifier subunit (GCLM)
Glutathione S-transferase M1 (GSTM1)
Glutathione S-transferase omega 1 (GSTO1)
Glutathione S-transferase omega 2 (GSTO2)
Glutathione S-transferase pi 1 (GSTP1)
Glutathione S-transferase theta 1 (GSTT1)
Glutathione S-transferase, C-terminal domain containing (GSTCD)
Hedgehog interacting protein (HHIP)
Heme oxygenase 1 (HMOX1)
Hemopoietic cell kinase (HCK)
Interferon, gamma (IFNG)
Interleukin 1 receptor antagonist (IL1RN)
Interleukin 1, alpha (IL1A)
Interleukin 1, beta (IL1B)
Interleukin 10 (IL10)
Interleukin 12B (IL12B)
Interleukin 13 (IL13)
Interleukin 13 receptor, alpha 1 (IL13RA1)
Interleukin 17F (IL17F)
Interleukin 2 (IL2)
Interleukin 27 (IL27)
Interleukin 4 (IL4)
Interleukin 4 receptor (IL4R)
Interleukin 5 (IL5)
Interleukin 6 (IL6)
Interleukin 8 (IL8)
Interleukin 8 receptor, alpha (IL8RA)
Interleukin 8 receptor, beta (IL8RB (CXCR2))
Iron-responsive element-binding protein 2 (IREB2)
Kelch-like ECH-associated protein 1 (KEAP1)
Latent transforming growth factor beta binding protein 4 (LTBP4)
Leptin (LEP)
Leptin receptor (LEPR)
Leukotriene A4 hydrolase (LTA4H)
Lymphotoxin alpha (LTA)
Macrophage scavenger receptor 1 (MSR1)
Mannose-binding lectin 2 (MBL2)

Table 4.1 (continued)

Matrix metallopeptidase 1 (MMP1)
Matrix metallopeptidase 12 (MMP12)
Matrix metallopeptidase 14 (MMP14)
Matrix metallopeptidase 2 (MMP2)
Matrix metallopeptidase 3 (MMP3)
Matrix metallopeptidase 9 (MMP9)
MHC class I polypeptide-related sequence B (MICB)
MicroRNA 196a-2 (MIR196A2)
MicroRNA 499a (MIR499A)
N-acetyltransferase 2 (NAT2)
NAD(P)H dehydrogenase, quinone 1 (NQO1)
Nitric oxide synthase 3 (NOS3)
Nuclear factor (erythroid-derived 2)-like 2 (NFE2L2)
Nuclear factor of kappa light polypeptide gene enhancer in B-cells inhibitor, beta (NFKBIB)
Nuclear receptor subfamily 3, group C, member 1 (NR3C1)
Olfactory receptor, family 4, subfamily X, member 1 (OR4X1)
Peroxisome proliferator-activated receptor gamma (PPARG)
Phosphatase and tensin homolog (PTEN)
Phosphodiesterase 4D (PDE4D)
Plasminogen activator, urokinase receptor (PLAUR)
Potassium large conductance calcium-activated channel, subfamily M, beta member 1 (KCNMB1)
Prostaglandin D2 receptor (PTGDR)
Prostaglandin-endoperoxide synthase 2 (PTGS2)
Serpin peptidase inhibitor A1 (SERPINA1)
Serpin peptidase inhibitor A3 (SERPINA3)
Serpin peptidase inhibitor E2 (SERPINE2)
Sex determining region Y-box 5 (SOX5)
Signal transducer and activator of transcription 1 (STAT1)
Signal transducer and activator of transcription 3 (STAT3)
Signal transducer and activator of transcription 6 (STAT6)
Sirtuin 2 (SIRT2)
SMAD family member 3 (SMAD3)
Solute carrier family 11 member 1 (SLC11A1)
Solute carrier family 6 member 4 (SLC6A4)
SPARC related modular calcium binding 2 (SMOC2)
Stress-induced-phosphoprotein 1 (STIP1)
Superoxide dismutase 2, mitochondrial (SOD2)
Superoxide dismutase 3, extracellular (SOD3)
Surfactant protein A1 (SFTPA1)
Surfactant protein A2 (SFTPA2)
Surfactant protein B (SFTPB)
Surfactant protein C (SFTPC)

(continued)

Table 4.1 (continued)

Surfactant protein D (SFTPD)
Tensin 1 (TNS1)
Thromboxane A2 receptor (TBXA2R)
Thymic stromal lymphopoietin (TSLP)
TIMP metallopeptidase inhibitor 1 (TIMP1)
TIMP metallopeptidase inhibitor 2 (TIMP2)
Toll-like receptor 4 (TLR4)
Transforming growth factor, beta 1 (TGFB1)
Transforming growth factor, beta receptor III (TGFBR3)
Transient receptor potential cation channel, subfamily V, member 4 (TRPV4)
Tumor necrosis factor member 2 (TNF2)
Tumor necrosis factor α (TNFA)
Tumor protein p53 (TP53)
Vascular endothelial growth factor A (VEGFA)
vitamin D binding protein (VDBP)
Vitamin D receptor (VDR)
X-ray repair complementing defective repair in Chinese hamster cells 1 (XRCC1)
X-ray repair complementing defective repair in Chinese hamster cells 5 (XRCC5)
5-hydroxytryptamine receptor 4 (HTR4)
8-oxoguanine DNA glycosylase (OGG1)

4.3 Popular Methods for Gene Analysis

4.3.1 Parametric Linkage Analysis

Parametric linkage analysis is the traditional analysis using the logarithm 10 of odds (LOD) score to assess the probability that a given pedigree has a certain trait. This method is useful when a valid model that is compliant to the Mendelian model is provided. The LOD score is given by logarithm 10 of probability of birth sequence with a given linkage value/probability of birth sequence with no linkage. A LOD score >3.0 suggests evidence of linkage, and a score <-2.0 suggests no such linkage [8–10].

4.3.2 Nonparametric Linkage Analysis

Nonparametric linkage analysis is another type of linkage analysis which is applicable even when the genetic model is unclear. For this analysis, we have to discriminate "identical by descent" and "identical by state." Affected sibling pair analysis is the most common style of nonparametric linkage analysis. A nonparametric LOD score >3.6 is often used as a cutoff [8–10].

Table 4.2 Case-control association analysis

	Cases with disease	Control without disease
MM genotype	a	b
Mm genotype	c	d
mm genotype	e	f
M allele	$2a + c$	$2b + d$
m allele	$c + 2e$	$d + 2f$

M major, *m* minor
a–f numbers of cases
Dominant model: odds ratio = $(c + e) \times b/(d + f)/a$
Recessive model: odds ratio = $e \times (b + d)/f/(a + c)$
Allelic model: odds ratio = $(c + 2e) \times (2b + d)/(d + 2f)/(2a + c)$

4.3.3 Case-Control Association Analysis

Both parametric and nonparametric linkage analyses have successfully identified only a few genetic linkages with traits. Instead, association analysis is more powerful in revealing the weak impact of polymorphism on disease development.

A case-control association analysis is currently the most common type of gene association analysis. In a case-control association analysis, the frequency of alleles and genotypes was compared between groups of individuals, usually diseased subjects and healthy controls. The magnitude of how each allele or genotype affects the risk of disease is usually expressed with odds ratios. Prior to the analysis, Hardy-Weinberg's equilibrium should be confirmed. Otherwise, the analysis provides biased results [11] (Table 4.2).

4.3.4 Genome-Wide Association Study (GWAS)

A GWAS, also known as a whole genome association study, is an examination of a genome-wide set of genetic variants in groups of individuals to see whether any variant is associated with a specific trait. A classical case-control association analysis test prespecified SNPs or alleles at a gene based on previous knowledge. Therefore, the analysis can just reconfirm the hypothesis that a SNP or allele is associated with some diseases. However, GWAS can test thousands of SNPs collectively without hypothesis. Thus, a key advantage of GWAS over the classical case-control association analysis is the possibility of identifying unrecognized genes. To avoid serious multiple comparisons, the cutoff value of the statistical test is set at the order of 10^{-8} instead of 0.05 [5, 12, 13]. The results are typically presented using Manhattan plot (Fig. 4.1) [37].

Some GWAS were done by an international study group. They repeatedly used data from previous large randomized controlled trials and large cohort studies

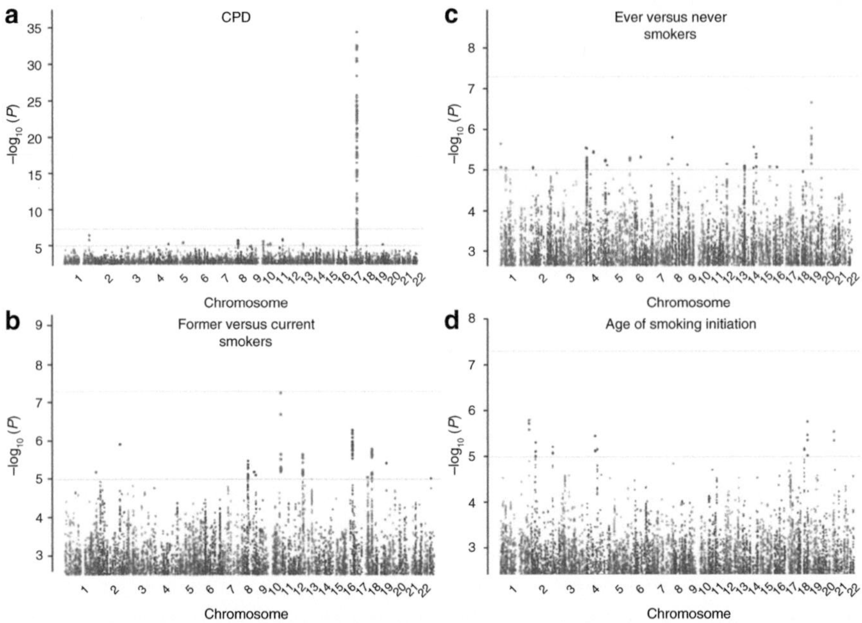

Fig. 4.1 Manhattan plot for of GWAS results identify multiple loci associated with smoking behavior. Presented with permission from Nature Publishing Group [37]

including the National Emphysema Treatment Trial, the Boston Early-Onset COPD Study, and the International COPD Genetics Network.

4.4 Candidate Risk Genes of A1-AT Deficiency

A1-AT is a protease inhibitor belonging to the serpin superfamily. A1-AT deficiency is a genetic autosomal codominant/recessive disease characterized by low serum levels of A1-AT [14–16]. The condition may lead to liver disease, early-onset pulmonary emphysema, and rare multi-organ vasculitis, necrotizing panniculitis, and fibromyalgia. A1-AT deficiency makes the lungs susceptible to smoking and results in emphysematous COPD. Although this disease is very rare in those of Asian descent, it affects about one in 2000–5000 Caucasians [4].

4.4.1 Serine Protease Inhibitors A1 (SERPINA1)

The SERPINA1 gene is located on the long arm of the 14th chromosome (14q32.1). More than one hundred types of variation of A1-AT have been detected in various populations. A normal population have homogenous M allele (PI*MM). Caucasians living in the Northwestern European Union are at high risk for carrying one of the common mutations of A1-AT, the Z mutation (Glu342Lys on M1A, rs28929474). The homogenous Z allele (PI*ZZ) causes severe A1-AT deficiency. This PI*ZZ genotype causes the protein to fold aberrantly and accumulate in the endoplasmic reticulum. This mutation reduces concentrations in serum of A1-AT by retaining polymerized molecules within hepatocytes. Heterogeneous M and Z alleles (PI*MZ) slightly increase the risk of emphysema.

A serum A1-AT level under the protective threshold increases the risk for emphysema. In addition to the Z mutation, some patients with A1-AT deficiency have the S mutation. The prevalences of COPD among each genotype are 91% for PI*MM, 6.1% for PI*MS, 2.7% for PI*MZ, 0.1% for PI*SS, 0.1% for PI*SZ, and 0.02% for PI*ZZ. When the serum A1-AT level is below 11 mmol/L, the risk of emphysema is elevated. Among patients who have PI*SZ, the A1-AT level was 8–16 mmol/L and 20–50% of these patients had risk of emphysema [4]. The A1-AT level of cases with PI*ZZ genotype was 2.5–7 mmol/L and more than 80% of these patients had emphysema [4].

Dalh et al. carried out a population-based cohort study in Copenhagen with a 21-year follow-up to evaluate the deteriorating effect of intermediate A1-AT deficiency (MZ genotype) on the lung. They recruited 9187 adults randomly selected from the Danish general population. Among this cohort, 4.9% of the participants carried the MZ genotype. Plasma A1-AT levels were 31% lower in MZ heterozygotes than in persons with the normal (MM) genotype. The annual decline of forced expiratory volume in 1 s was 25 and 21 ml in those with MZ heterozygotes and those with MM genotype, respectively ($P = 0.048$). In a logistic regression model adjusted for possible confounders such as age, sex, and tobacco consumption, the population with the MZ genotype had a higher risk of airway obstruction with an odds ratio of 1.3 (95% confidence interval 1.0–1.7) compared to the population with the MM genotype. The authors concluded that those with MZ heterozygotes had a slightly faster decline in forced expiratory volume in 1 s and that MZ heterozygosity may account for approximately 2% of COPD cases in the population in general [17].

4.5 Candidate Risk Genes of Non-hereditary COPD

In addition to emphysema-type COPD of severe A1-AT deficiency cases, researchers suspected that some genetic etiologies control lung susceptibility to tobacco smoking of non-hereditary COPD patients. This hypothesis is principally based on the fact that only 15% of smokers develop COPD. In this subsection, we will review famous identified genes related to gene-by-smoking interaction.

Note that most case-control studies and the GWAS had common limitations as regards revealing the link between smoking and COPD. This is because the suspected SNP may just change the smoking habit but not change the lung susceptibility to smoking irritation. In other words, confounding was not denied.

Furthermore, identified genes and SNPs may be just surrogates of nearby true causal genes. Thus, it is unclear whether identified genes and SNP are directly related to the COPD risk [1].

4.5.1 Serine Protease Inhibitor E2 (SERPINE2)

In 2006, DeMeo et al. identified SERPINE2 gene as a possible candidate susceptibility gene for COPD by integrating the results from mouse lung development and human COPD gene-expression microarray studies with human COPD linkage results on chromosome 2q to prioritize candidate-gene selection. They observed a meaningful association with COPD phenotypes and 18 SNPs at the SERPINE2 gene. Then, for 5 out of 18 SNPs, the link with COPD was further reconfirmed in case-control study [18].

The following year, Zhu et al. revealed the relationship between SERPINE2 polymorphisms and COPD-related phenotypes using data of 635 pedigrees with 1910 individuals. An independent case-control population consisted of 973 COPD cases, and 956 healthy subjects were also genotypes. Among 25 SNPs evaluated, a family-based study identified 6 SNPs that affect the risk of COPD. Five out of these six SNPs were then replicated in a case-control population [19].

Fujimoto et al. genotyped two SNPs located at SEPINE2 using samples obtained from 1335 consecutive autopsies of elderly Japanese people. Homozygous minor alleles of rs975278 were associated with emphysema with an odds ratio of 1.54 ($P = 0.037$) and the association was striking among smokers (odds ratio = 2.02, $P = 0.002$). This suggests the gene-by-smoking interaction [20].

4.5.2 Tumor Necrosis Factor Alpha (TNF-α)

TNF-α is a potent proinflammatory cytokine that may be involved in the development of COPD. A SNP at position -308 of TNF-α gene promoter (TNF-α-308 G/A) is known to adjust TNF-α secretion. Therefore, Sakao et al. conducted a case-control study with 106 COPD cases, 110 sex/age-matched asymptomatic smoker/ex-smokers, and 129 controls. The prevalence of minor alleles was 16.5% in patients with COPD, 8.2% in asymptomatic smoker/ex-smokers, and 7.8% in the control subjects [21].

Some similar studies were conducted over the next 10 years; however, the results were not consistent. A systematic review by Zhan et al. collected data from 24 eligible studies, comprising 2380 COPD cases and 3738 controls. Their analysis showed that the TNF-α-308 G/A SNP was significantly associated with an increased risk of COPD with a pooled odds ratio of 1.335 using the allelic model. However, a subgroup analysis showed that the association between the TNF-α-308 G/A SNP and COPD was observed only for the Asian population and not for the Caucasian population. Therefore, the authors concluded that the TNF-308 A allele is a more significant risk factor for developing COPD only among Asian populations [22].

4.5.3 Transforming Growth Factor-Beta1 (TGF-β1)

TGF-β1 is a polypeptide member of the TGF-β cytokine superfamily. This protein controls many cellular functions, including cell growth, cell proliferation, cell differentiation and apoptosis. Celedón et al. revealed that three SNPs at the TGF-β1 gene were significantly associated with pre- and post-bronchodilator forced expiratory volume in 1 s using data from family-based studies. In addition, they also showed that two SNPs in the promoter region of TGF-β1 and a SNP in exon 1 of TGF-β1 were significantly associated with COPD among smokers in the COPD cases and control subjects [23].

Wu et al. carried out another case-control study consisting of 165 subjects with COPD, 140 healthy blood donors, and 76 smokers with normal lung function. In this study, the distributions of the genotypes of Leu/Leu, Leu-Pro, and Pro-Pro were estimated using the polymerase chain reaction and restriction enzyme fragment length polymorphism. The Pro allele was less frequent in COPD patients than in blood donors (odds ratio 0.62, $P = 0.005$) and resistant smokers (odds ratio = 0.59, $P = 0.01$) [24].

4.5.4 Epoxide Hydratase (EPHX) 1

EPHXs, also known as epoxide hydratases, are a class of critical biotransformation enzymes that can convert epoxides from the degradation of aromatic compounds to trans-dihydrodiols which can be conjugated and excreted from the human body. Epoxide hydrolase functions in both the activation and detoxification of epoxides. A SNP, rs2234922 (A416G, H139R) is an A/G single-nucleotide variation on human chromosome 1 that influences EPHX1 activity in vitro.

A case-control study with 202 COPD cases and 136 controls by Vibhuti et al. revealed that the SNP A416G increases the risk of COPD with an odds ratio of 1.95 (95% confidence interval 1.16–4.53) [25]. Some similar case-control studies with an Asian population were published, most of which did not detect a significant impact of the SNP on COPD development. A meta-analysis by Smolonska showed that the SNP changes the risk of COPD with an odds ratio of 0.76 (95% confidence interval 0.61–0.96). This SNP was related to COPD only in an Asian population but not in a Caucasian population [26].

4.5.5 Glutathione S-transferase Mu 1 (GSTM1)

Glutathione S-transferases, formerly known as ligandins, are a family of eukaryotic and prokaryotic metabolic isozymes that catalyze the conjugation of the glutathione. Two forms of glutathione S-transferases, cytosolic and membrane-bound, are encoded by two distinct supergene families. There are eight distinct classes of the soluble cytoplasmic mammalian glutathione S-transferases: alpha, kappa, mu, omega, pi, sigma, theta, and zeta. The genes encoding the mu class of enzymes are in a gene cluster on chromosome 1p13.3. Null mutation of GSTM1 contributes a variety of malignancies by enhancing the susceptibility to environmental carcinogens.

Cheng et al. conducted a case-control study with 184 patients with COPD and 212 control subjects. GSTM1-null genotypes were significantly more frequent in patients with COPD (61.4%) than in control subjects (42.5%) [27]. According to a meta-analysis of 14 published original studies, the GSTM1 null allele increases the risk of COPD for both Caucasian (odds ratio 1.32) and Asian populations (odds ratio 1.24) [26].

4.5.6 Cholinergic Receptor Nicotinic Alpha 3/5 (CHRNA3/5)

In the last 10 years, GWAS has detected some genes that researchers could not have identified based on linkage analysis and case-control association analyses. An international group led by Pillai et al. conducted a GWAS using four large databases. First, 538,030 SNPs were screened in a Norway case-control population with 1643 subjects. Second, the top 100 SNPs in the Norway population were replicated in an International COPD Genetics Network family population with 1891 subjects. Among the 100 SNPs, 8 SNPs were successfully replicated at a cutoff *P* value of 0.05; however, 1 gene was excluded in this step because the SNP showed inconsistent results with that from the Norway population. The remaining 7 genes were then assessed in the third step using 389 National Emphysema Treatment Trial subjects and 472 Normative Aging Study. After this third step, rs8034191 and rs1051730 on chromosome 15 showed both a significant *P* value and a genome-wide significant combined *P* value ($P < 1 \times 10^{-7}$). The fourth step with the dataset of the Boston Early-Onset COPD families replicated these two SNPs [28].

CHRNA3/5 protein, also known as neuronal acetylcholine receptor subunit alpha-3/5, is ligand-gated ion channels that are believed to contribute to neurotransmission. Polymorphisms in CHRNA3/5 have been revealed to increase the risk of lung cancer and increase the risk of smoking initiation. The SNPs at CHRNA3/5 increase the risk of COPD with an odds ratio approximately in the range of 1.3–1.4. Given this, these SNPs are estimated to attribute the 12.2% of general COPD population. It is still not clear whether these SNPs change the risk of COPD by altering smoking behavior or the susceptibility of the lungs to smoking [28].

Another SNP, rs16969968, on chromosome 15q25.1 was also known to alter the risk of developing COPD. A systematic review and meta-analysis by Saccone et al. evaluated whether the SNP was related to risk of COPD, lung cancer, and smoking behavior. The risk of COPD was estimated using data from four databases. The pooled odds ratio of 1.12 (95% confidence interval 1.02–1.23, $P = 0.01$) indicated that the SNP increased the risk of COPD by approximately 12%. The odds ratio by the SNP, rs16969968, for lung cancer was 1.31 (95% confidence interval 1.24–1.38, $P = 2 \times 10^{-21}$). After smokers were divided into heavy and light smokers, how the SNP changes the smoking habit was estimated. Meta-analysis using data from 34 studies clearly showed a highly significant association between dichotomous smoking habit and the SNP. The pooled odds ratio to be a heavy smoker was 1.33 (95% confidence interval 1.26–1.39, $P = 6 \times 10^{-31}$). These results should be interpreted cautiously because there is clear interaction between smoking habit and developing COPD. After adjusting for the amount of smoking per day, the authors could not find evidence for an association between the SNP and smoking [29].

4.5.7 Hedgehog Interacting Protein (HHIP)

HHIP is involved in many fundamental processes in embryonic development and has been conserved during evolution. Human HHIP is like that of the mouse. The HHIP gene is located on chromosome 4.

The GWAS by Pillai et al. also identified two SNPs at the HHIP gene as risk factors of COPD (rs1828591, rs13118928). Although the two SNPs could not show genome-wide combined significance in the study, the SNPs showed consistent attribution to COPD. Previous GWAS using the Framingham Heart study by Wilk et al. and a few more recent case-control studies have also revealed the association between HHIP and COPD. Thus, it is plausible that the two SNPs are genetic risk factors [29].

4.5.8 Family with Sequence Similarity 13 Member A (FAM13A)

Cho et al. who were part of the same study group as Pillai performed another GWAS using COPD cases and controls from the Norway population, the National Emphysema Treatment Trial, the Normative Aging Study, and the Evaluation of COPD Longitudinally to Identify Predictive Surrogate Endpoints Study. In this primary dataset, two SNPs at 4q22.1 FAM13A (rs1903003 and rs7671167) were the most highly associated with COPD. Then the authors additionally reevaluated the two SNPs using the database of the COPD Gene Study, the Boston Early-Onset COPD Study, and the International COPD Genetics Network. The two polymorphisms were successfully replicated in all populations. The pooled P value was $<1 \times 10^{-10}$ (Table 4.3) [30].

The function of the FAM13A protein is not sufficiently clear. However, the GWAS and the replication studies proved that SNPs at FAM13A increase the development of COPD. FAM13A is also related to cystic fibrosis and adenocarcinoma of the bronchus.

Table 4.3 Association results in FAM13A

SNP	Location	Minor allele	Primary			COPD gene			EOCOPD		ICGN		Overall *P*
			MAF	OR (95%CI)	*P*	MAF	OR (95%CI)	*P*	MAF	*P*	MAF	*P*	
rs1903003	4:90105320	C	0.45	0.76 (0.68–0.84)	7.18×10^{-8}	0.46	0.78 (0.64–0.95)	7.19×10^{-3}	0.46	0.48	0.45	1.29×10^{-3}	9.47×10^{-11}
rs7671167	4:90103002	C	0.48	0.76 (0.68–0.84)	8.59×10^{-8}	0.49	0.77 (0.63–0.93)	3.93×10^{-3}	0.51	0.11	0.49	5.15×10^{-4}	1.22×10^{-11}
rs2869967	4:90088355	C	0.42	1.29 (1.16–1.44)	1.48×10^{-6}	0.4	1.24 (1.02–1.50)	1.72×10^{-2}					

The primary genome-wide meta-analysis includes 2940 cases and 1380 controls from 3 population cohorts. Replication results are shown for the case-control COPDGene, the family-based EOCOPD, and ICGN studies. All analyses are adjusted for age and pack-years of cigarette smoking; the primary analysis is also adjusted for population stratification using principal components. Minor allele frequencies are given for each cohort

Location: Chromosome/base position, referencing hg18

CI confidence interval, *OR* odds ratio

Presented with permission from Nature Publishing Group [30]

4.5.9 Iron-Responsive Element-Binding Protein 2 (IREB2)

The IREB2 protein binds to iron-responsive elements of ferritin and transferrin receptor mRNA sequences to control iron metabolism. The function of the IREB2 protein is regulated by the iron around the protein. Thus, IREB2 protein can produce an adequate amount of transferrin.

A GWAS by DeMeo et al. consisting of three steps identified seven SNPs on the IREB2 gene that control the risk of COPD. The first step evaluated 389 severe COPD cases from the National Emphysema Treatment Trial and 424 smoker controls from the Normative Aging Study. In this screening step, 71 out of 889 autosomal SNPs showed nominal significance with a cutoff value P of 0.05. In the next validation stage, the 71 SNPs that passed the screening were reevaluated in a family-based study of 127 probands with early-onset COPD and 822 of their family members from the Boston Early-Onset COPD Study. In this step, three SNPs in the IREB2 gene satisfied a conservative threshold for significance of combined $P = 5.6 \times 10^{-5}$. Four additional SNPs also demonstrated combined $P < 0.02$. The second validation step genotyped 3117 subjects from the International COPD Genetics Network family-based study. The combined P of the seven IREB2 SNPs ranged from 1.6×10^{-7} to 6.4×10^{-4}. In addition to the GWAS, IREB2 protein and its mRNA were increased in respiratory specimen of COPD cases when compared to normal controls. Thus, the authors concluded that the IREB2 gene and protein are related to COPD susceptibility. The results were further replicated in other case-control studies [31].

4.5.10 Vitamin D-Binding Protein (VDBP)

VDBP, also known as the group-specific component (GC) protein, is coded in chromosome 4q. VDBP has three major allele-level polymorphisms, GC-1F, GC-1S, and GC-2, based on the combination of two SNPs, rs7041 and rs4588. VDBP is a multifunctional protein found in plasma, ascitic fluid, cerebrospinal fluid, and on the surface of many cell types. VDBP binds to vitamin D and its plasma metabolites and transports them to target tissues [32].

We previously performed a systematic review and meta-analysis to evaluate the association between the VDBP variant and the risk of COPD including studies whose control satisfied Hardy-Weinberg equilibrium. Based on 472 cases and 1270 controls from 6 case-control studies, the GC-1F allele and the 1F-1F homo-genotype were risk factors of COPD with a pooled odds ratio of 1.44 (95% confidence interval 1.14–1.83, $P = 0.002$) and 2.64 (95% confidence interval 1.29–5.39, $P = 0.008$), respectively. This odds ratio of 2.64 suggested a much stronger impact than other risk genes of COPD (Fig. 4.2) [33].

Study or Subgroup	log[Odds Ratio]	SE	Weight	Odds Ratio IV, Fixed, 95% CI
1.1.1 Asian				
Ishii 2001	1.912	1.141184	10.2%	6.77 [0.72, 63.35]
Lu ming 2004	0.833	0.862252	17.9%	2.30 [0.42, 12.47]
Shen 2010	0.431	0.70594	26.7%	1.54 [0.39, 6.14]
Subtotal (95% CI)			**54.7%**	**2.31 [0.88, 6.07]**
Heterogeneity: Chi² = 1.22, df = 2 (P = 0.54): I² = 0%				
Test for overall effect: Z = 1.70 (P = 0.09)				
1.1.2 Caucasian				
Horne 1990	1.442	0.631474	33.3%	4.23 [1.23, 14.58]
Laufs 2004	−0.14	1.241107	8.6%	0.87 [0.08, 9.90]
Wood 2011	1.304	2.008031	3.3%	3.68 [0.07, 188.61]
Subtotal (95% CI)			**45.3%**	**3.10 [1.07, 8.96]**
Heterogeneity: Chi² = 1.30, df = 2 (P = 0.52): I² = 0%				
Test for overall effect: Z = 2.09 (P = 0.04)				
Total (95% CI)			**100.0%**	**2.64 [1.29, 5.39]**
Heterogeneity: Chi² = 2.68, df = 5(P = 0.75): I² = 0%				
Test for overall effect: Z = 2.66 (P = 0.08)				
Test for subgroub differences: Chi² = 0.16, df = 1(P = 0.69): I² = 0%				

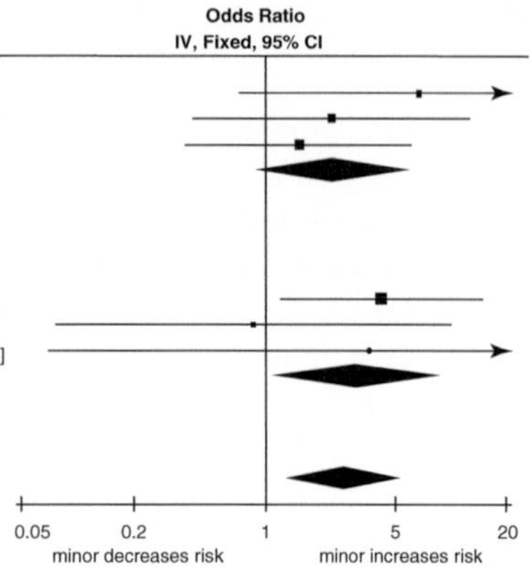

Fig. 4.2 1F-1F homo-genotype of VDBP was risk factor of COPD. Original data for the current review article

Nowadays, the VDBP phenotype is known to also alter the susceptibility to osteoporosis, Hashimoto's thyroiditis, Graves' disease, diabetes, multiple sclerosis, AIDS, sarcoidosis, and rheumatic fever [32].

4.5.11 Matrix Metalloproteinase (MMP) Family

MMP family members, especially MMP12, were considered to have an impact on COPD pathogenesis. The MMP protein plays important roles in tissue remodeling associated with various physiological or pathological pathways including morphogenesis, cirrhosis, arthritis, angiogenesis, tissue repair, and metastasis. MMP was also believed to be associated with COPD development. Therefore, many case-control studies were carried out. However, these results were highly inconsistent. Thus, Zhou et al. reported a systematic review to investigate whether MMP is associated with COPD risk. In this systematic review, they evaluated four SNPs (SNP, MMP1-16071G/2G, MMP3-11715A/6A, MMP9-1562C/T, MMP12-82 A/G). Among 123 potentially relevant reports, they finally included 21 studies including 4184 cases and 5716 controls. The pooled odds ratios were 0.99 (95% confidence interval 0.89–1.10, $P = 0.81$) for MMP1-1607 (rs1799750) 1G versus 2G, 0.88 (95% confidence interval 0.61–1.27, $P = 0.50$) for MMP3-1171 (rs35068180) 5A versus 6A, 0.83 (95% confidence interval 0.62–1.12, $P = 0.22$) for MMP9-1562 (rs3918242) C versus T, and 0.98 (95% confidence interval 0.80–1.20) for MMP12-82 (rs2276109) A versus G. Briefly, this meta-analysis did not detect an association between COPD susceptibility and MMP polymorphisms in the general population [34].

4.6 Genes Related to Smoking Behavior

In addition to the CHRNA3 gene [28], which we reviewed in the previous section, some genes are known to impact smoking behavior [35, 36]. The Tobacco and Genetics Consortium partnered with the European Network of Genetic and Genomic Epidemiology and Oxford-GlaxoSmithKline consortia to conduct a genome-wide meta-analysis to identify multiple loci associated with smoking behavior (Fig. 4.1). CHRNA3 SNP (rs1051730) showed the strongest link between smoking quantity ($P = 2.8 \times 10^{-73}$) followed by SNPs on 10q25 (rs1329650, $P = 5.7 \times 10^{-10}$; rs1028936, $P = 1.3 \times 10^{-9}$) and a SNP on the 9q13 EGLN2 gene (rs3733829, $P = 1.0 \times 10^{-8}$). Eight SNPs on brain derived neurotrophic factor had a genome-wide significant association with smoking initiation. A SNP (rs3025343) was associated with smoking cessation [37].

4.7 Future Direction

We reviewed many genes that can alter the risk of A1-AT deficient emphysema, non-hereditary COPD, and smoking behavior. However, these genes were just proved to be related to COPD and the mechanism by which the polymorphism of these genes impacts the development of COPD is still largely unclear. Clarifying the mechanism may teach us how to prevent and treat COPD [2, 38–40]. Personalized medicine for the high-risk population is also anticipated. Potential drug targets are listed and discussed in depth elsewhere [41]. If a genetic test that can judge whether subjects had COPD risk genes and smoking-prone genes can be developed in a clinical setting, a selective smoking cessation intervention might be possible. People generally think that smoking behavior is determined by individual will, education, and environment. However, we should recognize that part of smoking behavior is congenitally decided. We hope a future genetic study will clarify the mechanism of COPD development leading to innovation in COPD treatment and prevention [2, 38–40].

References

1. Vogelmeier CF, Criner GJ, Martinez FJ, et al. Global strategy for the diagnosis, management, and prevention of chronic obstructive lung disease 2017 Report: GOLD executive summary. Eur Respir J. 2017;49(3)
2. Mannino DM, Buist AS. Global burden of COPD: risk factors, prevalence, and future trends. Lancet. 2007;370(9589):765–73.
3. Siafakas NM, Vermeire P, Pride NB, et al. Optimal assessment and management of chronic obstructive pulmonary-disease (COPD). Eur Respir J. 1995;8(8):1398–420.

4. Stoller JK, Aboussouan LS. Alpha1-antitrypsin deficiency. Lancet. 2005;365(9478):2225–36.
5. Visscher PM, Brown MA, McCarthy MI, Yang J. Five Years of GWAS Discovery. Am J Hum Genet. 2012;90(1):7–24.
6. Bosse Y. Updates on the COPD gene list. Int J Chron Obstruct Pulmon Dis. 2012;7:607–31.
7. Berndt A, Leme AS, Shapiro SD. Emerging genetics of COPD. EMBO Mol Med. 2012;4(11):1144–55.
8. Kruglyak L, Daly MJ, ReeveDaly MP, Lander ES. Parametric and nonparametric linkage analysis: a unified multipoint approach. Am J Hum Genet. 1996;58(6):1347–63.
9. Gu C, Province M, Todorov A, Rao DC. Meta-analysis methodology for combining nonparametric sibpair linkage results: genetic homogeneity and identical markers. Genet Epidemiol. 1998;15(6):609–26.
10. Strauch K, Fimmers R, Kurz T, Deichmann KA, Wienker TF, Baur MP. Parametric and nonparametric multipoint linkage analysis with imprinting and two-locus-trait models: application to mite sensitization. Am J Hum Genet. 2000;66(6):1945–57.
11. Thomas DC, Witte JS. Point: population stratification: a problem for case-control studies of candidate-gene associations? Cancer Epidemiol Biomarkers Prev. 2002;11(6):505–12.
12. Cantor RM, Lange K, Sinsheimer JS. Prioritizing GWAS results: a review of statistical methods and recommendations for their application. Am J Hum Genet. 2010;86(1):6–22.
13. Xu ZL, Taylor JA. SNPinfo: integrating GWAS and candidate gene information into functional SNP selection for genetic association studies. Nucleic Acids Res. 2009;37:W600–5.
14. Holme J, Stockley RA. Radiologic and clinical features of COPD patients with discordant pulmonary physiology - lessons from alpha(1)-antitrypsin deficiency. Chest. 2007;132(3):909–15.
15. Rodriguez F, de la Roza C, Jardi R, Schaper M, Vidal R, Miravitlles M. Glutathione S-transferase P1 and lung function in patients with alpha(1)-antitrypsin deficiency and COPD. Chest. 2005;127(5):1537–43.
16. Wood AM, de Pablo P, Buckley CD, Ahmad A, Stockley RA. Smoke exposure as a determinant of autoantibody titre in alpha(1)-antitrypsin deficiency and COPD. Eur Respir J. 2011;37(1):32–8.
17. Dahl M, Tybjaerg-Hansen A, Lange P, Vestbo J, Nordestgaard BG. Change in lung function and morbidity from chronic obstructive pulmonary disease in alpha1-antitrypsin MZ heterozygotes: a longitudinal study of the general population. Ann Intern Med. 2002;136(4):270–9.
18. Demeo DL, Mariani TJ, Lange C, et al. The SERPINE2 gene is associated with chronic obstructive pulmonary disease. Am J Hum Genet. 2006;78(2):253–64.
19. Zhu G, Warren L, Aponte J, et al. The SERPINE2 gene is associated with chronic obstructive pulmonary disease in two large populations. Am J Respir Crit Care Med. 2007;176(2):167–73.
20. Fujimoto K, Ikeda S, Arai T, et al. Polymorphism of SERPINE2 gene is associated with pulmonary emphysema in consecutive autopsy cases. BMC Med Genet. 2010;11:159.
21. Sakao S, Tatsumi K, Igari H, Shino Y, Shirasawa H, Kuriyama T. Association of tumor necrosis factor alpha gene promoter polymorphism with the presence of chronic obstructive pulmonary disease. Am J Respir Crit Care Med. 2001;163(2):420–2.
22. Zhan P, Wang J, Wei SZ, et al. TNF-308 gene polymorphism is associated with COPD risk among Asians: meta-analysis of data for 6,118 subjects. Mol Biol Rep. 2011;38(1):219–27.
23. Celedon JC, Lange C, Raby BA, et al. The transforming growth factor-beta1 (TGFB1) gene is associated with chronic obstructive pulmonary disease (COPD). Hum Mol Genet. 2004;13(15):1649–56.
24. Wu L, Chau J, Young RP, et al. Transforming growth factor-beta1 genotype and susceptibility to chronic obstructive pulmonary disease. Thorax. 2004;59(2):126–9.
25. Vibhuti A, Arif E, Deepak D, Singh B, Qadar Pasha MA. Genetic polymorphisms of GSTP1 and mEPHX correlate with oxidative stress markers and lung function in COPD. Biochem Biophys Res Commun. 2007;359(1):136–42.
26. Smolonska J, Wijmenga C, Postma DS, Boezen HM. Meta-analyses on suspected chronic obstructive pulmonary disease genes: a summary of 20 years' research. Am J Respir Crit Care Med. 2009;180(7):618–31.

27. Cheng SL, Yu CJ, Chen CJ, Yang PC. Genetic polymorphism of epoxide hydrolase and glutathione S-transferase in COPD. Eur Respir J. 2004;23(6):818–24.
28. Pillai SG, Ge D, Zhu G, et al. A genome-wide association study in chronic obstructive pulmonary disease (COPD): identification of two major susceptibility loci. PLoS Genet. 2009;5(3):e1000421.
29. Saccone NL, Culverhouse RC, Schwantes-An TH, et al. Multiple independent loci at chromosome 15q25.1 affect smoking quantity: a meta-analysis and comparison with lung cancer and COPD. PLoS Genet. 2010;6(8)
30. Cho MH, Boutaoui N, Klanderman BJ, et al. Variants in FAM13A are associated with chronic obstructive pulmonary disease. Nat Genet. 2010;42(3):200–2.
31. DeMeo DL, Mariani T, Bhattacharya S, et al. Integration of genomic and genetic approaches implicates IREB2 as a COPD susceptibility gene. Am J Hum Genet. 2009;85(4):493–502.
32. Speeckaert M, Huang G, Delanghe JR, Taes YE. Biological and clinical aspects of the vitamin D binding protein (Gc-globulin) and its polymorphism. Int J Clin Chem. 2006;372(1-2):33–42.
33. Horita N, Miyazawa N, Tomaru K, Inoue M, Ishigatsubo Y, Kaneko T. Vitamin D binding protein genotype variants and risk of chronic obstructive pulmonary disease: a meta-analysis. Respirology. 2015;20(2):219–25.
34. Zhou H, Wu Y, Jin Y, et al. Genetic polymorphism of matrix metalloproteinase family and chronic obstructive pulmonary disease susceptibility: a meta-analysis. Sci Rep. 2013;3:2818.
35. Caporaso N, Gu FY, Chatterjee N, et al. Genome-Wide and Candidate Gene Association study of cigarette smoking behaviors. PLoS One. 2009;4(2):e4653.
36. Li MD, Ma JZ, Beuten J. Progress in searching for susceptibility loci and genes for smoking-related behaviour. Clin Genet. 2004;66(5):382–92.
37. Tobacco and Genetics Consortium. Genome-wide meta-analyses identify multiple loci associated with smoking behavior. Nat Genet. 2010;42(5):441–7.
38. Barnes PJ. Future advances in COPD therapy. Respiration. 2001;68(5):441–8.
39. Cazzola M, Hanania NA, MacNee W, Rudell K, Hackford C, Tamimi N. A review of the most common patient-reported outcomes in COPD - revisiting current knowledge and estimating future challenges. Int J Chron Obstruct Pulmon Dis. 2015;10:725–38.
40. Konigshoff M, Kneidinger N, Eickelberg O. TGF-beta signalling in COPD: deciphering genetic and cellular susceptibilities for future therapeutic regimens. Swiss Med Wkly. 2009;139(39-40):554–63.
41. Wain LV, Shrine N, Artigas MS, Erzurumluoglu AM, Noyvert B, Bossini-Castillo L, et al. Genome-wide association analyses for lung function and chronic obstructive pulmonary disease identify new loci and potential druggable targets. Nat Genet. 2017;49:416–25.

Chapter 5
Smoking Behavior and Cessation (Nicotine Addiction): Are Genetic Factors Involved in Smoking Behavior?

Tetsuya Kubota and Akihito Yokoyama

Abstract Tobacco smoking is a major risk factor for a number of health problems, including cancer, chronic obstructive pulmonary disease, lung fibrosis, and cardiovascular disease. Tobacco smoke contains thousands of harmful, carcinogenics and toxic substances. Particularly, nicotine is the causative substance in tobacco smoke that leads to dependence. Smoking behavior is addictive, and this addiction is categorized among the behavioral and neurodevelopmental disorders in the tenth revision of the *International Classification of Diseases*. Once absorbed, nicotine directly affects the nervous system. However, the sensitivity for developing nicotine addiction varies between individuals. Affinity to nicotinic receptors and related enzymatic activity can influence the metabolism of nicotine. Although environmental factors are associated with nicotine addiction, meta-analyses of genome-wide association studies have revealed that genetic factors contribute to the risks of developing such clinical conditions. Regarding genetic factors, single nucleotide polymorphisms of nicotinic acetylcholine receptors and cytochrome P450 (CYP) family 2 subfamily A polypeptides are associated with nicotine dependence. Smoking cessation would help prevent the numerous health problems associated with smoking. An effective smoking cessation strategy would be to combine both behavioral and pharmacological therapies, including nicotine replacement therapy and a partial nicotinic receptor agonist.

Keywords Smoking behavior · Smoking cessation · Nicotine addiction
Genetic factor

T. Kubota (✉) · A. Yokoyama
Department of Hematology and Respiratory Medicine, Kochi University,
Nankoku, Kochi, Japan
e-mail: kubotat@kochi-u.ac.jp

T. Kaneko (ed.), *Clinical Relevance of Genetic Factors in Pulmonary Diseases*,
Respiratory Disease Series: Diagnostic Tools and Disease Managements,
https://doi.org/10.1007/978-981-10-8144-6_5

5.1 Introduction

5.1.1 Tobacco

Tobacco (made from the leaves of *Nicotiana tabacum*) was originally used by ancient Central Americans as early as 1400 BC [1]. After the arrival of the Europeans to Central America, tobacco smoking grew in popularity worldwide. Current sex and regional differences in smoking rates around the world are shown in Table 5.1. Although tobacco is mostly consumed in the form of manufactured cigarettes, it is also smoked in other products, such as hand-rolled cigarettes, cigars, cigarillos, pipes, water pipes, and e-cigarettes. The accumulation of scientific evidence pointing toward the hazardous effects of tobacco smoking led to a drastic change in thinking in the twentieth century. Tobacco is now recognized as a leading contributor to health disorders. The World Health Organization estimates that the global population of smokers totals one billion people and that six million people, including 600,000 exposed to secondhand smoke, die from tobacco-related illnesses each year [2]. If current trends continue, more than eight million people will die from tobacco-related illness each year worldwide by the year 2030. Tobacco smoke is a complex mixture of chemicals and includes at least 60 carcinogens [3, 4]. Harmful compounds are included in both the gas phase and the solid phase. For example, the gas phase contains acetone, acetonitrile, ammonia, carbon monoxide, methane, propane, pyridine, and propionaldehyde. The solid phase contains aniline, benzopyrene, naphthalene, nicotine, phenol, pyrene, and quinolone. The chemical compositions of mainstream smoke and sidestream smoke are qualitatively similar, although quantitatively different. In this chapter, concerns about tobacco will be discussed, including its harmful components, diseases, addiction, cessation, and genetic factors.

Table 5.1 Global prevalence of tobacco smoking

	Prevalence (% of the population ≥15 years of age)		
WHO region	Men	Women	Total
African	24.7	2.3	13.4
Region of the Americas	21.9	12.7	17.1
Eastern Mediterranean	36.8	2.8	20.4
European	37.8	18.7	27.8
South-East Asian	31.7	2.4	17.2
Western Pacific	47.9	3.2	25.9
World	35.8	6.6	21.1

WHO World Health Organization
Cited from WHO report on global tobacco epidemic 2015

5.2 Harmful Components of Tobacco

5.2.1 Nicotine

Nicotine is a natural ingredient and a principal alkaloid in tobacco. An average tobacco rod contains 10–14 mg of nicotine, and approximately 1–1.5 mg of nicotine is absorbed systemically during smoking [5]. Nicotine is distilled from burning tobacco and is carried proximately on inhaled tar droplets. As much as 90% of inhaled nicotine is rapidly absorbed when the smoke reaches the small airways and alveoli [6]. Blood concentrations of nicotine increase quickly, reaching the brain via the systemic arterial circulation within 10–20 s after a single puff of a cigarette [5]. Nicotine activates nicotinic acetylcholine receptors (nAChRs) on neurons that cause the release of many chemical messengers, such as dopamine, acetylcholine, norepinephrine, epinephrine, and serotonin, resulting in the smoker experiencing a feeling of relaxation [7]. Nicotine also activates the sympathetic nervous system, acting via splanchnic nerves innervating the adrenal medulla, stimulating the release of epinephrine. Acetylcholine released by preganglionic sympathetic fibers of these nerves acts on nAChRs, causing the release of epinephrine and norepinephrine into the bloodstream [8]. Nicotine exhibits several harmful effects on the cardiovascular system, including coronary vasoconstriction, increased hypercoagulability, dyslipidemia, and endothelial dysfunction. Nicotine is extensively metabolized to a number of metabolites by enzymes in the liver, including cytochrome P450 (CYP). Six primary metabolites of nicotine have been identified: nornicotine, nicotine glucuronide, nicotine isomethonium ion, 1′(*S*)-2′(*S*)-*trans*-nicotine-*N*′-oxide, 2′-hydroxynicotine, and nicotine-$\Delta^{1'(5')}$-iminium ion [5]. Of these, the nicotine-$\Delta^{1'(5')}$-iminium ion is then converted to cotinine by aldehyde oxidase. The most important metabolite of nicotine in most mammalian species is cotinine, a lactam derivative. In humans, approximately 70–80% of nicotine is converted to cotinine [5]. Cotinine is further metabolized into other compounds through oxidation, glucuronidation, and methylation before excretion. Because of the long half-life of cotinine, it has been used as a biomarker for daily intake of nicotine.

5.2.2 Carcinogens

Tobacco contains a high number of carcinogenic compounds both in the gas phase and the solid phase [3, 4]. The carcinogenicity of at least 60 substances has been scientifically evaluated in laboratory animals by the International Agency for Research on Cancer (IARC). For instance, benzo[*a*]pyrene, furan, *N*-nitrosamines, 2-toluidine, 1,3-butadiene, 2-naphthylamine, formaldehyde, benzene, nitrobenzene,

Table 5.2 Target sites associated with some carcinogenic chemical compounds and metals present in tobacco smoke

Agent	Tumor sites or types for which there is *sufficient* evidence in humans	Tumor sites or types for which there is *limited* evidence in humans
Chemicals		
1,3-Butadiene	Hematolymphatic organs	
2-Naphthylamine	Urinary bladder	
4-Aminobiphenyl	Urinary bladder	
Benzene	Acute nonlymphocytic leukemia	Acute lymphocytic leukemia, chronic lymphocytic leukemia, multiple myeloma, non-Hodgkin lymphoma
Ethylene oxide		Breast, lymphoid tumors
Formaldehyde	Nasopharynx, leukemia (particularly myeloid leukemia)	Sinonasal cancer
O-Toluidine	Urinary bladder	
Vinyl chloride	Hepatocellular carcinoma, hepatic angiosarcoma	
Metals		
Arsenic and inorganic arsenic compounds	Lung, skin, urinary bladder	Kidney, liver prostate
Beryllium and beryllium compounds	Lung	
Cadmium and cadmium compounds	Lung	Kidney, prostate
Chromium (VI) compounds	Lung	Nasal cavity and paranasal sinuses
Lead		Stomach
Nickel compounds	Lung, nasal cavity, and paranasal sinuses	

Reference [3]

vinyl chloride, arsenic, cadmium, chromium (hexavalent), and others are present in cigarette smoke. Representative examples of over 60 carcinogens are summarized in Table 5.2 [3]. The same carcinogens are also present in secondhand cigarette smoke. Tissues like the lung and larynx that are directly exposed to tobacco smoke, as well as tissue like the bladder that is directly exposed to tobacco metabolites, show significantly elevated levels of DNA adducts in smokers. Cumulative DNA damage can lead to mis-replication and cancer [9].

5.2.3 Reactive Oxygen Species

Oxygen (O_2) is essential for living; however, highly concentrated oxygen is hazardous to cells. Although humans have antioxidant mechanisms, aberrations in oxidant and antioxidant balance can lead to a variety of diseases. The most physiologically significant reactive oxygen species (ROS) are the superoxide anion ($O_2\cdot^-$), hydroxyl radical ($\cdot OH$), nitric oxide (NO), and hydrogen peroxide (H_2O_2). In the gas phase, tobacco smoke contains high concentrations of oxidants/free radicals ($>10^{15}$ molecules per puff) and short-lived oxidants such as the $O_2\cdot^-$ and NO [10]. NO and $O_2\cdot^-$ immediately react to form the highly reactive peroxynitrite ($ONOO^-$) molecule, which is highly injurious to cells. The tar phase of cigarette smoke contains organic radicals, such as the long-lived semiquinone radicals, which can react with molecular oxygen in a redox-dependent manner to form $O_2\cdot^-$, $\cdot OH$ and H_2O_2. H_2O_2 is then converted to water by catalase. Neutrophils also use myeloperoxidase, which uses H_2O_2 produced by dismutation of $O_2\cdot^-$ to oxidize chloride ions into hypochlorous acid (HCLO), a powerful antibacterial agent. Oxidant stress can lead to peroxidation of membrane lipids, depletion of nicotinamide nucleotides, increases in intracellular calcium ion concentrations, cytoskeleton disruption, and DNA damage [11].

5.2.4 Carbon Monoxide

Incomplete combustion of tobacco produces carbon monoxide, a colorless, odorless, and tasteless gas that is highly toxic. However, the hazardous effects of carbon monoxide are underestimated, as compared to nicotine and carcinogens. It binds with hemoglobin (Hb) to produce carboxyhemoglobin (COHb), which takes the place of oxyhemoglobin that normally delivers bound oxygen to the tissues throughout the body. Carbon monoxide binds to hemoglobin at the same sites as oxygen but much more tightly. Tobacco smoking increases the blood levels of COHb, thereby decreasing the amount of oxygen reaching bodily tissues. The level of COHb is approximately 5% per pack smoked per day in smokers and approximately 1% in nonsmokers. Exposure to carbon monoxide may severely damage the cardiovascular system [12].

5.3 Respiratory Diseases

5.3.1 Leading Cause of Illness

Tobacco smoking is one of the biggest risks not only for respiratory diseases but also for systemic diseases. Tobacco smoking exposes cells in the respiratory system to multiple harmful components, which can cause diseases in almost every organ and part of the body. The three major causes of smoking-related mortality are chronic obstructive pulmonary disease (COPD), lung cancer, and atherosclerotic cardiovascular disease [13]. As for pulmonary diseases, smoking is highly associated with chronic lung diseases, such as desquamative interstitial pneumonia, respiratory bronchitis-associated interstitial lung disease, combined pulmonary fibrosis and emphysema, and Langerhans cell histiocytosis. Smoking also exacerbates lung conditions, including asthma, bronchitis, bronchiectasis, and several types of infection, such as the common cold, influenza, tuberculosis, and pneumonia. Moreover, the number of cigarettes smoked daily is associated with an increased risk of developing type 2 diabetes mellitus. Smoking also accelerates the progression of osteoporosis, periodontal disease, gastric ulcers, and postoperative complications.

5.3.2 COPD

Epidemiological studies indicate that tobacco smoking is overwhelmingly the most significant cause of COPD. Especially, smoking-induced oxidative stress plays a key role in driving COPD-related inflammation. Inflammatory and structural cells, including neutrophils, macrophages, and epithelial cells, produce ROS. Oxidative stress occurs when ROS are produced in excess of the antioxidant defense. Oxidative stress may result in impaired antiprotease defenses; damage to lipids, proteins, and DNA; cellular senescence; autoantibody generation; and corticosteroid resistance [14]. Oxidative stress leads to oxidation of arachidonic acid and formation of a new series of prostanoid mediators, which can exert significant functional effects, inducing bronchoconstriction and plasma exudation. Oxidative stress also increases the inflammatory response and reduces the expression of *sirtuin-1*, a key repair molecule implicated in aging [14]. The majority of smokers with cough and sputum production associated with COPD show an improvement in symptoms after smoking cessation, and their prognosis also improves [15]. Recently, genome-wide association studies (GWAS) identified multiple novel genetic risk factors for COPD. One of these risk loci is located on chromosome 15q24/25 in the region that contains nAChRs [16]. A previous cohort study demonstrated that genetic variations in nAChRs in the 15q24/25 locus, which play an important role in nicotine addiction, are also associated with lung function levels and COPD [17]. However, another study showed that the variants are related to smoking habits, and not directly to COPD [18]. The genetic factors in nicotine dependence are discussed in Sect. 5.

5.3.3 Lung Cancer

As mentioned above, tobacco smoke contains at least 60 carcinogens [3], and tobacco smoking drastically increases the risk of lung cancer. Many other cancer types also occur more frequently in smokers than in nonsmokers, including cancers of the oral cavity, larynx, pharynx, esophagus, liver, cervix, pancreas, bladder, and kidney. Considerable evidence supports that polycyclic aromatic hydrocarbons and *N*-nitrosamines are two of the major causative factors in lung cancer [19]. Although specific driver oncogene mutations, such as epidermal growth factor receptor (*EGFR*) gene mutation, and *EML4/ALK* gene translocation, play important roles in carcinogenesis on adenocarcinoma, the classic mechanisms of carcinogens are still of importance in lung cancer development. Carcinogens induce activation of DNA adducts, leading to miscoding and mutations in critical growth control genes. Previous studies have demonstrated that smoking increases the total mutation burden. A pack of cigarettes a day for a year accumulates approximately 150 mutations in lung tissues [20]. Tobacco has also been shown to have an adverse impact on chemotherapy for lung cancer. In fact, some lung cancer cells express nAChRs; nicotine stimulates the phosphorylation of Akt, STAT3, and EGFR expressed by lung cancer cells, which exhibit resistance to anticancer agents [21]. To enhance the effectiveness of chemotherapy, lung cancer patients who currently smoke must stop smoking when receiving anticancer therapies.

5.4 Nicotine Addiction

5.4.1 Withdrawal

One of the biggest health problems associated with tobacco is the strong dependence that users develop. Tobacco dependence is as strong as that for heroin or cocaine [22]. Among the many compounds in tobacco, nicotine plays a central role in inducing the dependence. When regular smokers abstain from smoking for a while, they develop unpleasant symptoms, including anxiety, irritability, depression, insomnia, restlessness, increasing stressfulness, difficulty in concentration, and increased appetite. These symptoms are part of the dependence syndrome, also called withdrawal. When nicotine dependence has developed, smoking cessation produces an unpleasant withdrawal state, which promotes the continuation of smoking. Withdrawal is a powerful incentive to take up smoking again. A smoker empirically learns that smoking is the easiest way to escape the withdrawal state, which includes both physical dependence and psychological dependence. Smoking cessation decreases the brain function of the smoker, and brain function is temporarily improved by smoking again. Smoking does not resolve a smoker's stress; it only alleviates a smoker's withdrawal symptoms. In this way, withdrawal strongly enhances the psychological dependence. The number of cigarettes smoked per day and the severity of the urge to smoke are good indicators for assessing the degree of dependence. The Fagerström test is commonly used for assessing nicotine dependence, due to its accuracy, reproducibility, and ease of use.

5.4.2 Reward System and Addiction Development

Addiction is characterized by the craving for a substance, with goal-directed behavior toward excessive substance intake and a loss of control in limiting intake. Nicotine is a very strong addiction-forming substance that acts via dopamine release in the reward system of the brain. Dopaminergic neurons in the mesolimbic system, which project from A10 cells of the midbrain ventrotegmental area to the nucleus accumbens of the limbic system, are part of the reward system in the brain. When this system is activated, the person experiences feelings of satisfaction, euphoria, hyperthymia, awakening, and relaxation. Because nicotine has a similar structure to acetylcholine chloride, which is an innate neurotransmitter, nicotine directly binds to and activates nAChRs in the midbrain. Activation of nAChRs results in the release of dopamine, serotonin, glutamate, and gamma aminobutyric acid (GABA). Thus, as shown in Fig. 5.1, nicotine activates the reward system in the brain, causing the release of dopamine which makes smokers feel good [23]. However, the satisfaction and sense of pleasure gained from smoking are fleeting. Repeated tobacco smoking decreases the number of dopamine receptors in the limbic system, resulting in reduced neural responses. In such a condition, the brain's reward system becomes unstable without nicotine. As a result, smokers feel unpleasant withdrawal symptoms including feelings of anxiousness, disconcertedness, and stressed. To avoid withdrawal and regain the sense of satisfaction and pleasure, smokers replenish their nicotine levels by adjusting the volume of puffs and the depth of inhalation when smoking. As described above, smokers develop a strong addiction to nicotine. The very short time interval between puffing and nicotine reaching the brain allows smokers to titrate the dose of nicotine to achieve a desired pharmacological effect, thereby promoting the addiction.

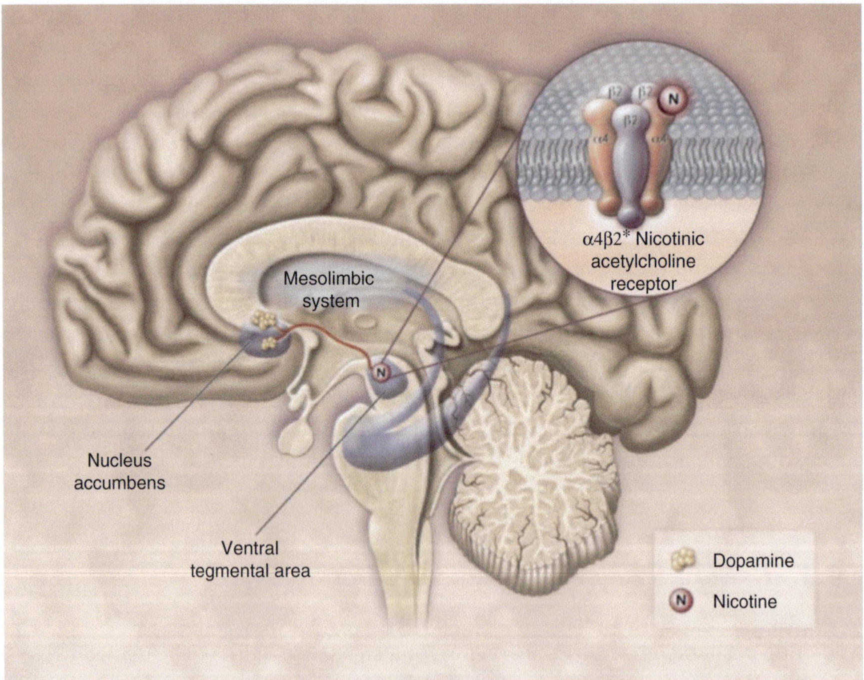

Fig. 5.1 Reward system in the brain. Role of the mesolimbic dopamine system in nicotine activity. Nicotine activates $\alpha_4\beta_2$ receptors in the ventral tegmental area, resulting in dopamine release in the shell of the nucleus accumbens. From New Engl J Med. Benowitz NL. Nicotine addiction. 362: 2295–2303. Copyright © (2010) Massachusetts Medical Society. Reprinted with permission from Massachusetts Medical Society

5.5 Genetic Factors

5.5.1 Genetic Factors Associated with Nicotine Addiction

Many factors are associated with developing nicotine addiction. Previous studies demonstrated that gender and race could be correlated with nicotine dependence [24, 25]. Genetic factors are also involved in the formation of tobacco addiction. Meta-analysis of twin studies showed that both the environment and genes are important in smoking-related behaviors, with an estimated mean heritability of 50% for smoking initiation and 59% for nicotine dependence [26]. It seems that the heritability of addictions itself is not well defined, but it is possible to inherit the susceptibility to these behaviors. The genetic influence on addiction is not due to a contribution of a single gene but the result of the interaction of different genes that induce a condition of susceptibility to the disorder together with environmental factors. It is evident that nicotine exerts its biological function by binding to nAChRs, and nicotine is extensively metabolized by the liver to form cotinine. The most important enzyme of nicotine metabolism is cytochrome P450 2A6 (CYP2A6). Genetic factors associated with nicotine addiction are mainly related to components of dopaminergic pathways and metabolism. Such is the case for nAChRs and CYP2A6. Representative genetic factors associated with nicotine addiction are summarized in Table 5.3.

5.5.2 Nicotinic Receptor Subunit Polymorphism

Previous studies have demonstrated that nicotinic receptor subunit polymorphism is strongly associated with nicotine dependence. The nAChRs are a family of receptors with multiple subunits. The mammalian nervous system is known to express 12 neuronal subunits, including nine alfa subunits (α_2–α_{10}), three beta subunits (β_2–β_4), and five muscular subunits ($\alpha1$, $\beta1$, γ, δ, and ε). These subunits are encoded by different genes [27]. For instance, the *CHRNA4* gene on chromosome 20 encodes

Table 5.3 Genetic factors associated with nicotine addiction

Receptors	
nAChR	
CHRNA5–CHRNA3–CHRNB4 cluster	SNPs
CHRNB3–CHRNA6 cluster	SNPs
CHRND–CHRNG cluster	SNPs
GABAR2	variant
Cell surface protein	
neurexin 1	SNPs
Metabolic enzyme	
CYP2A6	SNPs, duplication, deletion, conversion
CYP2B6	SNPs, duplication, deletion, conversion

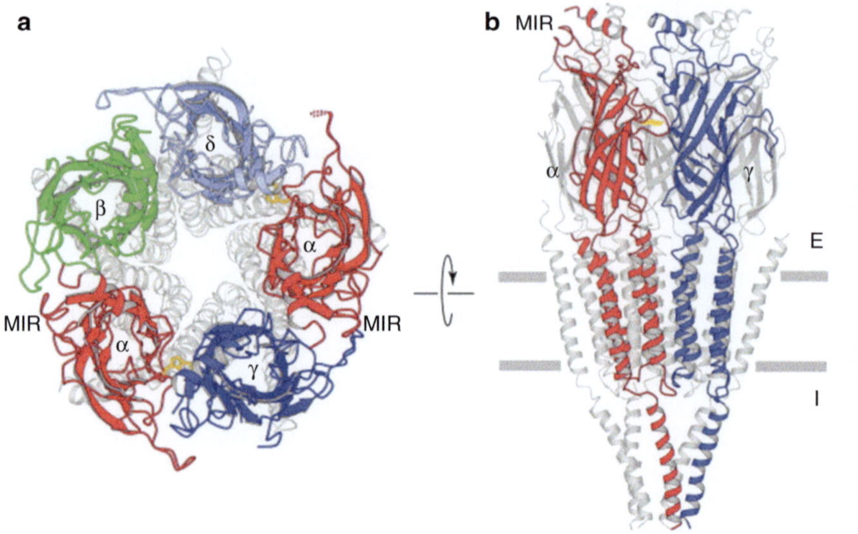

Fig. 5.2 Ribbon diagrams of the nicotinic acetylcholine receptor structure, as viewed (**a**) from the synaptic cleft and (**b**) parallel with the membrane plane. For clarity, only the ligand-binding domain is highlighted in (**a**), and only the front two subunits are highlighted in (**b**) (α, red; β, green; γ, blue; δ, light blue). Also shown are the locations of αTrp149 (gold), the main immunogenic region (MIR), and the membrane (horizontal bars; *E* extracellular, *I* intracellular). The dotted lines on the right denote the three main zones of subunit–subunit contacts. The apex of the C-loop of αδ (broken trace in (**a**)) was not visible in the densities. Reprinted from J Mol Biol 346 Unwin N. Refined structure of the nicotinic acetylcholine receptor at 4A resolution. pp. 967–989, 2005, with permission from Elsevier

the α_4 subunit, and the *CHRNB2* gene on chromosome 1 encodes the β_2 subunit. The nAChRs have pentagonal structures, and different combinations of subunits result in different receptor subtypes that have various pharmacological properties [28] (Fig. 5.2). The most commonly expressed nAChR subtypes in the human brain are composed of $\alpha_4\beta_2$ subunits, which play a central role in the physiological effects of nicotine. Previous studies demonstrated that α_4-containing nAChRs are associated with nicotine dependence. Labarca et al. reported that knock-in mice harboring an α_4 nAChR point mutation exhibited an approximately 30-fold increase in nAChR sensitivity to acetylcholine and nicotine, suggesting that genetic variability in the α_4 subunit can produce dramatic changes in nicotine sensitivity [29]. Recently, GWAS meta-analyses have revealed that nicotine dependence is significantly associated with some single-nucleotide polymorphisms (SNPs) in three different clusters of genes: 12 SNPs in the *CHRNA5–CHRNA3–CHRNB4* gene cluster on chromosome 15, eight SNPs in the *CHRNB3–CHRNA6* gene cluster on chromosome 8, and one SNP in the *CHRND–CHRNG* gene cluster on chromosome 2. The *CHRNA5–CHRNA3–CHRNB4* gene cluster on chromosome 15q25, which encodes the α_5, α_3, and β_4 subunits, has showed the most prominent evidence [30]. Among many SNPs in nAChRs, functional SNP rs16969968 is the most well-established locus on chromosome 15q25 [30]. The presence of SNP rs16969968 causes a change in the amino acid sequence (D398N) in the α_5 subunit, leading to a change in the charge of the intracellular domain of the subunit, requiring more nicotine to activate the dopaminergic pathway.

5.5.3 Synaptic Transmissions

Neurexin is a small cell surface adhesion molecule that is responsible for stabilizing synaptic GABAergic and glutamatergic communication. Neurexin is necessary for the normal release of neurotransmitters. The SNPs in neurexin 1 (*NRXN1*) are believed to be involved in nicotine dependence [27]. According to previous studies other genes are also implicated in nicotine dependence. Different variants in GABAR2 (located on chromosome 9q22) are associated with smoking behavior [31]. The dopamine receptor D4 (*DRD4*) gene and dopamine transporter *SLC6A3* gene have variable number tandem repeat polymorphisms, showing changes in the length of the receptor. Although it is still controversial, these tandem repeat polymorphisms may be associated with nicotine dependence [27]. Nicotine affects the release of serotonin, a neurotransmitter in the brain related to anxiety and depression. The serotonin transporter protein (5-HTT) regulates the concentration of serotonin in the synaptic cleft. The gene that encodes 5-HTT contains a polymorphism with short and long alleles. The short allele is associated with decreased transcriptional efficiency, as compared to the long allele, which may be associated with tobacco consumption [27].

5.5.4 Nicotine Metabolic Factors

Nicotine is extensively metabolized in the liver, and there is considerable individual variability in the rate of nicotine metabolism. Approximately 80% of nicotine is converted to cotinine in a two-step process. The first step is mediated by the CYP system, mainly by CYP2A6. The second step is induced by cytoplasmic aldehyde oxidase [5]. To date, more than 60 distinct *CYP2A6* alleles have been identified, including SNPs, deletions, duplications, and conversions. Phenotypic differences in metabolism include slow, intermediate, and fast metabolizers [30]. A GWAS showed that SNPs of the *CYP2A6* gene are significantly associated with nicotine metabolism [32]. Allele frequencies are significantly different among ethnic groups and people with *CYP2A6* alleles exhibiting reduced activity are less likely to develop nicotine dependence. People who metabolize nicotine quickly are generally heavy smokers, who are more dependent on nicotine. Thus, they have a harder time quitting than people who metabolize nicotine slowly. Similarly, the second most active enzyme CYP2B6 is involved in nicotine metabolism and has approximately 10% of the catalytic efficiency of CYP2A6 [30]. Of note, CYP2B6 is expressed at higher levels in the brain than in the liver, suggesting possible association with localized metabolism of nicotine in the brain of smokers. Additionally, CYP2D6 and CYP2E1 may be partly involved in nicotine dependence [30].

5.6 Smoking Cessation

5.6.1 Benefit of Smoking Cessation

Smokers who stop smoking reduce their risks of developing and dying from smoking-related diseases, including COPD, lung cancer, cardiovascular diseases, and recurrent stroke. The extent of the benefit from smoking cessation partly depends on the intensity and duration of prior exposure to tobacco smoke. Male and female smokers of all ages who quit smoking can be expected to live longer and are less likely to develop smoking-related diseases. Quitting smoking at younger ages is associated with a larger decrease in premature mortality than stopping at a later age. However, quitting smoking at older ages, even over 80, is still beneficial for reducing mortality [33]. How can smokers stop smoking? Habitual tobacco smoking is not just a person's favorite behavior; it is essentially an addiction, categorized as a mental disease, which should be treated. Smokers may develop a strategy such as reducing the number of cigarettes smoked to stop smoking but often find it difficult to quit on their own. Reducing the nicotine in cigarettes may lead to lower levels of addiction; however, this strategy does not solve the problem. Smokers may compensate for the lower levels of nicotine by smoking more cigarettes or by smoking more intensively. The most effective interventions consist of medication and counseling. Medication includes nicotine replacement therapy (NRT), varenicline, and bupropion.

5.6.2 Nicotine Replacement Therapy (NRT)

The United States Food and Drug Administration (FDA) has approved five nicotine replacement medications, including a patch, gum, lozenge, inhaler, and nasal spray, which can be used in combination. Some NRT medications can be obtained as over-the-counter drugs. NRT reduces the cravings due to nicotine addiction and increases the rate of quitting by 50–70%, regardless of the setting [34]. Overall risks of NRT medications, including nicotine poisoning and continued addiction, remain, but these medications do not appear to increase the risk of heart attack. Common side effects with the patch include skin irritation and dry mouth.

5.6.3 Varenicline

Varenicline, a partial nAChR agonist, was made available for sale in 2006, in the United States and Europe. It binds selectively and competitively to nAChRs and works by stimulating nAChRs more weakly than nicotine. Varenicline has less effect on dopamine release than nicotine and reduces the ability of nicotine to stimulate the mesolimbic reward system. As a partial agonist, it reduces cravings and decreases the satisfaction and sense of pleasure gained by tobacco smoking. Varenicline is the most effective medication for smoking cessation, more efficacious than bupropion or NRT, and as effective as combined NRT for smoking cessation [35]. Nausea is a common side effect of taking varenicline. Although post-marketing reports included suicide thoughts and occasional suicidal behavior, the FDA removed the black box warning in 2016. A recent review concluded that varenicline does not increase the risk of neuropsychiatric side effects [35]. Since varenicline reacts with nAChRs, genetic factors, including SNPs in nAChR genes, may be involved in not only nicotine dependence but also smoking cessation.

5.6.4 *Bupropion*

Bupropion was originally used as an antidepressant and is now also used as a smoking cessation aid. Although it is one of the most frequently prescribed antidepressants in North America, it is not available in Japan. Bupropion reduces the severity of nicotine cravings and withdrawal [36]. The effectiveness of bupropion is comparable to NRT; however, it is less effective than varenicline [36]. Since bupropion is metabolized to hydroxybupropion by CYP2B6, genetic factors, including SNPs, may be associated with bupropion and smoking cessation. Further studies may clarify the genetic factors associated with smoking cessation when taking bupropion.

5.6.5 *Counseling*

Although NRT or medication with either varenicline or bupropion is effective, the smoking cessation rate is unsatisfactory [36]. It is important to combine medication, guidance, counseling, and behavioral therapy to improve the cessation results.

5.7 Conclusions

As described above, genetic factors are involved in nicotine addiction. Although nicotine addiction is a complex process influenced by multiple factors, including the family environment, sociocultural factors, and an individual's own biology, genetic factors are associated with nicotine sensitivity and metabolism. The most effective way to promote smoking cessation is to combine both behavioral and pharmacological therapies. Because smoking cessation is associated with a mortality benefit for smokers of all ages, physicians must give patients guidance in smoking cessation. In the near future, genetic tests will predict patients at high risk for developing nicotine addiction.

References

1. Goodman J. Timeline. In: Tobacco in history and culture. An encyclopedia. Farmington Hills, MI: Thomson Gale; 2005. p. xiii–xvi.
2. WHO. Tobacco fact sheet. Geneva: World Health Organization Media Centre; 2016. http://www.who.int/mediacentre/factsheets/fs339/en/. Accessed 1 Jan 2017.
3. International Agency for Research on Cancer IARC. Monographs on the evaluation of carcinogenic risks to humans. Personal habits and indoor combustions, vol. 100E. Lyon: WHO press; 2012.
4. Cogliano VJ, Baan R, Straif K, Grosse Y, Lauby-Secretan B, Ghissassi FE, Bouvard V, et al. Preventable exposures associated with human cancers. J Natl Cancer Inst. 2011;103:1827–39. https://doi.org/10.1093/jnci/djr483.
5. Hukkanen J, Jacob P III, Benowitz NL. Metabolism and disposition kinetics of nicotine. Pharmacol Rev. 2005;57:79–115. https://doi.org/10.1124/pr.57.1.3.
6. Armitage A, Dollery C, Houseman T, Kohner E, Lewis PJ, Turner D. Absorption of nicotine from small cigars. Clin Pharmacol Ther. 1978;23:143–51.
7. Fattinger K, Verotta D, Benowitz NL. Pharmacodynamics of acute tolerance to multiple nicotinic effects in humans. J Pharmacol Exp Ther. 1997;281:1238–46.
8. Yoshida T, Sakane N, Umekawa T, Kondo M. Effect of nicotine on sympathetic nervous system activity of mice subjected to immobilization stress. Physiol Behav. 1994;55:53–7. https://doi.org/10.1016/0031-9384(94)90009-4.
9. Phillips DH. Smoking-related DNA and protein adducts in human tissues. Carcinogenesis. 2002;23:1979–2004. https://doi.org/10.1093/carcin/23.12.1979.
10. Church DF, Prior WA. Free-radical chemistry of cigarette smoke and its toxicologyical implications. Environ Health Perspect. 1985;64:111–26.
11. Rahman I, Biswas SK, Kode A. Oxidant and antioxidant balance in the airways and airway diseases. Eur J Pharmacol. 2006;533:222–39.
12. Ludvig J, Miner B, Eisenberg MJ. Smoking cessation in patients with coronary artery disease. Am Heart J. 2005;149:565–72. https://doi.org/10.1016/j.ahj.2004.09.040.
13. Centers for Disease Control and Prevention (CDC). Smoking-attributable mortality, years of potential life lost, and productivity losses---United States, 2000--2004. Morb Mortal Wkly Rep. 2008;57:1226–8.
14. Barnes PJ. Inflammatory mechanisms in patients with chronic obstructive pulmonary disease. J Allergy Clin Immunol. 2016;138:16–27.
15. Fletcher C, Peto R. The natural history of chronic airflow obstruction. Br Med J. 1977;1:1645–8. https://doi.org/10.1136/bmj.1.6077.1645.
16. Pillai SG, Ge D, Zhu G, Kong X, Shianna KV, Need AC, Feng S, et al. A genome –wide association study in chronic obstructive pulmonary disease (COPD): identification of two major susceptibility loci. PLoS Genet. 2009;5:e1000421. https://doi.org/10.1371/journal.pgen.1000421.
17. Mohamed Hoesein FAA, Wauters E, Janssens W, Groen HJM, Smolonska J, Wijmenga C, Postma DS, et al. Variants in the 15q24/25 locus associate with lung function decline in active smokers. PLoS One. 2013;8:e53219. https://doi.org/10.1371/journal.pone.0053219.
18. Budulac SE, Vonk JM, Postma DS, Siedlinski M, Timens W, Boezen MH. Nicotinic acetylcholine receptor variants are related to smoking habits, but not directly to COPD. PLoS One. 2012;7:e33386. https://doi.org/10.1371/journal.pone.0033386.
19. Hecht SS. Lung carcinogenesis by tobacco smoke. Int J Cancer. 2012;131:2724–32. https://doi.org/10.1002/ijc.27816.
20. Alexandrov LB, Ju YS, Haase K, Loo PV, Martincorena I, Nik-Zainal S, Totoki Y, et al. Mutational signatures associated with tobacco smoking in human cancers. Science. 2016;354:618–22. https://doi.org/10.1126/science.aag0299.
21. Wang S, Takayama K, Tanaka K, Takeshita M, Nakagaki N, Ijichi K, Li H, et al. Nicotine induces resistance to epidermal growth factor receptor tyrosine kinase inhibitor by α_1 nicotinic

acetylcholine receptor-mediated activation in PC9 cells. J Thorac Oncol. 2013;8:719–25. https://doi.org/10.1097/JTO.0b013e31828b51d4.
22. Nutt D, King LA, Saulsbury W, Blakemore C. Development of a rational scale to assess the harm of drugs of potential misuse. Lancet. 2007;369:1047–53. https://doi.org/10.1016/S0140-6736(07)60464-4.
23. Benowitz NL. Nicotine addiction. N Engl J Med. 2010;362:2295–303.
24. Pogun S, Yararbas G, Nesil T, Kanit L. Sex differences in nicotine preference. J Neurosci Res. 2017;95:148–62. https://doi.org/10.1002/jnr.23858.
25. Pérez-Stable EJ, Herrera B, Jacob P III, Benowitz NL. Nicotine metabolism and intake in black and white smokers. JAMA. 1998;280:152–6.
26. Li MD, Ma JZ, Cheng R, Dupont RT, Williams NJ, Crews KM, Payne TJ, et al. A genome-wide scan to identify loci for smoking rate in the Framingham Heart Study population. BMC Genet. 2003;4(Suppl 1):S103.
27. Pérez-Rubio G, Sansores R, Ramírez-Venegas A, Camarena Á, Pérez-Rodríguez ME, Falfán-Valencia R. Nicotin addiction development: from epidemiology to genetic factors. Rev Invest Clin. 2015;67:333–43.
28. Unwin N. Refined Structure of the nicotinic acetylcholine receptor at 4A resolution. J Mol Biol. 2005;346:967–89. https://doi.org/10.1016/j.jmb.2004.12.031.
29. Labarca C, Schwarz J, Deshpande P, Schwarz S, Nowak MW, Fonck C, Nashmi R, et al. Point mutant mice with hypersensitive α4 nicotinic receptors show dopaminergic deficits and increased anxiety. Proc Natl Acad Sci. 2001;98:2786–91. https://doi.org/10.1073/pnas.041582598.
30. Loukola A, Hällfors J, Korhonen T, Kaprio J. Genetics and smoking. Curr Addict Rep. 2014;1:75–82. https://doi.org/10.1007/s40429-013-0006-3.
31. Li MD. The genetics of nicotine dependence. Curr Psychiatry Rep. 2006;8:158–64.
32. Loukola A, Buckwald J, Gupta R, Palviainen T, Hällfors J, Tikkanen E, Korhonen T, et al. A genome-wide association study of a biomarker of nicotine metabolism. PLoS Genet. 2015;11:e1005498. https://doi.org/10.1371/journal.pgen.1005498.
33. Gellert C, Scöttker B, Brenner H. Smoking and all-cause mortality in old people. Arch Intern Med. 2012;172:837–44.
34. Stead LF, Perera R, Bullen C, Mant D, Hartmann-Boyce J, Cahill K, Lancaster T. Nicotine replacement therapy for smoking cessation. Cochrane Database Syst Rev. 2013;11:CD000146. https://doi.org/10.1002/14651858.CD000146.pub4.
35. Cahill K, Stevens S, Perera R, Lancaser T. Pharmacological intervenetions for smoking cessation: an overview and network meta-analysis. Cochrane Database Syst Rev. 2013;(5):CD009329. https://doi.org/10.1002/14651858.CD009329.pub2.
36. Wu P, Wilson K, Dimoulas P, Mills EJ. Effectiveness of smoking cessation therapies: a systematic review and meta-analysis. BMC Public Health. 2006;6:300. https://doi.org/10.1186/1471-2458-6-300.

Chapter 6
Cystic Fibrosis, Primary Ciliary Dyskinesia, and Diffuse Panbronchiolitis: Hereditary and Non-hereditary—What Are the Roles of Genetic Factors in the Pathogenesis of These Diseases?

Masaharu Shinkai

Abstract Cystic fibrosis (CF), primary ciliary dyskinesia (PCD), and diffuse panbronchiolitis (DPB) are rare airway diseases. CF is the most common life-shortening genetic disorder in Caucasians, caused by mutations in a single gene on the long arm of chromosome 7 that encodes the cystic fibrosis transmembrane conductance regulator (CFTR). The predominant CFTR mutation is Phe508del, yet more than 2000 variants in this gene have been identified, which can be divided into six classes. Class II mutations, including Phe508del, cause retention of a misfolded protein in the endoplasmic reticulum and subsequent degradation in the proteasome. Patients with Class I, II, and III mutations, which are associated with loss of CFTR function, typically have a severe phenotype, whereas individuals with Class IV, V, and VI mutations, which retain residual CFTR function, have mild lung phenotypes and pancreatic sufficiency. PCD is usually inherited in an autosomal recessive manner and is genetically heterogeneous. Of the 30 mutations that are known to cause PCD, those affecting the *DNAH5*, *DNAI1*, *DNAAF1 (LRRC50)*, *LRRC6*, *CCDC39*, *CCDC40*, and *DNAH11 genes are found in* 15–21%, 2–9%, 4–5%, 3%, 2–10%, 2–8%, and 6% of patients, respectively. In terms of the relationship between phenotype and genotype, mutation of *DNAH5*, *DNAI1*, *DNAI2*, *DNAL1*, *CCDC114*, *TXNDC3 (NME8)*, *or ARMC4* results in loss of the outer dynein arms. In regard to DPB, an interaction of environmental and genetic factors is thought to underpin the disease. The most probable location for DPB susceptibility genes is thought to lie in a 200 kb major histocompatibility complex (MHC) class I region between *HLA-A* and *HLA-B*. This contains the DPB critical region 1 gene (*DPCR1*, chromosome 6p21.33), as well as *MUC21*, and the panbronchiolitis-related mucin-like genes 1 and 2 (*PBMUCL1* and *PBMCL2*). The fact that *DPCR1*, *MUC21*, *PBMUCL1*, and

M. Shinkai
Tokyo Shinagawa Hospital, Tokyo, Japan

T. Kaneko (ed.), *Clinical Relevance of Genetic Factors in Pulmonary Diseases*, Respiratory Disease Series: Diagnostic Tools and Disease Managements, https://doi.org/10.1007/978-981-10-8144-6_6

PBMUCL2 are all mucin or mucin-like genes is highly relevant for the excessive airway mucus secretion that is typical in DPB. In summary, CF and PCD are both hereditary disorders of mucociliary clearance that result in chronic upper and lower airways disease, while in DPB, it is thought that genetic factors may determine disease susceptibility.

Keywords Cystic fibrosis · Phe508del · Primary ciliary dyskinesia · *DNAH5* Diffuse panbronchiolitis · PBMUCL · Hereditary · Genetic factor

6.1 Introduction

Cystic fibrosis (CF), primary ciliary dyskinesia (PCD), and diffuse panbronchiolitis (DPB) are rare airway diseases. CF is the most common life-shortening genetic disorder in Caucasians in the United States. CF affects approximately 30,000 individuals in the United States and 70,000 individuals worldwide [1]. The functional failure of CFTR results in mucus retention and chronic infection. Early in life, airway infections are most commonly caused by *Staphylococcus aureus* and *H. influenzae*. As patients age, *P. aeruginosa* becomes the predominant infecting organism, and about 80% of patients with CF are infected with this organism by adulthood [2]. Subsequently, airway inflammation becomes harmful to the lungs. The development and delivery of drugs that improve the clearance of mucus from the lungs and treat the associated infection, in combination with the correction of pancreatic insufficiency and undernutrition by multidisciplinary teams, have resulted in remarkable improvements in quality of life and clinical outcomes in patients with CF, with median life expectancy now >40 years [3]. Innovative and transformational therapies that target the basic defect in CF have recently been developed and are effective in improving lung function and reducing pulmonary exacerbations [4].

PCD is a genetic disease that causes abnormalities in ciliary function, leading to impaired mucociliary clearance. PCD is rare, with an estimated prevalence of one in 20,000 live births (range, 1/10,000 to 1/40,000) [5]. Congenital abnormality of the primary cilia results in situs inversus in 50% of patients [6]. Cases with situs inversus are considered to show "Kartagener's syndrome" [7]. Decreased function of motile cilia causes chronic rhinosinusitis, otitis media with effusion, bronchiectasis, and infertility. The clinical features usually start with neonatal respiratory distress, with early-onset persistent rhinosinusitis and serous otitis media with hearing impairment and persistent daily wet cough [8]. PCD without situs inversus is underdiagnosed because prolonged chronic cough represents an important symptom that is seen in most patients. Diagnosis of PCD requires the presence of characteristic clinical phenotypes, in addition to either the identification of mutation in one of the genes known to be associated with PCD [9] or specific ciliary ultrastructural defects identified by transmission electron microscopy in biopsy samples of the respiratory epithelium [10]. Nasal nitric oxide concentration is extremely low in PCD and may also therefore be useful for screening of the disease [11]. Diagnosis in the early stages is important to prevent progression of bronchiectasis and deterioration of lung function, by providing lifestyle guidance in regard to immunization, cessation of smoking, and the need for prompt therapy at the time of respiratory tract infection. Genetic counseling is necessary after definitive diagnosis since it is inherited in an autosomal recessive manner.

DPB has many similarities with CF, in that it is an inflammatory lung disease characterized by the chronic inflammation of bronchioles (small airways) in both lungs [12]. DPB can also present as one of the characteristic features of the lung in PCD [13]. The term *diffuse* means that lesions appear throughout both lungs, while *panbronchiolitis* refers to the inflammation that is found in the respiratory bronchioles. DPB causes severe coughing, large amounts of sputum, and exertional breathlessness, often associated with chronic sinusitis. Histopathologically, thickening of the terminal bronchiole walls with infiltration of lymphocytes, plasma cells, and foamy macrophages, leading to chronic neutrophilic inflammatory airway disease, are the predominant features [14]. The disease was first described by a Japanese group of clinicians as a new entity in the 1960s but was not accepted internationally because the disease had been reported predominantly in East Asia. Introduced to Western countries in the 1980s, cases were then recognized throughout Asia, as well as in Europe and the USA [15, 16]. According to a nationwide survey conducted in Japan [17], there appears to be no remarkable gender or age predominance for DPB, and a history of smoking or exposure to toxic fumes do not seem to be involved. In many cases, symptoms of chronic sinusitis first appear in the transition from child to adulthood, followed by the development of symptoms in the lower airways. In 1980, the prevalence of DPB was 11.1 cases per 100,000 people [18], but the number was reported to have decreased to only 3.4 cases per 100,000 in an unofficial survey conducted in 1995 [9]. The reason for this drop is presumed to be the positive effect of macrolide therapy given at an early stage [19], resulting in the appearance only of chronic sinusitis symptoms.

In patients with these three diseases, the associated infections and intense neutrophilic inflammatory responses lead to airway destruction, bronchiectasis, and obstructive lung disease, ultimately resulting in respiratory failure, which if left untreated, is fatal. This chapter is a discussion on the roles of genetic factors in the pathogenesis of these three diseases.

6.2 Genetic Factors in the Pathogenesis of CF

CF is a common autosomal recessive disorder caused by mutations in a single gene on the long arm of chromosome 7 that encodes the cystic fibrosis transmembrane conductance regulator (CFTR) protein [20–23]. The predominant mutation is Phe508del, although more than 2000 gene variants have been identified [24]. CFTR is a chloride-conducting transmembrane channel that regulates anion transport and mucociliary clearance in the airways (Fig. 6.1a) [25]. Wildtype CFTR is also involved in the regulation of the inflammasome and the epithelial sodium channel (ENaC) [26]. The functional failure of CFTR results in hyper-inflammation, proteasome stress, reduced or absent anion transport, and hyper-reabsorption of Na+, which in turn leads to impaired innate immunity, mucus abnormalities, and reduced airway surface liquid (ASL) hydration and suboptimal mucociliary clearance. Together, these factors subsequently result in mucus retention, chronic infection, and local airway inflammation that is harmful to the lungs [25] (Fig. 6.1b). CFTR dysfunction mainly affects epithelial cells, although there is also evidence of a role for this protein in immune cells. CF affects several body systems; however, morbidity and mortality are mostly related to bronchiectasis, small airway obstruction, and progressive respiratory impairment. Important comorbidities caused by epithelial cell dysfunction present in the pancreas as malabsorption, in the liver as biliary cirrhosis, in the sweat glands as heat shock, and in the vas deferens as infertility. Mutations in the *CFTR* gene have different effects on the either production of the CFTR protein, its stability at the cell membrane, or functional defects in regard to chloride and bicarbonate transport. Most mutations in *CFTR* are missense alterations, but frameshift, splicing, and nonsense mutations, as well as in-frame deletions and insertions, have all been reported [27]. About 15% of identified genetic variants are not associated with clinical disease.

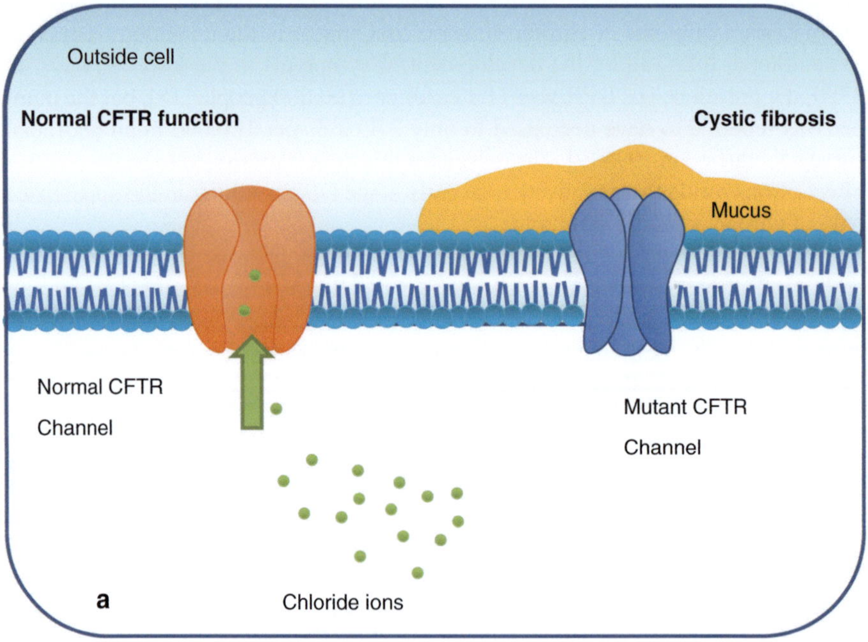

Fig. 6.1 (**a**) Schematic representation of pathology of cystic fibrosis. (**b**) Effects of CFTR dysfunction. ASL = airway surface liquid. CFTR = cystic fibrosis transmembrane conductance regulator. ENaC = epithelial sodium channel. Adapted from J Stuart Elborn [25]

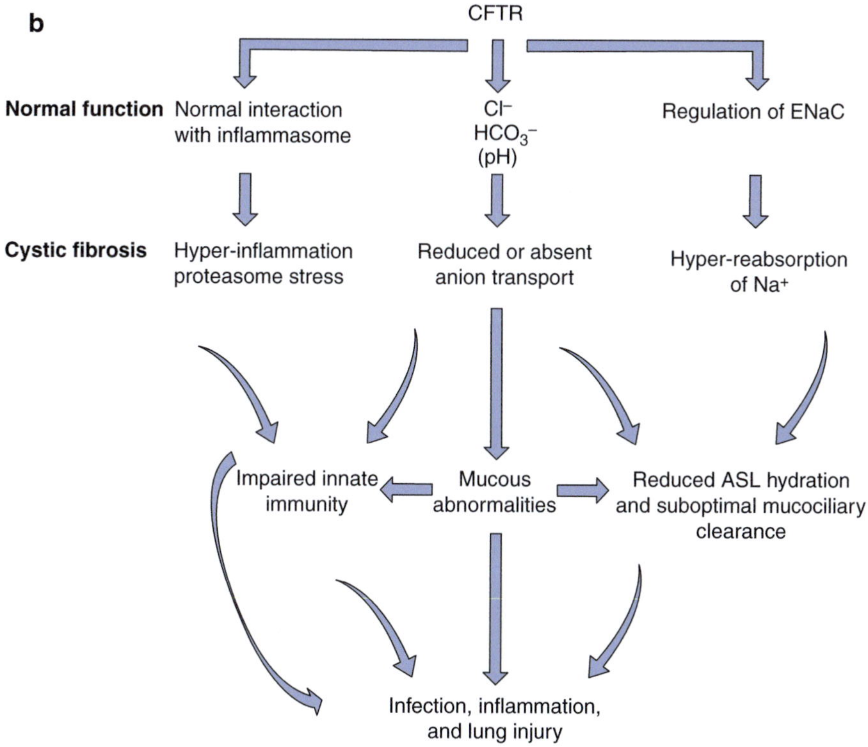

Fig. 6.1 (continued)

As shown in Fig. 6.2, mutations of the *CFTR* gene can be divided into six classes. Class I mutations, including Gly542X, Trp1282X, and Arg553X, result in no protein production. Class II mutations, including the most prevalent Phe508del variation, cause retention of a misfolded protein at the endoplasmic reticulum and subsequent degradation in the proteasome. Class III mutations, including Gly551Asp, Gly178Arg, and Gly551Ser, affect channel regulation, impairing the channel opening. Class IV mutants, including Arg117His, Arg347Pro, and Arg117Cys, show reduced conduction and a decreased flow of ions. Class V mutations cause substantial reduction in mRNA or protein or both. Class VI mutations, including 4326delTC, gln1412X, and 4279insA, cause substantial plasma membrane instability [28]. This classification system is helpful because it relates to the molecular and cellular processes in gene translation and protein processing and has some useful clinical correlates (Fig. 6.3). Patients with Class I, II, or III mutations are associated with no residual CFTR function and generally have a severe phenotype, whereas individuals with Class IV, V, or VI mutations have some residual CFTR function, with a mild lung phenotype and pancreatic sufficiency [29]. However, as with any system of classification, there are several oversimplifications with this approach. Phe508del, for example, is predominantly a Class II trafficking

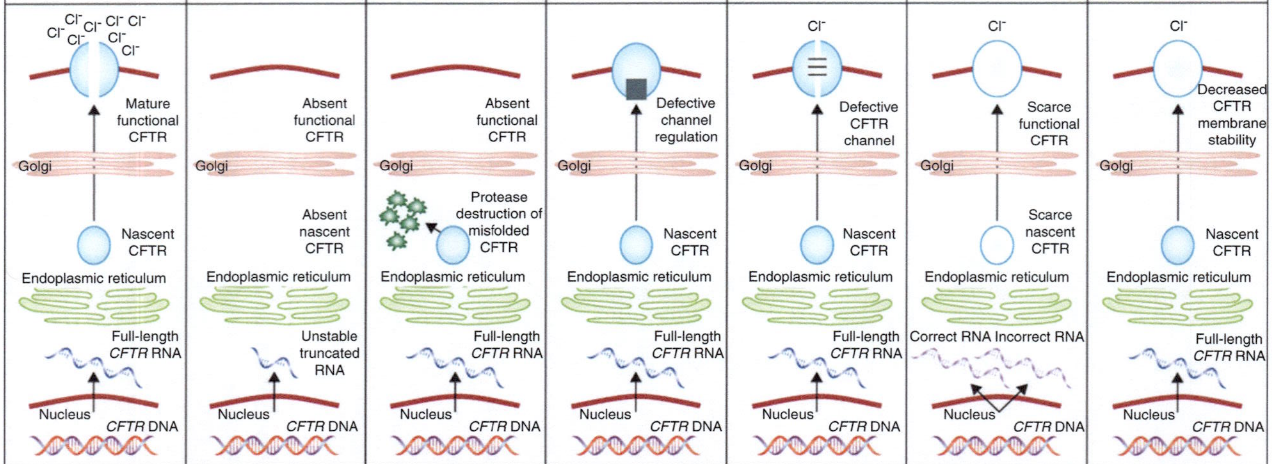

Normal	I	II	III	IV	V	VI
CFTR defect	No functional CFTR protein	CFTR trafficking defect	Defective channel regulation	Decreased channel conductance	Reduced synthesis of CFTR	Decreased CFTR stability
Type of mutations	Nonsense; frameshift; canonical splice	Missense; aminoacid deletion	Missense; aminoacid change	Missense; aminoacid change	Splicing defect; missense	Missense; aminoacid change
Specific mutation examples	Gly542X Trp1282X Arg553X 621+1G→T	Phe508del Asn1303Lys Ile507del Arg560Thr	Gly551Asp Gly178Arg Gly551Ser Ser549Asn	Arg117His Arg347Pro Arg117Cys Arg334Trp	3849+10kbC→T 2789+5G→A 3120+1G→A 5T	4326delTC Gln1412X 4279insA

Fig. 6.2 Classes of CFTR mutations. Mutations in the cystic fibrosis transmembrane conductance regulator (CFTR) gene can be divided into six classes. Class I mutations result in no protein production. Class II mutations (including the most prevalent, Phe508del) cause retention of a misfolded protein at the endoplasmic reticulum and subsequent degradation in the proteasome. Class III mutations affect channel regulation, impairing channel opening (e.g., Gly551Asp). Class IV mutants show reduced conduction, i.e., decreased flow of ions (e.g., Arg117His). Class V mutations cause substantial reduction in mRNA or protein or both. Class VI mutations cause substantial plasma membrane instability and include Phe508del when rescued by most correctors (rPhe508del). Reproduced from Boyle and De Boeck. Adapted from J Stuart Elborn [25]

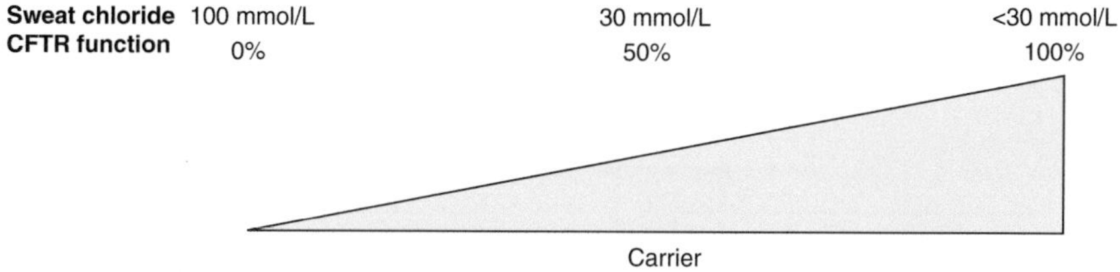

Sweat chloride	100 mmol/L	30-60 mmol/L	<30 mmol/L
Lung phenotype	Bronchiectasis	Airway wall thickening	Normal airways
Bacteriology	*Pseudomonas aeruginosa*	*Staphylococcus aureus*	Normal microbiome
Pancreatic function	None	50% pancreatic insufficiency	Normal pancreatic function
Male fertility	Infertile	Infertile	Fertile
Typical mutations	Gly542X	Arg117His (5T)	
	Phe508del	Arg334Trp	
	Gly551Asp	Ala55Glu	
	Class I-III mutations	Class IV-VI mutations	Healthy

Heterozygote carrier

Fig. 6.3 Relation between phenotype, genotype, and CFTR function in patients with cystic fibrosis, carriers, and healthy individuals. CFTR = cystic fibrosis transmembrane conductance regulator. Adapted from J Stuart Elborn [25]

mutation, with only around 3% of protein being trafficked to the cell membrane; however, the channel is not functional and thus has properties of a Class III gating mutation, in addition to having the decreased stability of a Class VI mutation [30]. Gene-based small-molecule therapies are currently being developed to restore CFTR function and thus improve the clinical outcomes of people with CF.

6.3 Genetic Factors in the Pathogenesis of PCD

As shown in Fig. 6.4 [9], pathogenesis associated with PCD begins with a defect in genes related to ciliary motility. PCD is usually inherited in an autosomal recessive manner, but the disorder is genetically heterogeneous, and cases of autosomal dominant or X-linked inheritance have also been reported [31]. In their review, Takeuchi et al. [9] described how impaired ciliary motility in embryos results in the *NODAL* gene being randomly expressed either to the right or the left of the body in this disease [32]. *NODAL* expressed to the right results in situs inversus *totalis* which is a known feature of Kartagener syndrome. When *NODAL* is expressed to the left, however, the heart develops in the normal location and PCD instead develops without situs inversus *totalis*. Decreased ciliary movement in motile cilia results in decreased mucociliary clearance, manifesting as rhinosinusitis, otitis media, pneumonia, bronchiectasis, infertility, and ectopic pregnancy. Mutations known to cause PCD have

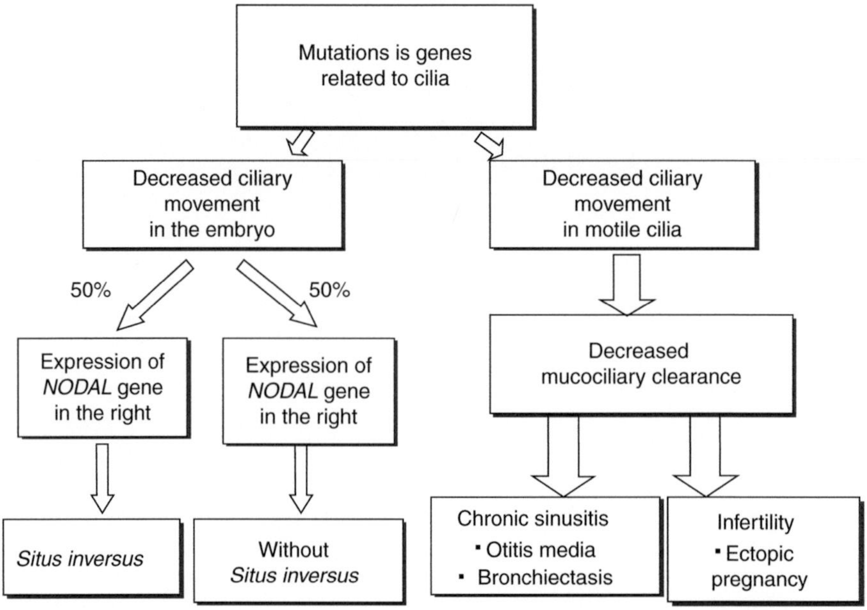

Fig. 6.4 Etiology of primary ciliary dyskinesia. All abnormalities start with mutations in genes related to cilia or ciliary movement. Decreased movement of primary cilia in the embryo results in expression of the *NODAL* gene on the right in approximately 50% of patients, causing situs inversus. Decreased movement of motile cilia causes decreased mucociliary clearance, which results in chronic sinusitis, otitis media, bronchiectasis, infertility, and ectopic pregnancy. Adapted from K Takeuchi [9]

been identified in 30 genes, as reviewed by Knowles et al. [33] and Takeuchi et al. [9]. These are shown in Table 6.1 [9] with the prevalence of *DNAH5*, *DNAI1*, *DNAAF1 (LRRC50)*, *LRRC6*, *CCDC39*, *CCDC40*, and *DNAH11 mutations among patients with PCD being* 15–21%, 2–9%, 4–5%, 3%, 2–10%, 2–8%, and 6%, respectively. Mutations in 30 of these genes account for the genetic etiology in approximately 70% of individuals affected with PCD [9, 34]; however, disease-causing mutations have yet to be identified for many patients with PCD.

Numerous mutations can arise in each of the genes involved in ciliary movement. This fact may help explain the wide variation in the degree of mucociliary dysfunction and disease severity among patients. In terms of the relationship between phenotype and genotype, mutation of *DNAH5*, *DNAI1*, *DNAI2*, *DNAL1*, *CCDC114*, *TXNDC3 (NME8)*, or *ARMC4* results in the loss of the outer dynein arms. Mutations in *DNAAF1 (LRRC50)*, *DNAAF2 (KTU)*, *DNAAF3 (C19orf51)*, *CCDC103*, *HEATR2*, *LRRC6*, *ZMYND10*, *DYX1C1*, *C21orf59*, *SPAG1*, or *CCDC151*, which code for proteins associated with the assembly of cilia, result in the loss of both outer and inner dynein arms. *CCDC39* and *CCDC40* mutations result in the loss of the inner dynein arms and abnormalities in axoneme structure. *RSPH1*, *RSPH4A*, and *RSPH9* code for radial spork proteins, with mutations resulting in the loss of central microtubules. Eighty-five percent of mutations represent loss-of-function

Table 6.1 List of genes causing primary ciliary dyskinesia and the relation to phenotypes

Locus name	Gene symbol	Structure of cilia	Percentage of PCD	Laterality defects
CILD3	*DNAH5*	Loss of outer dynein arms	15–21%	Possible
CILD1	*DNAI1*		2–9%	
CILD9	*DNAI2*		2%	
CILD16	*DNAL1*		NA	
CILD20	*CCDC114*		6% of outer dynein loss	
CILD06	*TXNDC3(NME8)*		NA	
CILD23	*ARMC4*		NA	
CILD13	*DNAAF1(LRRC50)*	Loss of inner and outer dynein arms	4–5%	
CILD10	*DNAAF2(KTU)*		~2%	
CILD2	*DNAAF3 (C19orf51)*		NA	
CILD17	*CCDC103*		NA	
CILD18	*HEATR2*		NA	
CILD19	*LRRC6*		3%	
CILD22	*ZMYND10*		NA	
CILD25	*DYX1C1*		NA	
CILD26	*C21orf59*		NA	
CILD28	*SPAG1*		NA	
CILD30	*CCDC151*		NA	
CILD14	*CCDC39*	Loss of inner dynein arm and abnormalities of axoneme structure	2–10%	
CILD15	*CCDC40*		2–8%	
CILD24	*RSPH1*	Loss of central microtubules	NA	Absent
CILD11	*RSPH4A*		NA	
CILD12	*RSPH9*		NA	
CILD5	*HYDIN*	Occasional loss of central microtubules	NA	
CILD21	*DRC1(CCDC164,C2orf39)*	Loss of nexin link axonemal disorganization	NA	
CILD27	*CCDC65*		NA	
CILD29	*CCNO*	Decrease of cilia, centriole and basal bodies	NA	
	RPGR	Various	NA	
CILD7	*DNAH11*	Normal	6%	Possible
	OFD1	Not determined	NA	Absent

Adapted from K Takeuchi [9]

variants, while 15% are conservative missense mutations [33]. In 30% of PCD patients, cilial structures are normal under electron microscopy, meaning that genetic analysis represents the ultimate method of diagnosis in some patients. Takeuchi et al. [9], for example, have reported that they initially screen mutation hot spots on *DNAI1* and *DNAH5* by direct sequencing, but if no variants are detected in these loci, they then screen for variants in other genes using whole-exome sequencing.

6.4 Genetic Factors in the Pathogenesis of DPB

Although the cause of DPB remains unknown, the interaction of environmental and genetic factors appears to underpin the disease. Since DPB has been reported mainly in Japan and East Asia, it was initially suspected that a genetic predisposition unique to Asian descendants might determine disease susceptibility. Now, studies have shown that specific human leukocyte antigen (HLA) haplotypes are strongly associated with the development of DPB, such as HLA-B54 for Japanese patients [35] and HLA-A11 for Korean patients [36]. With this in mind, the most probable location for DPB susceptibility genes is thought to lie in a 200 kb major histocompatibility complex (MHC) class I region between *HLA-A* and *HLA-B* on chromosome 6, as shown in Fig. 6.5a [37]. This contains the DPB critical region 1 gene (*DPCR1*, chromosome 6p21.33) [38], as well as *MUC21*, and the panbronchiolitis-related

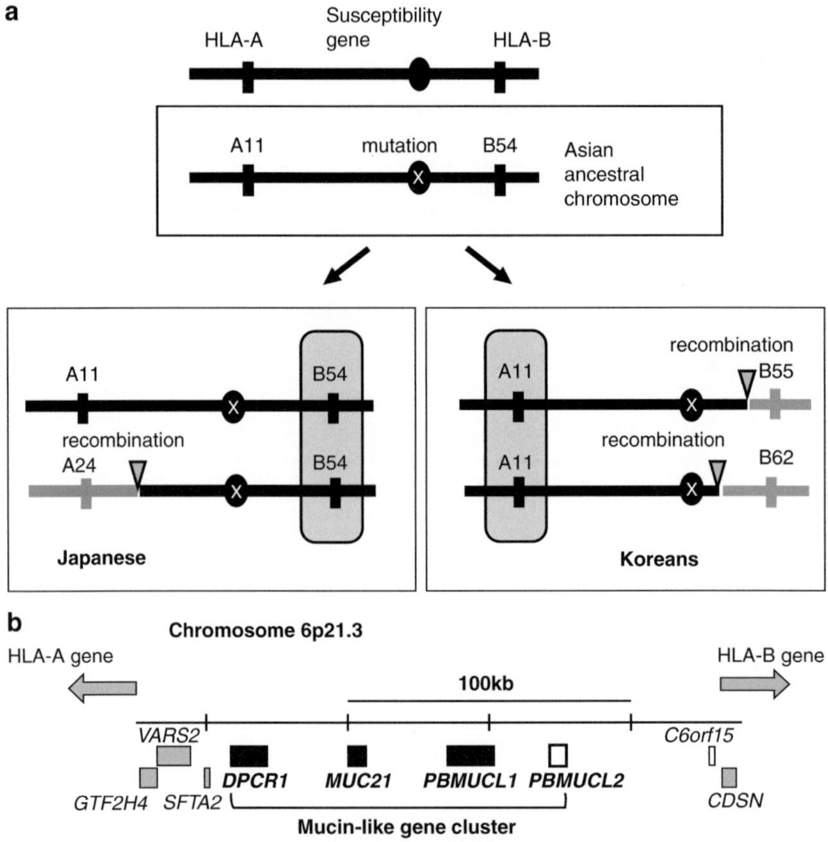

Fig. 6.5 (**a**) A hypothesis that may explain the findings that diffuse panbronchiolitis is associated with different HLA types in Japanese and Koreans. A disease susceptibility gene may be located between HLA-A locus and the HLA-B locus (see text for details). Adapted from: N Keicho [15]. (**b**) A novel mucin or mucin-like gene cluster in the HLA class I region on the short arm of chromosome 6 (6p21.3), members of which showed associations with diffuse panbronchiolitis. *DPCR1*, *MUC21*, *PBMUCL1*, and *PBMUCL2* are all mucin or mucin-like genes. Adapted from N Keicho [15]

mucin-like genes 1 and 2 (*PBMUCL1* and *PBMCL2*) [39] (Fig. 6.5b). The fact that *DPCR1*, *MUC21*, *PBMUCL1*, and *PBMUCL2* are all mucin or mucin-like genes [38, 40, 41] is highly relevant for the excessive airway mucus secretion that is typical in DPB. The HLA system contributes to appropriate immune responses through T-cell receptors, and thus, genetic predisposition in this disease may also involve defective immunity in the airways. Together with the number of familial cases, the high rate observed for current or past history of chronic sinusitis, and systematic failure of respiratory defense mechanisms, genetic susceptibility in the development and progression of DPB is quite possible.

Transmural and peribronchial infiltration by lymphocytes, the presence of plasma cells and lipid-engulfed foamy macrophages around the small airways, and large numbers of neutrophils and hypersecretion of mucus due to persistent bacterial infection in the large airways are the major characteristic aspects of DPB (Fig. 6.6). It is assumed that defective immunity caused by genetic predisposition results in both the persistent bacterial infection and the associated inflammatory disorders. It is generally accepted that key players in the development of DPB are neutrophils and T-lymphocytes, especially CD8+ cells, and cytokines such as interleukin 8 (IL-8) and macrophage inflammatory protein 1 (MIP-1). Cross sections of autopsied lung tissue from DPB patients show yellow nodules, mainly in the respiratory bronchioles [42]. Interstitial accumulation of foamy macrophages in the walls of the respiratory bronchioles and the surrounding interalveolar spaces (Fig. 6.7a) and thickened bronchiolar walls infiltrated by inflammatory cells (Fig. 6.7b) are found

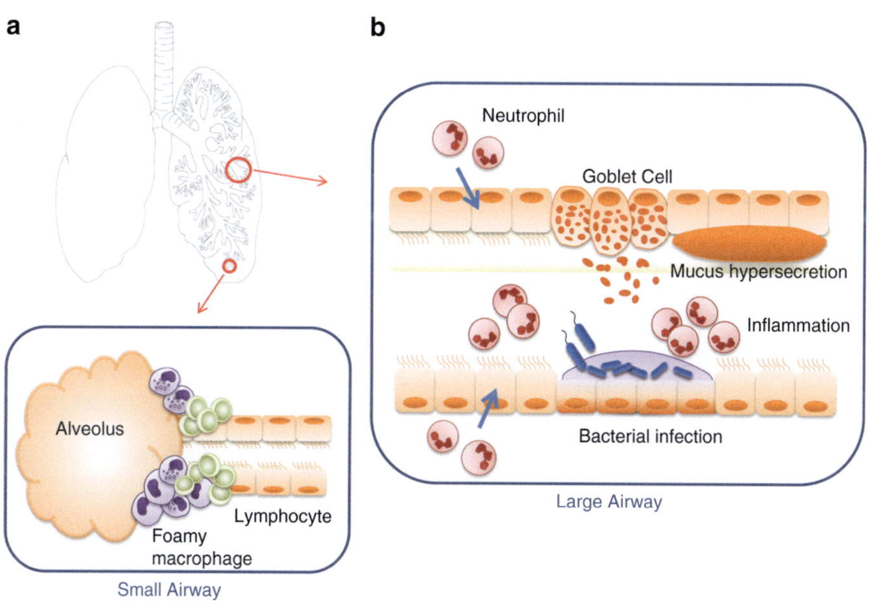

Fig. 6.6 Schematic representation of pathology of diffuse panbronchiolitis. Typical features seen include transmural accumulations of foamy macrophages, lymphocytes, and plasma cells in the small airways. The adjacent alveolar area tends not to be affected. Bacterial infections, along with a large number of neutrophils and mucus hypersecretion, are seen in large airways

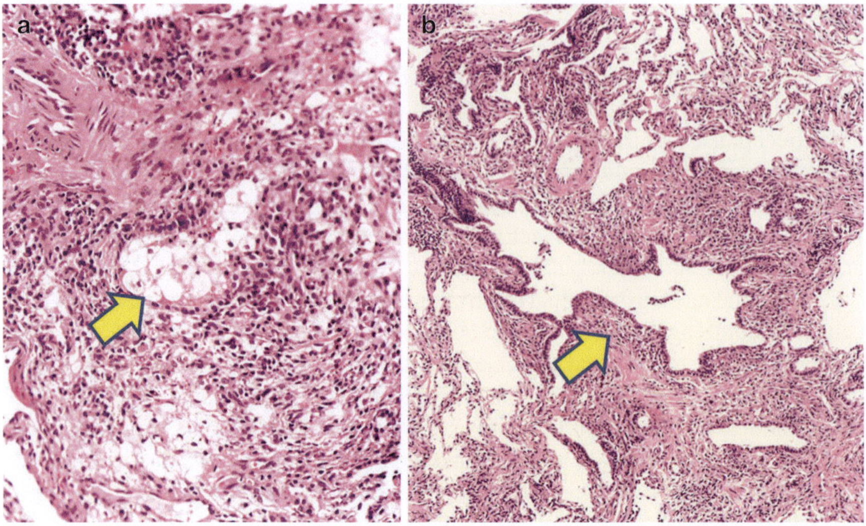

Fig. 6.7 (**a**) A respiratory bronchiole with the thickened wall infiltrated by inflammatory cells. (**b**) Interstitial accumulations of foamy macrophages in the wall of the respiratory bronchiole

in transbronchial lung biopsies from DPB patients. These histological features represent one of the distinctive characteristics of DPB [35], but their clinical significance remains uncertain.

6.5 Conclusion

CF and PCD are both hereditary disorders of mucociliary clearance that result in chronic upper and lower airways disease. In DPB, it is thought that genetic factors may determine disease susceptibility.

References

1. Hamosh A, FitzSimmons SC, Macek M Jr, Knowles MR, Rosenstein BJ, Cutting GR. Comparison of the clinical manifestations of cystic fibrosis in black and white patients. J Pediatr. 1998;132(2):255–9.
2. Gibson RL, Emerson J, McNamara S, Burns JL, Rosenfeld M, Yunker A, et al. Significant microbiological effect of inhaled tobramycin in young children with cystic fibrosis. Am J Respir Crit Care Med. 2003;167(6):841–9.
3. Burgel PR, Bellis G, Olesen HV, Viviani L, Zolin A, Blasi F, et al. Future trends in cystic fibrosis demography in 34 European countries. Eur Respir J. 2015;46(1):133–41.
4. VanDevanter DR, Kahle JS, O'Sullivan AK, Sikirica S, Hodgkins PS. Cystic fibrosis in young children: a review of disease manifestation, progression, and response to early treatment. J Cyst Fibros. 2016;15(2):147–57.

5. Kuehni CE, Frischer T, Strippoli MP, Maurer E, Bush A, Nielsen KG, et al. Factors influencing age at diagnosis of primary ciliary dyskinesia in European children. Eur Respir J. 2010;36(6):1248–58.
6. Carlen B, Stenram U. Primary ciliary dyskinesia: a review. Ultrastruct Pathol. 2005;29(3-4):217–20.
7. Kartagener M. Zur pathogenese der bronkiectasien. Bronkiectasien bei situs viscerum inversus. Beitr Klin Tuberk Spezif Tuberkuloseforsch. 1933;1933(83):489–501.
8. Goutaki M, Meier AB, Halbeisen FS, Lucas JS, Dell SD, Maurer E, et al. Clinical manifestations in primary ciliary dyskinesia: systematic review and meta-analysis. Eur Respir J. 2016;48(4):1081–95.
9. Takeuchi K, Kitano M, Ishinaga H, Kobayashi M, Ogawa S, Nakatani K, et al. Recent advances in primary ciliary dyskinesia. Auris Nasus Larynx. 2016;43(3):229–36.
10. Holzmann D, Ott PM, Felix H. Diagnostic approach to primary ciliary dyskinesia: a review. Eur J Pediatr. 2000;159(1-2):95–8.
11. Collins SA, Gove K, Walker W, Lucas JS. Nasal nitric oxide screening for primary ciliary dyskinesia: systematic review and meta-analysis. Eur Respir J. 2014;44(6):1589–99.
12. Homma H, Yamanaka A, Tanimoto S, Tamura M, Chijimatsu Y, Kira S, et al. Diffuse panbronchiolitis. A disease of the transitional zone of the lung. Chest. 1983;83(1):63–9.
13. Chen W, Shao C, Song Y, Bai C. Primary ciliary dyskinesia complicated with diffuse panbronchiolitis: a case report and literature review. Clin Respir J. 2014;8(4):425–30.
14. Homma S, Sakamoto S, Kawabata M, Kishi K, Tsuboi E, Motoi N, et al. Comparative clinicopathology of obliterative bronchiolitis and diffuse panbronchiolitis. Respiration. 2006;73(4):481–7.
15. Keicho N, Hijikata M. Genetic predisposition to diffuse panbronchiolitis. Respirology. 2011;16(4):581–8.
16. Anthony M, Singham S, Soans B, Tyler G. Diffuse panbronchiolitis: not just an Asian disease: Australian case series and review of the literature. Biomed Imaging Interv J. 2009;5(4):e19.
17. Izumi T, Doi O, Nobechi A, et al. Nation-wide survey of diffuse panbronchiolitis. Annual report on the study of interstitial lung disease in 1982. Grant-in Aid from the Ministry of Health and Welfare of Japan, Tokyo; 1983. p. 3–41.
18. Okada M, Saito N, Hosoda Y, et al. An epidemiological study of DPB in a large company. Annual report on the study of interstitial lung disease in 1980. Grant-in Aid from the Ministry of Health and Welfare of Japan, Tokyo; 1980. p. 25–8.
19. Shinkai M, Henke MO, Rubin BK. Macrolide antibiotics as immunomodulatory medications: proposed mechanisms of action. Pharmacol Ther. 2008;117(3):393–405.
20. Robinson P, Schechter MS, Sly PD, Winfield K, Smith J, Brennan S, et al. Clarithromycin therapy for patients with cystic fibrosis: a randomized controlled trial. Pediatr Pulmonol. 2012;47(6):551–7.
21. Riordan JR, Rommens JM, Kerem B, Alon N, Rozmahel R, Grzelczak Z, et al. Identification of the cystic fibrosis gene: cloning and characterization of complementary DNA. Science. 1989;245(4922):1066–73.
22. Kerem B, Rommens JM, Buchanan JA, Markiewicz D, Cox TK, Chakravarti A, et al. Identification of the cystic fibrosis gene: genetic analysis. Science. 1989;245(4922):1073–80.
23. Rommens JM, Iannuzzi MC, Kerem B, Drumm ML, Melmer G, Dean M, et al. Identification of the cystic fibrosis gene: chromosome walking and jumping. Science. 1989;245(4922):1059–65.
24. Castellani C, Cuppens H, Macek M Jr, Cassiman JJ, Kerem E, Durie P, et al. Consensus on the use and interpretation of cystic fibrosis mutation analysis in clinical practice. J Cyst Fibros. 2008;7(3):179–96.
25. Elborn JS. Cystic fibrosis. Lancet. 2016;388(10059):2519–31.
26. Stoltz DA, Meyerholz DK, Welsh MJ. Origins of cystic fibrosis lung disease. N Engl J Med. 2015;372(4):351–62.
27. Bell SC, De Boeck K, Amaral MD. New pharmacological approaches for cystic fibrosis: promises, progress, pitfalls. Pharmacol Ther. 2015;145:19–34.

28. Boyle MP, De Boeck K. A new era in the treatment of cystic fibrosis: correction of the underlying CFTR defect. Lancet Respir Med. 2013;1(2):158–63.
29. Wilschanski M, Zielenski J, Markiewicz D, Tsui LC, Corey M, Levison H, et al. Correlation of sweat chloride concentration with classes of the cystic fibrosis transmembrane conductance regulator gene mutations. J Pediatr. 1995;127(5):705–10.
30. Boucher RC. Bronchiectasis: a continuum of ion transport dysfunction or multiple hits? Am J Respir Crit Care Med. 2010;181(10):1017–9.
31. Narayan D, Krishnan SN, Upender M, Ravikumar TS, Mahoney MJ, Dolan TF Jr, et al. Unusual inheritance of primary ciliary dyskinesia (Kartagener's syndrome). J Med Genet. 1994;31(6):493–6.
32. Hirokawa N, Tanaka Y, Okada Y, Takeda S. Nodal flow and the generation of left-right asymmetry. Cell. 2006;125(1):33–45.
33. Knowles MR, Daniels LA, Davis SD, Zariwala MA, Leigh MW. Primary ciliary dyskinesia. Recent advances in diagnostics, genetics, and characterization of clinical disease. Am J Respir Crit Care Med. 2013;188(8):913–22.
34. Knowles MR, Ostrowski LE, Leigh MW, Sears PR, Davis SD, Wolf WE, et al. Mutations in RSPH1 cause primary ciliary dyskinesia with a unique clinical and ciliary phenotype. Am J Respir Crit Care Med. 2014;189(6):707–17.
35. Sugiyama Y. Diffuse panbronchiolitis. Clin Chest Med. 1993;14(4):765–72.
36. Park MH, Kim YW, Yoon HI, Yoo CG, Han SK, Shim YS, et al. Association of HLA class I antigens with diffuse panbronchiolitis in Korean patients. Am J Respir Crit Care Med. 1999;159(2):526–9.
37. Keicho N, Ohashi J, Tamiya G, Nakata K, Taguchi Y, Azuma A, et al. Fine localization of a major disease-susceptibility locus for diffuse panbronchiolitis. Am J Hum Genet. 2000;66(2):501–7.
38. Rose MC, Voynow JA. Respiratory tract mucin genes and mucin glycoproteins in health and disease. Physiol Rev. 2006;86(1):245–78.
39. Hijikata M, Matsushita I, Tanaka G, Tsuchiya T, Ito H, Tokunaga K, et al. Molecular cloning of two novel mucin-like genes in the disease-susceptibility locus for diffuse panbronchiolitis. Hum Genet. 2011;129(2):117–28.
40. Voynow JA, Gendler SJ, Rose MC. Regulation of mucin genes in chronic inflammatory airway diseases. Am J Respir Cell Mol Biol. 2006;34(6):661–5.
41. Mishina K, Shinkai M, Shimokawaji T, Nagashima A, Hashimoto Y, Inoue Y, et al. HO-1 inhibits IL-13-induced goblet cell hyperplasia associated with CLCA1 suppression in normal human bronchial epithelial cells. Int Immunopharmacol. 2015;29(2):448–53.
42. Poletti V, Casoni G, Chilosi M, Zompatori M. Diffuse panbronchiolitis. Eur Respir J. 2006;28(4):862–71.

Chapter 7
Pulmonary Fibrosis: Hereditary and Non-hereditary—What Are the Role of Genetic Factors in the Pathogenesis of Pulmonary Fibrosis?

Takafumi Suda

Abstract Pulmonary fibrosis is a diverse group of disorders with various etiologies and characterized by varying patterns of lung inflammation and fibrosis. To date, familial aggregation has been noted even in idiopathic pulmonary fibrosis (IPF), suggesting genetic background of pulmonary fibrosis. Over the past decade, remarkable progress has been made in understanding the genetic causes of pulmonary fibrosis. For instance, investigations of familial interstitial pneumonia (FIP) have identified rare genetic variants in genes related to surfactant and telomere biology. Large genome-wide association and linkage studies have also uncovered common genetic variants that confer the risk of pulmonary fibrosis, including genes associated with mucus secretion, telomerase function, and immunity. Further, functional studies of these rare as well as common genetic variants have provided novel insights into pathophysiology of pulmonary fibrosis. More importantly, genetic factors also determine response to treatment and outcome in patients with pulmonary fibrosis. Moving forward, next-generation and high-throughput sequencing will probably identify additional causative genes and pathways. Ultimately, combined analysis of genetic and environmental factors, including epigenetic modifications, will further improve our understanding of this disease, possibly leading to the development of novel, more effective therapies.

Keywords Pulmonary fibrosis · Familial interstitial pneumonia · Surfactant Telomerase · Mucin

---

T. Suda
Second Division, Department of Internal Medicine, Hamamatsu University School of Medicine, Shizuoka, Japan
e-mail: suda@hama-med.ac.jp

T. Kaneko (ed.), *Clinical Relevance of Genetic Factors in Pulmonary Diseases*, Respiratory Disease Series: Diagnostic Tools and Disease Managements, https://doi.org/10.1007/978-981-10-8144-6_7

7.1 Introduction

Pulmonary fibrosis is a diverse group of disorders with various etiologies and characterized by varying patterns of lung inflammation and fibrosis. For example, idiopathic pulmonary fibrosis (IPF), the most common form in the practice, is a chronic, progressive, and fatal disease of unknown cause that generally affects adults over 50 years old [1]. Nevertheless, forms of pulmonary fibrosis share common clinical, radiological, and physiological features regardless of etiology and are thought to develop from an interplay of genetic, epigenetic, and environmental factors. For instance, several defined genetic disorders such as dyskeratosis congenita and Hermansky-Pudlak syndrome are associated with inherited pulmonary fibrosis, and not a few IPF patients have been shown to have familiar clustering [2–5], suggesting a genetic component. Indeed, recent advances in genomic technologies, including whole-exosome sequencing, have uncovered a number of such genetic factors, greatly advancing our understanding of underlying molecular mechanisms. In a first breakthrough, Nogee and colleagues described in 2001 a heterozygous mutation in surfactant protein C (*SFTPC*) in a young mother and her infant with idiopathic interstitial pneumonia (IIP) [6]. Other *SFTPC* mutations were identified shortly thereafter [7–12]. Additional genetic mutations that confer risk of pulmonary fibrosis have now been discovered, including in *SFTA2* (surfactant protein A2) [13], *ABCA3* (ATP-binding cassette member A3) [14, 15], *TERC* (telomerase RNA component) [16, 17], *TERT* (telomerase reverse transcriptase) [16, 17], *RTEL1* (regulator of telomere elongation helicase 1) [18, 19], and *PARN* (poly(A)-specific ribonuclease) [18]. Interestingly, some of these mutations are present in a small population of patients with sporadic pulmonary fibrosis, suggesting a common set of pathogenic processes among all forms of pulmonary fibrosis. In addition, large-scale genome-wide association studies recently identified a number of common genetic variants in *MUC5B* and *TOLLIP* (*Toll-interacting protein*) as potentially causative [20, 21]. To date, mutations in more than seven genes, as well as variants in more than ten loci, are associated with pulmonary fibrosis (Table 7.1). In this chapter, current evidence on genetic factors that confer risk of pulmonary fibrosis are reviewed, and potential implications of recent genetic discoveries are described.

7.2 Defined Rare Genetic Diseases

Pulmonary fibrosis often develops in defined genetic disorders such as dyskeratosis congenita [16], Hermansky-Pudlak syndrome [22], Niemann-Pick's disease [23], and Gaucher's disease [24]. Of these, Hermansky-Pudlak syndrome is the most well-known and is characterized by oculocutaneous albinism, bleeding tendency due to platelet defects, and accumulation of ceroid lipofuscin, an abnormal fat-protein compound, in lysosomes [25]. The syndrome is autosomal recessive and

Table 7.1 Genetic variants linked to pulmonary fibrosis

Gene function	Gene	Chromosome	Variation	Risk of pulmonary fibrosis	Reference
Surfactant	*SFTPC*	8p21	c.460+1G>A	Yes (FIP)	[6]
			+128T>A	Yes (FIP)	[10]
			+1286T>C	Yes (Infant NSIP)	[9]
				Yes (Child ILD)	[8]
			+6108T>C	Yes* (UIP)	[11]
			c.211A>G c.435+2T>C	Yes (FIP)	[12]
	SFTPA2	10q22	c.692G>T g.593T>C	Yes (FIP)	[13]
	ABCA3	16p13	C1-28A>G IVS9+11C>T C3765C>G	Yes (UIP)	[60]
			c.875A>T, e.g.	Yes (CPFE)	[15, 61]
Telomerase	*TERT*	5p15	CTG>CAG IVS+1G>A Codon112 delC IVS9-2A>C	Yes (FIP)	[16]
			c.3346_3522del c.2594G>A c.2240delT c.1456C>T c.97C>T c.430G>A c.2593C>T	Yes (IPF)	[17]
			g.12799426G>A, e.g.	Yes (IPF)	[63]
			rs2736100	Yes (IPF)	[20, 69]
	TERC	3p26	98G>A	Yes (FIP)	[16]
			r.37a>g	Yes (IPF)	[17]
			rs6793295	Yes (IPF)	[20]
	RTEL1	20q13	c.146C>T, e.g.	Yes (FIP)	[18, 72]
			g.6232456C>T, e.g.	Yes (IPF)	[63]
	PARN	16q13	IVS4-2a>g, e.g.	Yes (FIP)	[18]
			g.14698077G>A, e.g.	Yes (IPF)	[63]
	DKC1	Xq28	+1213A>G, e.g.	Yes (FIP)	[45, 46]
Mucus secretion	*MUC5B*	11p15	rs35705950	Yes (IPF)	[74, 76–81]

(continued)

Table 7.1 (continued)

Gene function	Gene	Chromosome	Variation	Risk of pulmonary fibrosis	Reference
Innate immunity	*TLR3*	4q35	rs3775291	Disease progression (IPF)	[92]
	ELMOD	4q31	Unknown	Yes (FIP)	[97]
	TOLLIP	11p15	rs11521887	Yes (IPF)	[21]
			rs5743894	Yes (IPF)	
			rs5743890	Yes (IPF) protective	
Inflammation and cytokine	*IL1RN*	2q14	+2018C>T	Yes (FA)	[100]
			rs408392 rs419598	Yes (IPF)	[104]
			rs2637988	Yes (IPF)	[103]
	TNFA	6p21.	-308G>A	Yes (FA)	[100]
	IL4	5q31	-590C>T -33C>T	Yes (IPF)	[106]
	TGFB1	19q13	rs1800470	Disease progression (IPF) Yes (IPF)	[107, 108] [108]
	IL8	4q13	rs4073	Yes (IPF)	[112]
	CR1	1q32	+5507C>G	Yes (IPF)	[116]
	FcγR IIIb	1q23	rs1801274	Yes (IPF)	[119]
Extracellular matrix	*MMP1*	11q22	-1607I/D	Yes (FIP)	[124]
			-1562C>T	Yes (CPFE)	[125]
HLA	*MHC*	6p21	HLA-DRB1*1501	Yes (IPF)	[129]
			HLA-B*15-DRB*0101-DQB1*0501 HLA-B*52-DRB*1402-DQB1*0301 HLA-B*35-DRB1*0407-DQB1*0302	Yes (IPF)	[128]

FIP familial interstitial pneumonia, *ILD* interstitial lung disease, *NSIP* nonspecific interstitial pneumonia, *UIP* usual interstitial pneumonia, *CPFE* combined pulmonary fibrosis and emphysema, *FA* fibrosing alveolitis

associated with highly penetrant pulmonary fibrosis in young adults. So far, ten genetically distinct subtypes have been identified, including type 1 (due to mutations in *HPS1*), type 2 (*AP3B1*), type 3 (*HPS3*), type 4 (*HPS4*), type 5 (*HPS5*), type 6 (*HPS6*), type 7 (*DTNBP1*), type 8 (*BLOC1S3*), type 9 (*BLOC1S6*), and type 10 (*AP3D1*) [26–29]. Most of these gene products assemble into distinct protein complexes called biogenesis of lysosome-related organelle complexes (BLOCs), which cooperate to form and/or traffic lysosome-related endosomal compartments [30].

Although the precise mechanisms by which defects in these complexes cause pulmonary fibrosis are unknown, patients with pulmonary fibrosis due to Hermansky-Pudlak syndrome have increased production of cytokines and chemokines in alveolar macrophages [31], elevated expression of galectin-3 in fibroblasts [32], and increased number of circulating fibrocytes that express C-X-C chemokine receptor type 4 (CXCR-4) [33]. In addition, pulmonary fibrosis due to Hermansky-Pudlak syndrome, especially subtypes 1, 2, and 4, has similar clinical, radiological, and histologic features to IPF but manifests at a younger age. While prognosis is variable, most patients follow a progressive course. There are no established specific therapies. Indeed, although pirfenidone was initially reported to be effective [34], efficacy was not corroborated in a second controlled trial [35]. Figures 7.1 and 7.2 show a patient with a homozygous IVS5+5 G>A mutation in *HPS1*.

On the other hand, dyskeratosis congenita is characterized by a classic triad of dysplastic nails, reticulated skin hyperpigmentation, and oral leukoplakia [16]. Pulmonary fibrosis occurs in up to 20% of patients and is the second leading cause of death [36]. Patients also have abnormally short telomeres for their age, and the disease has been thought to be a form of telomerase disorders. Recent studies show that the most common genetic causes are mutations in *DKC1* (20–25%) [37, 38] and *TINF2* (12–20%) [39, 40]. *DKC1* encodes dyskeratin, a component of the telomerase complex, while *TINF2* encodes TIN2, a critical subunit of the shelterin complex that protects telomeres. Accordingly, mutations in these two genes result in telomerase defects and shortened telomeres. Rare genetic variants in *TERT* and *TERC* also account for a small fraction of dyskeratosis congenita patients [38, 41, 42]. Of note, *DKC1* mutations are X-linked, while *TERT* and *TERC* mutations are autosomal dominant.

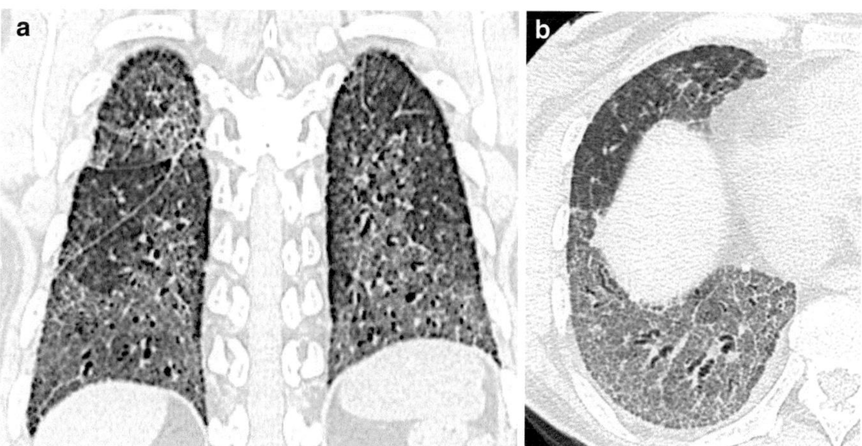

Fig. 7.1 A 58-year-old woman with Hermansky-Pudlak syndrome (IVS5+5, homozygous). (**a**) Coronal reformation of a CT scan shows extensive bilateral ground-glass opacities. (**b**) High-resolution CT scan shows diffuse ground-glass opacities with superimposed reticular opacities. Traction bronchiectasis is also present

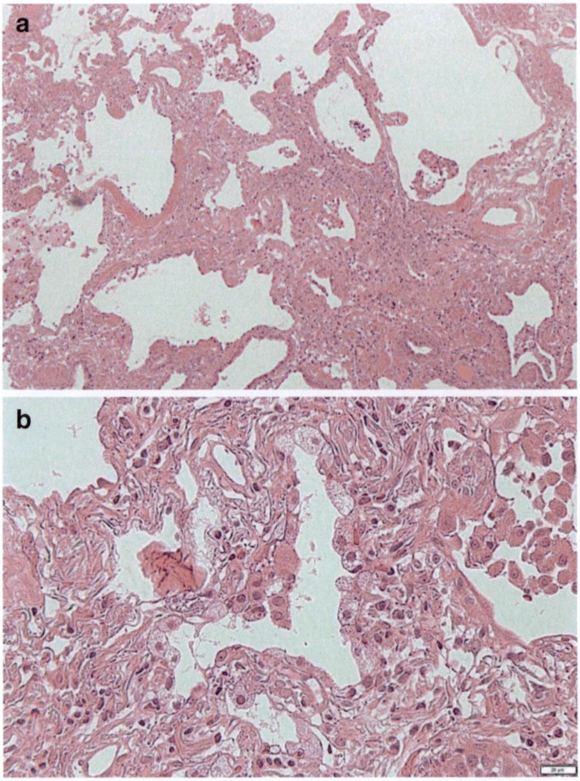

Fig. 7.2 A 58-year-old woman with Hermansky-Pudlak syndrome (IVS5+5, homozygous). (**a**) Surgical lung biopsies show diffuse interstitial collagen deposits with mild mononuclear cell infiltration. The lung lesion is temporally uniform, consistent with nonspecific interstitial pneumonia (hematoxylin and eosin staining, ×25). (**b**) Foamy brown-pigmented macrophages are focally aggregated in the alveolar air space. Foamy type 2 alveolar epithelial cells are also present (hematoxylin and eosin staining, ×400)

7.3 Familial Interstitial Pneumonia (FIP)

While IIPs are essentially sporadic, familial forms have also been observed and are recognized as FIP [2–5]. Indeed, FIP was initially thought to be a rare subset of IIP [2, 3] but has since been demonstrated to account for as much as 20% of IIP cases [5, 43]. FIP is typically diagnosed when a proband with IIPs has at least one other first-degree relative with IIPs, and/or carries a known genetic variant associated with FIP [44]. Importantly, FIP is clinically, radiologically, and histologically indistinguishable from IIPs, except for younger age of onset. As noted, rare genetic variants in three genes linked to surfactant function (*SFTPC*, *SFTPA2*, and *ABCA3*) have been associated with FIP, along with four genes linked to telomere maintenance (*TERT*, *TERC*, *RTEL1*, and *PARN*). In addition, a novel mutation in *DKC1* was found in two IPF patients without features of dyskeratosis congenita, suggesting that *DKC1* may also be associated with FIP [45, 46]. In any case, pathogenic variants in *TERT* and *TERC* account for most cases of FIP, while an *SFTC* mutation accounts for 1–25% (Table 7.2). Although FIP inheritance is not yet fully defined, complex inheritance, e.g., multifactorial and autosomal dominant inheritance with reduced penetrance, is likely. Nevertheless, autosomal recessive inheritance has not

Table 7.2 Proportion of familial interstitial pneumonia (FIP) attributed to mutations in various genes

Gene	Reported % of FIP	Reference
TERT	8–15	[16, 17]
TERC	<1	[16, 17]
DKC1	<1	[45, 46]
SFTPC	2–25	[6, 10, 12, 130]
SFTPA2	<1	[13]
ABCA3	<1	[14, 15]
Unknown	75–85	

been definitively ruled out. Notably, histologic features of interstitial pneumonias, including usual interstitial pneumonia (UIP) and nonspecific interstitial pneumonia (NSIP), differ among families with the same genetic mutation [47]. In addition, symptoms in individuals with the same mutation may range from absent to respiratory failure requiring lung transplantation [48]. Taken together, these observations suggest that additional environmental or genetic factors contribute to phenotypic heterogeneity. For example, smoking is an independent risk factor for pulmonary fibrosis among individuals with pathogenic gene variants [47].

7.4 Genes Linked to Surfactant Biology

Surfactant proteins are secreted by alveolar type II cells to maintain alveolar structure and function. Thus, defects in surfactant biology may compromise lung homeostasis. Accordingly, genes encoding surfactant proteins have been investigated extensively as potentially causative of pulmonary fibrosis.

7.4.1 SFTPC

In a mother with desquamative interstitial pneumonia (DIP) and an affected daughter with NSIP, Nogee and colleagues identified a heterozygous c.460+1 G/A mutation in *SP-C* that results in skipping of exon 4 and deletion of 37 amino acids from the C-terminal domain of the immature prosurfactant protein C (proSP-C) [6]. As a result, the mature protein was absent from the lung of these patients. Subsequently, Thomas et al. identified, in a large kindred of 11 individuals with IPF and three individuals with biopsy-proven NSIP, a heterozygous missense +128T>A mutation in exon 5 of *SFTPC*, which mutates leucine to glutamine at position 188 [10]. Brash and colleagues also found in an infant with NSIP a heterozygous missense g.1286T>C mutation in the same gene, resulting in a substitution of threonine for isoleucine at position 73 [9]. To date, more than 40 pathogenic mutations in *SFTPC* have been discovered in humans [7–12]. Figures 7.3 and 7.4 show a patient with a c.365A>G and Y122C *SFTC* mutation.

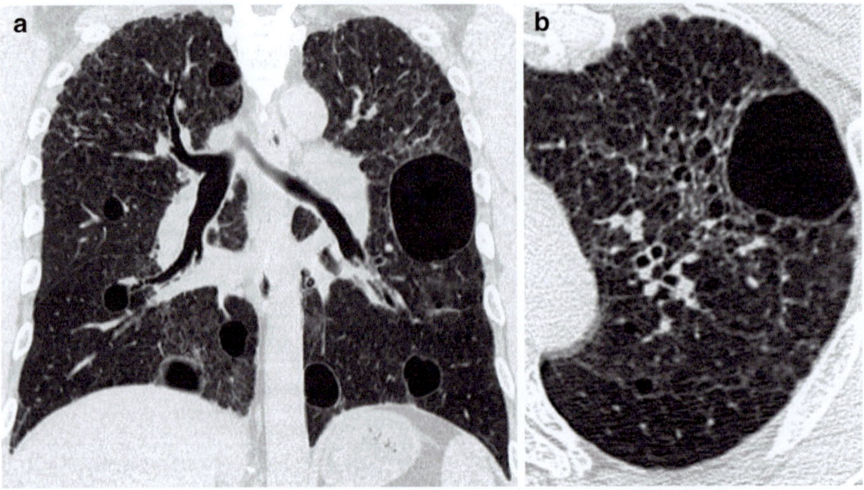

Fig. 7.3 A 45-year-old man with an *SFTC* mutation (c.365 A>G, Y122C). (**a**) Coronal reformation of a CT scan shows multiple cystic lesions of variable size. Reticular opacities are predominantly present in the upper lung. Focal ground-glass opacities are also seen. (**b**) High-resolution CT scan shows a large cyst surrounded by reticular opacities

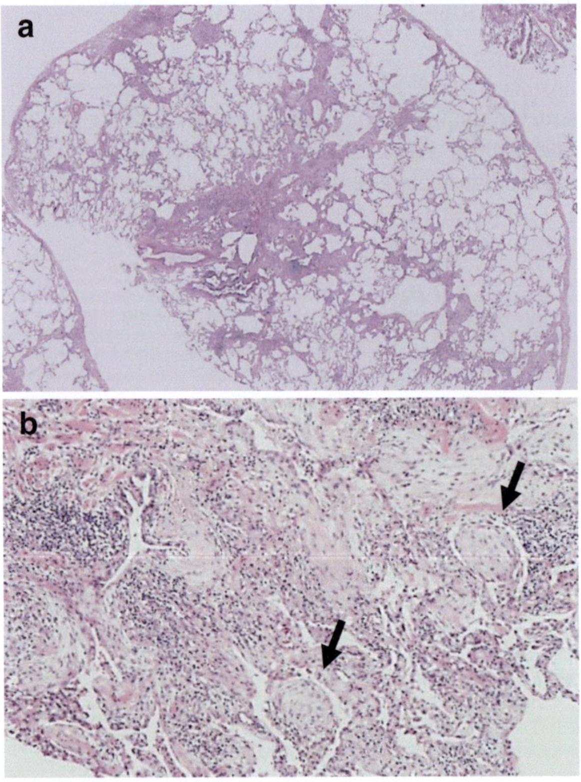

Fig. 7.4 A 45-year-old man with an *SFTC* mutation (c.365 A>G, Y122C). Surgical lung biopsies show patchy fibrosis with microscopic honeycombing (**a**, hematoxylin and eosin staining, ×12.5). Although fibroblastic foci are occasionally found (**b**, arrows, hematoxylin and eosin staining, ×400), histologic features are consistent with unclassifiable interstitial pneumonia because of centrilobular predominance and focal organizing pneumonia

In type II alveolar epithelial cells, immature proSP-C undergoes several proteolytic cleavages to form mature SP-C, which is then secreted to the alveolar space. In contrast, mutated SP-C accumulates in the endoplasmic reticulum (ER), induces ER stress, and activates the unfolded protein response (UPR) [49–51]. For example, the c.460+1G/A mutation impedes trafficking of proSP-C and causes it to misfold, aggregate [52, 53], and trigger ER stress. Subsequently, ER stress may induce apoptosis and epithelial-mesenchymal transition [54, 55], both of which accelerate the development of pulmonary fibrosis. Interestingly, only one *SFTPC* mutation was found in a cohort of 135 individuals with sporadic IIPs, indicating that such mutations are rare in IIPs [11]. Nevertheless, ER stress and unfolded protein response are observed in the lung of patients with noninherited sporadic IIPs, suggesting that both are common pathways in pulmonary fibrosis, regardless of genetic background [51, 56].

7.4.2 *SFTPA2*

After *SPFTC* mutations were discovered, other surfactant proteins (SP-A, -B, and -D) were extensively surveyed for similarly pathogenic mutations. In 2009, Wang and colleagues reported for the first time missense mutations in *SP-A* in two families with FIP [13]. In particular, linkage analysis of one of these families identified a susceptibility locus in chromosome 10q22, which was subsequently found to contain a substitution of valine for a highly conserved glycine at codon 231 in *SFTPA2*. A mutation in codon 198, which substitutes serine for phenylalanine, was also identified in the other FIP family. Like *SFTPC* mutations, these mutations are likely to impair protein trafficking, cause misfolding and accumulation of immature SP-A, and thereby elicit ER stress [13, 57].

7.4.3 *ABCA3*

ATP-binding cassette (ABC) transporters are transmembrane proteins that transport a wide variety of substrates across biological membranes. ABCA3, a subclass A transporter, is abundantly expressed in type II alveolar epithelial cells and maintains cellular homeostasis through biosynthesis, assembly, intracellular trafficking, and metabolism of resident proteins, organelles, and surfactants. In 2004, *ABCA3* mutations were associated for the first time with severe, fatal respiratory distress in early infancy in a group of racially and ethnically diverse full-term infants [58]. These mutations consisted of homozygous missense, nonsense, and frameshift mutations, as well as heterozygous insertion and splice-site mutations, and caused the formation of abnormal lamellar bodies in type II alveolar epithelial cells [59]. To date, more than 150 distinct *ABCA3* mutations have been identified, of which those that cause lung disease are inherited in autosomal recessive fashion. Mutations in

ABCA3 have also been identified in older patients with pulmonary fibrosis, such as in a 15-year-old boy with biopsy-proven UIP [60], in young and adult members of a large kindred [14], and in patients with combined pulmonary fibrosis and emphysema (CPFE) [15, 61]. Intriguingly, patients heterozygous for both an *ABCA3* mutation and the *SFTPC* I73T mutation develop more severe fibrosis than family members with only the I73T mutation, suggesting that *ABCA3* may affect the course of pulmonary fibrosis with *SFTPC* mutations [62].

7.5 Telomere-Associated Genes

Telomeres are repeated DNA segments with sequence 5′-TTAGGG-3′ and that protect chromosome ends from end-to-end fusions. However, telomeres shorten with each cycle of cell division, so that chromosomes become unstable and fuse with age, resulting in cell apoptosis. To maintain integrity and impede progressive shortening, telomeres are replenished by the telomerase complex, the two major components of which are telomerase reverse transcriptase (TERT) and telomerase RNA component (TERC). TERC is a noncoding RNA that serves as template for telomere replication by TERT, the catalytic subunit. In humans, the telomerase complex is expressed exclusively in germ cells, stem cells, and certain cancer cells. Accumulating evidence now imply that abnormal telomere biology, including shortened telomeres and mutations in the telomerase complex, may lead to pulmonary fibrosis. For example, pulmonary fibrosis in dyskeratosis congenita is, as noted earlier, attributable to mutations in dyskerin, especially *DKC1* [16], which is also a component of the telomerase complex. Notably, rare variants of telomere-related genes previously implicated in FIP were also identified in more than 10% of patients with sporadic pulmonary fibrosis [63]. More recently, 12 (11.9%) of 101 patients with interstitial lung disease secondary to rheumatoid arthritis were found to carry heterozygous mutations in coding regions in *TERT*, *RTEL1*, *PARN*, or *SFTPC* [64].

7.5.1 TERT and TERC

Armanios and colleagues reported a pedigree with autosomal dominant dyskeratosis congenita and a null *TERT* allele, in which pulmonary fibrosis was transmitted without the mucocutaneous features typical of dyskeratosis congenita [41]. A subsequent screen in 2007 of 73 probands from the Vanderbilt Familial Pulmonary Fibrosis Registry revealed that five families carried mutations in *TERT* and one family carried a mutation in *TERC* [16], all of which were shown to decrease telomerase activity. Five of these six families had none of the classic hallmarks of dyskeratosis congenita, although the mutated telomerases led to short telomeres in peripheral blood lymphocytes even in asymptomatic subjects. Shortly thereafter, Tsakiri and colleagues identified, by linkage analysis of chromosome 5 in two families, seven mutations in *TERT* and one mutation in *TERC* [17] that also markedly decreased telomerase activity and, even in the heterozygous state, shortened telomeres in peripheral blood lymphocytes. Collectively, these observations provide strong evidence that telomerase defects confer susceptibility to adult-onset pulmonary fibrosis.

Remarkably, shortened telomeres are not limited to patients with pulmonary fibrosis who have mutated telomerase. For instance, Alder and colleagues found that, as in carriers of telomerase mutations, telomeres in peripheral blood leukocytes and alveolar cells are shortened in 84 patients with IPF and 16 patients with IIPs other than IPF [65]. Similarly, short telomeres (<10th percentile) in circulating leukocytes were found in 37% of cases of sporadic pulmonary fibrosis in the absence of telomerase mutations [66]. More importantly, shortened telomeres were shown to be independently associated with worse survival in IPF [67, 68]. Taken together, these studies suggest that short telomeres are an important predictor not only of susceptibility to sporadic pulmonary fibrosis but also its prognosis.

In 2008, 159 Japanese patients with IPF and 934 controls were surveyed for single nucleotide polymorphisms (SNPs) to find a susceptibility gene [69]. A significant association was noted between IPF and the rs2736100 variant in intron 2 of *TERT*. A later, much larger study of 1616 non-Hispanic whites with IPF and 4683 controls demonstrated genetic associations between IPF and *TERC* at 3q26 and *TERT* at 5p15 [20]. Another survey of 10,379 individuals confirmed that the *TERT* locus is associated with susceptibility to pulmonary fibrosis [70]. These findings suggest that a common genetic variation in TERT and/or TERC may contribute to the risk of sporadic pulmonary fibrosis.

7.5.2 *RTEL1*

RTEL1 is an essential iron-sulfur DNA helicase crucial for telomere maintenance and DNA repair. Germline mutations in this gene were observed along with short telomeres in patients with Hoyeraal-Hreidarsson syndrome [71], a clinically severe variant of dyskeratosis congenita characterized by cerebellar hypoplasia, severe immunodeficiency, enteropathy, and intrauterine growth retardation. Interestingly, whole-exome sequencing of 78 patients with FIP and 2816 controls identified five heterozygous loss-of-function variants in *RTEL1*, and noted shortened leukocyte telomeres, but not mucocutaneous features of DC [18]. Kannengiesser and colleagues also sequenced the exome in 35 families with FIP but without *TERT* or *TERC* mutations and found heterozygous mutations in *RTEL1* in four families; carriers of which presented shorter telomeres against age-matched controls [72].

7.5.3 *PARN*

PARN is an exoribonuclease that regulates the stability of a large number of mRNA transcripts, and governs several key cellular processes, including cell growth, differentiation, and DNA damage response. In 2015, Stuart identified by whole-exome sequencing heterozygous loss-of-function *PARN* mutations in six unrelated families with pulmonary fibrosis [18]. These mutations were eventually demonstrated to cause defective telomere maintenance [73]. Heterozygous *PARN* mutations were also identified in five of 262 cases of sporadic IPF [63].

7.6 Mucus-Associated Genes

7.6.1 *MUC5B*

In 2001, linkage analysis by genome-wide positional cloning in 82 patients with FIP, 492 patients with IPF, and 322 controls revealed an association between pulmonary fibrosis and a 3.4 Mb region in chromosome 11q15 [74]. Consequently, fine mapping of SNPs in the cluster of mucin genes in chromosome 11 identified rs35705950, a common variant in the putative promoter of mucin 5B (*MUC5B*), to be strongly associated with pulmonary fibrosis. This minor allele was present in 34% of FIP cases and 38% of sporadic IPF cases but only in 9% of controls. However, like common polymorphisms associated with other rare diseases, rs35705950 only has a small predictive value for the future development of IPF in the general population. Nevertheless, rs35705950 is thought to be exclusively associated with FIP and IPF, but not other interstitial lung diseases, because it does not increase the risk of sarcoidosis or scleroderma-associated interstitial lung disease [75–77]. This association has been confirmed in independent cohorts in the USA, Europe, and Mexico [76, 78, 79]. In Asia, however, the association does not appear to be as definitive. For example, the T allele of rs35705950 is significantly more frequent in Chinese patients than in controls but is still considerably less frequent (3.33%) than in Caucasians with IPF [80]. Similarly, rs35705950 was rare even in Korean patients with IPF and was not associated with pulmonary fibrosis [79]. In Japan, Horimasu and colleagues found that rs35705950 was significantly associated with IPF but at a much lower frequency than in Germany [81]. Indeed, the rs35705950 allele frequencies in patients with IPF, NSIP, and unaffected controls were 3.4%, 1.7%, and 0.8% in Japan but 33.1%, 27.4%, and 4.3%, respectively, among Germans. Collectively, these observations suggest that, although polymorphisms in the *MUC5B* promoter may be significantly associated with IPF, its impact varies widely with race or ethnicity.

Recently, interstitial lung abnormality (ILA) was proposed as a term to encompass specific patterns of increased lung densities observable on computed tomography but that are seemingly without clinical significance. These include focal, unilateral, or patchy ground-glass opacity and focal or unilateral reticulation [82]. Hunninghake and colleagues first demonstrated in 2013 an association between rs35705950 and ILA in the general population, based on data from the Framingham Heart Study [83]. In particular, ILA increased in prevalence with an allele copy dependence of rs35705950, especially among older individuals. Subsequently, Araki et al. found, in 1847 participants in the same cohort, that increased copies of rs35705950 were independently associated with long-term progression of ILA [84].

Taken together, these observations suggest that polymorphisms in the *MUC5B* promoter may confer risk of ILA and its progression in individuals with clinically unrecognized interstitial lung disease.

MUC5B is a member of a family of mucins, which are conserved, structurally related glycoproteins, and are the principal macromolecules in airway mucus [85]. How rs35705950 contributes to the development of pulmonary fibrosis is poorly understood. Of note, rs35705950 is a gain-of-function variant in the *MUC5B* promoter that boosts MUC5B production >30-fold even in unaffected carriers [74] and in the distal airways of the IPF lung [86]. Strikingly, excessive MUC5B expression is observed in metaplastic epithelia lining honeycomb cysts, as well as in terminal airway epithelia [74], in patients with IPF. Ectopic MUC5B expression was also reported in atypically differentiated cells in the bronchiolized distal airspaces of the IPF lung [87]. Taken together, the data suggest that MUC5B overexpression in the distal airway space is likely to be involved in pulmonary fibrosis. Indeed, excessive MUC5B production is hypothesized to reduce mucociliary clearance in the distal airway, cause retention of inhaled particles, and thereby enhance epithelial injury and probably impair epithelial repair in the alveoli. Thus, elucidating the precise mechanistic role of MUC5B in IPF may greatly advance our understanding of the pathogenesis of pulmonary fibrosis and identify novel therapeutic targets.

The *MUC5B* promoter variant also has prognostic value. Peljto and colleagues unexpectedly found, in two large independent cohorts, that rs35705950 is significantly associated with better survival, independent of age, sex, pulmonary function, and treatment [88]. One possibility for the increased susceptibility but also increased survival is that IPF phenotypes are heterogeneous and that other genetic and/or environmental factors modify IPF phenotypes. Nevertheless, why mucus hypersecretion in the distal airway promotes survival in IPF is still unclear, and further investigation is required.

7.7 Genes Associated with Innate Immunity

Recent studies imply that the innate immune system plays a pivotal role in pulmonary fibrosis. For example, activation of Toll-like receptors (TLRs) 2 and 9 promote lung fibrogenesis [89–91], while TLRs 3 and 4 inhibit fibrosis [92, 93]. In addition, type 2 innate lymphoid cells accumulate in the IPF lung and are actively involved in fibrosis [94]. Several variants of genes linked to innate immunity have also been associated with pulmonary fibrosis [21, 92, 95].

7.7.1 TLR3

O'Dwyer and colleagues hypothesized that defective TLR3 signaling may contribute to IPF [92] and investigated the role of rs3775291, a loss-of-function L412F variant in the TLR3 promoter, which was recently shown to be ineffective at activating NFκB and IRF3 [96]. In two separate IPF cohorts, the L412F polymorphism was associated with rapid progression and higher mortality. In addition, the activity TLR3 ligands that significantly inhibit proliferation in lung fibroblasts from wild-type IPF patients was markedly attenuated in cells from L412F heterozygous and homozygous IPF patients, possibly because of reduced production of type 1 interferon. This study suggests that the L412F polymorphism in TLR3 is a potential marker of rapidly progressive IPF and that rescue of defective TLR3 signaling may be therapeutic.

7.7.2 *ELMOD2*

Genome-wide association studies of six multiplex Finnish FIP families identified *ELMOD2*, a protein with engulfment and motility (ELMO) motifs, as a candidate susceptibility gene for IPF [97]. Indeed, one-third of affected family members shared a haplotype encompassing *ELMOD2* and spanning 110 kb to 13 Mb on chromosome 4q31.1. In contrast, this haplotype was present in only 7.7% of controls. ELMOD2 is expressed in alveolar macrophages and epithelium but is severely diminished in the IPF lung. Interestingly, Pulkkinen et al. demonstrated that ELMOD2 is involved in TLR3-mediated antiviral response through type I and II interferon [95], suggesting that an ELMOD2-TLR3 axis against viral infection is associated with individual susceptibility to pulmonary fibrosis.

7.7.3 *TOLLIP*

A recent three-stage genome-wide study by Noth and colleagues identified an association between IPF susceptibility and three SNPs in *TOLLIP* (rs111521887, rs5743894, and rs5743890) that lower TOLLIP expression to varying degrees in lung tissues [21]. Of these, the novel variant rs5743890 lowers the risk of IPF but also increases mortality. As TOLLIP is an inhibitory adaptor protein that suppresses TLR-mediated signaling and innate immunity, immune dysregulation due to SNPs may contribute to IPF susceptibility as well as disease course. Importantly, SNPs in *TOLLIP* may also determine the response to *N*-acetylcysteine therapy, which was reported by Oldham and collaborators to be beneficial to IPF patients with an rs3750920 TT genotype but harmful to those with a CC genotype [98].

7.8 Genes Associated with Pro- or Anti-inflammatory Cytokines and Chemokines

7.8.1 IL-1/IL-1 Receptor Antagonist and TNF-α

IL-1 and TNF-α are potent proinflammatory cytokines that mediate fibrotic processes and are abundantly secreted by alveolar macrophages in the lung [99]. Whyte and colleagues found that the *TNF-α* allele -308G>A is associated with susceptibility to fibrosing alveolitis, as is the +2018C>T allele of *IL-1 receptor antagonist (IL-1RN)*, a naturally occurring inhibitor that suppresses the proinflammatory properties of IL-1 [100]. However, these associations were not observed in other studies [101, 102], although Barlo et al. also demonstrated that the rs2637988 SNP in *IL1RN* confers risk of IPF [103]. Similarly, meta-analysis of five case-control studies of Caucasians [104] established conclusively that polymorphisms in the variable number tandem repeat in *IL1RN* (rs408392 and rs419598) increase susceptibility to IPF [104], suggesting that its reduced expression due to these polymorphisms predisposes individuals to fibrogenesis.

7.8.2 IL-4

Pulmonary fibrosis is characterized by bias toward Th2 cytokines such as IL-4 and IL-13 [105]. Although the latter is the central player in pulmonary fibrosis, the former induces and maintains the observed shift to Th2. Vasakova et al. reported that two polymorphisms in the IL-4 promoter (-590C>T and -33C>T) are more common in IPF patients than in healthy controls [106].

7.8.3 TGF-β

TGF-β is a key cytokine that promotes pulmonary fibrosis via multiple mechanisms, including enhanced proliferation and differentiation of fibroblasts, collagen production, and mesenchymal-epithelial transition. Xaubet and colleagues demonstrated that *TGF-β1* polymorphisms in codons 10 and 25 (+869 T>C and +915 G>C) do not confer risk of IPF but affect disease progression in Spanish patients [107]. Recently, the *TGF-β1* polymorphism T869C was shown in Koreans to be associated with IPF susceptibility and disease severity [108].

7.8.4 IL-8

IL-8 is a C-X-C chemokine with potent angiogenic properties as well as chemotactic activity for neutrophils. In IPF patients, an increase in IL-8 protein in bronchoalveolar lavage fluid (BALF) and mRNA expression in alveolar macrophages has been demonstrated [109–111]. In a survey of Koreans, Ahn and colleagues detected an association between IPF risk and a promoter SNP (rs4073T>A) in a common *IL-8* allele, possibly via increased IL-8 production [112].

7.8.5 IL-10

IL-10, an anti-inflammatory cytokine with potent immunosuppressive activity, effectively resolves inflammation, although its role in pulmonary fibrosis is controversial. *IL-10* gene delivery was shown to attenuate bleomycin-induced pulmonary fibrosis by inhibiting TGF-β [113], but overexpression also induced pulmonary fibrosis by recruitment of fibrocytes and activation of M2 macrophages [114]. Whittington and colleagues identified a novel *IL-10* polymorphism (+43G>A) associated with reduced expression in IPF patients [115].

7.9 Other Inflammation-Associated Genes

7.9.1 CR-1

Complement receptor 1 (CR1), also known as C3b/C4b or CD35, is a type 1 transmembrane glycoprotein that mediates transport of immune complexes. Zorzetto and coworkers detected an association between the *CR1* polymorphism +5507C>G and IPF susceptibility in white Italians [116]. However, subsequent studies indicated that this association is absent in Finnish, Czech, and English populations [117, 118].

7.9.2 IgG Fc Receptor

Fcγ receptors (FcγR) are immunoglobulins that induce phagocytosis of opsonized microbes. Bournazos and colleagues demonstrated that polymorphisms in *FcγR IIa* (*CD32*) and *FcγR IIIb* (*CD16b*) are associated with IPF susceptibility [119, 120]. In particular, R131H polymorphism in the former (rs1801274) affects disease severity and progression [119], while copy number of the latter elevates IPF susceptibility [121].

7.10 Genes Associated with the Extracellular Matrix

7.10.1 MMPs

Matrix metalloproteinases (MMPs) are zinc- and calcium-dependent enzymes that degrade virtually all extracellular matrix components and are implicated in many physiological and pathological processes, including wound healing and fibrosis. In pulmonary fibrosis, certain MMPs accumulate in the lung, possibly leading to degradation of alveolar epithelial basement membranes and enhanced fibroblast invasion into alveolar spaces [122]. Checa and colleagues demonstrated that the 2G polymorphism at -1607 in the *MMP-1* promoter not only boosts transcriptional activity [123] but also confers risk of IPF in a case-control study of 130 patients and 305 healthy controls [124]. Interestingly, a recent study found that the T allele in *MMP-9* (-1562C>T) possibly predisposes IPF patients to CPFE [125].

7.11 HLA

In humans, major histocompatibility complex (MHC) genes are located on chromosome 6p, and encode class I and II human leukocyte antigens (HLA). *HLA* genes are highly polymorphic, and the *HLA* haplotype essentially determines the repertoire of antigens that stimulate T-cells. To date, several studies have reported associations between various HLA alleles and IPF [126–128]. For instance, Xue and colleagues demonstrated that the prevalence of *DRB1*1501* at the HLA-DR locus was significantly higher in IPF patients than in healthy controls [129]. Collectively, these data suggest that immunogenetic processes contribute to IPF susceptibility.

7.12 Conclusion

Over the past decade, tremendous progress has been achieved in understanding the genetic causes of pulmonary fibrosis (Fig. 7.5). For instance, investigations of FIP have identified rare genetic variants in genes related to surfactant and telomere biology. Large genome-wide association and linkage studies have also uncovered common genetic variants that confer risk, including in *MUC5B* and *TERT*. Further, functional studies of these rare as well as common genetic variants have provided novel insights into pathophysiology. More importantly, genetic factors that influence response to treatment and patient outcome have also been detected. Moving forward, next-generation and high-throughput sequencing will probably identify additional causative genes and pathways. Ultimately, combined analysis of genetic and environmental factors, including epigenetic modifications, will further improve our understanding of this disease, possibly leading to the development of novel, more effective therapies.

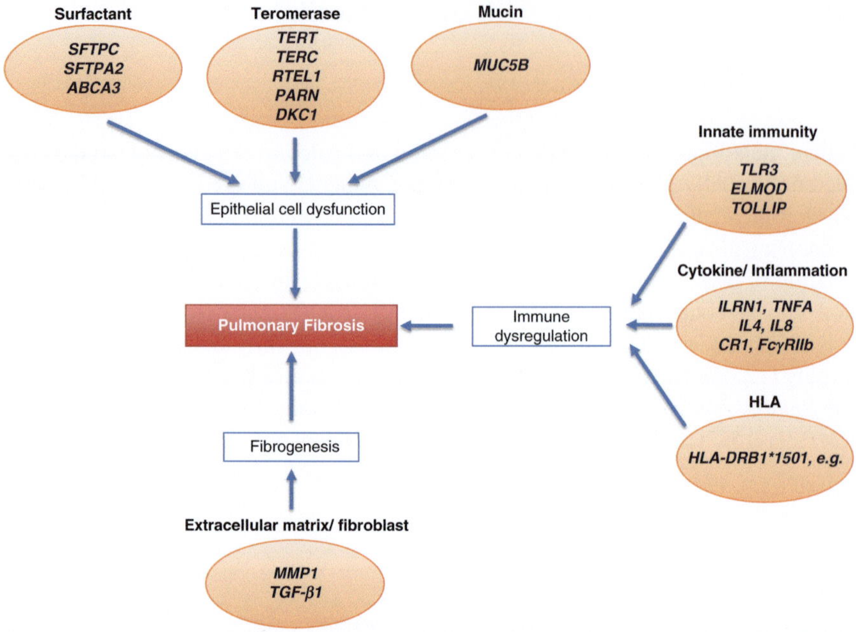

Fig. 7.5 Genes and their functions associated with the development of pulmonary fibrosis. *SFTPC* surfactant protein C, *SFTA2* surfactant protein A2, *ABCA3* ATP-binding cassette member A3, *TERT* telomerase reverse transcriptase, *TERC* telomerase RNA component, *RTEL1* regulator of telomere elongation helicase 1, *PARN* poly(A)-specific ribonuclease, *DKC1* dyskeratosis congenita 1, *MUC5B* mucin 5B, *TLR3* Toll-like receptor 3, *ELMOD2* ELMO domain-containing protein 2, *TOLLIP* Toll-interacting protein, *ILRN1* IL-1 receptor antagonist, *TNFA* TNF-α, *IL4* IL-4, *IL8* IL-8, *CR1* complement receptor 1, *FcγR IIb* Fcγ receptor IIb, *MMP1* Matrix metalloproteinase 1, *TGF-β1* transforming growth factor-β1

Acknowledgement I thank Prof. Tamio Suzuki (Department of Dermatology, Yamagata University School of Medicine) and Prof. Yasuhiro Setoguchi (Department of Pulmonary Medicine, Tokyo Medical University) for performing genetic analysis.

References

1. Raghu G, Collard HR, Egan JJ, Martinez FJ, Behr J, Brown KK, Colby TV, Cordier JF, Flaherty KR, Lasky JA, Lynch DA, Ryu JH, Swigris JJ, Wells AU, Ancochea J, Bouros D, Carvalho C, Costabel U, Ebina M, Hansell DM, Johkoh T, Kim DS, King TE Jr, Kondoh Y, Myers J, Muller NL, Nicholson AG, Richeldi L, Selman M, Dudden RF, Griss BS, Protzko SL, Schunemann HJ, Fibrosis AEJACIP. An official ATS/ERS/JRS/ALAT statement: idiopathic pulmonary fibrosis: evidence-based guidelines for diagnosis and management. Am J Respir Crit Care Med. 2011;183:788–824.
2. Marshall RP, Puddicombe A, Cookson WO, Laurent GJ. Adult familial cryptogenic fibrosing alveolitis in the United Kingdom. Thorax. 2000;55:143–6.

3. Hodgson U, Laitinen T, Tukiainen P. Nationwide prevalence of sporadic and familial idiopathic pulmonary fibrosis: evidence of founder effect among multiplex families in Finland. Thorax. 2002;57:338–42.
4. Loyd JE. Pulmonary fibrosis in families. Am J Respir Cell Mol Biol. 2003;29:S47–50.
5. Garcia-Sancho C, Buendia-Roldan I, Fernandez-Plata MR, Navarro C, Perez-Padilla R, Vargas MH, Loyd JE, Selman M. Familial pulmonary fibrosis is the strongest risk factor for idiopathic pulmonary fibrosis. Respir Med. 2011;105:1902–7.
6. Nogee LM, Dunbar AE III, Wert SE, Askin F, Hamvas A, Whitsett JA. A mutation in the surfactant protein C gene associated with familial interstitial lung disease. N Engl J Med. 2001;344:573–9.
7. Nogee LM, Dunbar AE III, Wert S, Askin F, Hamvas A, Whitsett JA. Mutations in the surfactant protein C gene associated with interstitial lung disease. Chest. 2002;121:20S–1S.
8. Cameron HS, Somaschini M, Carrera P, Hamvas A, Whitsett JA, Wert SE, Deutsch G, Nogee LM. A common mutation in the surfactant protein C gene associated with lung disease. J Pediatr. 2005;146:370–5.
9. Brasch F, Griese M, Tredano M, Johnen G, Ochs M, Rieger C, Mulugeta S, Muller KM, Bahuau M, Beers MF. Interstitial lung disease in a baby with a de novo mutation in the SFTPC gene. Eur Respir J. 2004;24:30–9.
10. Thomas AQ, Lane K, Phillips J III, Prince M, Markin C, Speer M, Schwartz DA, Gaddipati R, Marney A, Johnson J, Roberts R, Haines J, Stahlman M, Loyd JE. Heterozygosity for a surfactant protein C gene mutation associated with usual interstitial pneumonitis and cellular nonspecific interstitial pneumonitis in one kindred. Am J Respir Crit Care Med. 2002;165:1322–8.
11. Lawson WE, Grant SW, Ambrosini V, Womble KE, Dawson EP, Lane KB, Markin C, Renzoni E, Lympany P, Thomas AQ, Roldan J, Scott TA, Blackwell TS, Phillips J III, Loyd JE, du Bois RM. Genetic mutations in surfactant protein C are a rare cause of sporadic cases of IPF. Thorax. 2004;59:977–80.
12. van Moorsel CH, van Oosterhout MF, Barlo NP, de Jong PA, van der Vis JJ, Ruven HJ, van Es HW, van den Bosch JM, Grutters JC. Surfactant protein C mutations are the basis of a significant portion of adult familial pulmonary fibrosis in a dutch cohort. Am J Respir Crit Care Med. 2010;182:1419–25.
13. Wang Y, Kuan PJ, Xing C, Cronkhite JT, Torres F, Rosenblatt RL, DiMaio JM, Kinch LN, Grishin NV, Garcia CK. Genetic defects in surfactant protein A2 are associated with pulmonary fibrosis and lung cancer. Am J Hum Genet. 2009;84:52–9.
14. Campo I, Zorzetto M, Mariani F, Kadija Z, Morbini P, Dore R, Kaltenborn E, Frixel S, Zarbock R, Liebisch G, Hegermann J, Wrede C, Griese M, Luisetti M. A large kindred of pulmonary fibrosis associated with a novel ABCA3 gene variant. Respir Res. 2014;15:43.
15. Epaud R, Delestrain C, Louha M, Simon S, Fanen P, Tazi A. Combined pulmonary fibrosis and emphysema syndrome associated with ABCA3 mutations. Eur Respir J. 2014;43:638–41.
16. Armanios MY, Chen JJ, Cogan JD, Alder JK, Ingersoll RG, Markin C, Lawson WE, Xie M, Vulto I, Phillips JA III, Lansdorp PM, Greider CW, Loyd JE. Telomerase mutations in families with idiopathic pulmonary fibrosis. N Engl J Med. 2007;356:1317–26.
17. Tsakiri KD, Cronkhite JT, Kuan PJ, Xing C, Raghu G, Weissler JC, Rosenblatt RL, Shay JW, Garcia CK. Adult-onset pulmonary fibrosis caused by mutations in telomerase. Proc Natl Acad Sci U S A. 2007;104:7552–7.
18. Stuart BD, Choi J, Zaidi S, Xing C, Holohan B, Chen R, Choi M, Dharwadkar P, Torres F, Girod CE, Weissler J, Fitzgerald J, Kershaw C, Klesney-Tait J, Mageto Y, Shay JW, Ji W, Bilguvar K, Mane S, Lifton RP, Garcia CK. Exome sequencing links mutations in PARN and RTEL1 with familial pulmonary fibrosis and telomere shortening. Nat Genet. 2015;47:512–7.
19. Cogan JD, Kropski JA, Zhao M, Mitchell DB, Rives L, Markin C, Garnett ET, Montgomery KH, Mason WR, McKean DF, Powers J, Murphy E, Olson LM, Choi L, Cheng DS, Blue EM, Young LR, Lancaster LH, Steele MP, Brown KK, Schwarz MI, Fingerlin TE, Schwartz DA,

Lawson WE, Loyd JE, Zhao Z, Phillips JA III, Blackwell TS. Rare variants in RTEL1 are associated with familial interstitial pneumonia. Am J Respir Crit Care Med. 2015;191:646–55.
20. Fingerlin TE, Murphy E, Zhang W, Peljto AL, Brown KK, Steele MP, Loyd JE, Cosgrove GP, Lynch D, Groshong S, Collard HR, Wolters PJ, Bradford WZ, Kossen K, Seiwert SD, du Bois RM, Garcia CK, Devine MS, Gudmundsson G, Isaksson HJ, Kaminski N, Zhang Y, Gibson KF, Lancaster LH, Cogan JD, Mason WR, Maher TM, Molyneaux PL, Wells AU, Moffatt MF, Selman M, Pardo A, Kim DS, Crapo JD, Make BJ, Regan EA, Walek DS, Daniel JJ, Kamatani Y, Zelenika D, Smith K, McKean D, Pedersen BS, Talbert J, Kidd RN, Markin CR, Beckman KB, Lathrop M, Schwarz MI, Schwartz DA. Genome-wide association study identifies multiple susceptibility loci for pulmonary fibrosis. Nat Genet. 2013;45:613–20.
21. Noth I, Zhang Y, Ma SF, Flores C, Barber M, Huang Y, Broderick SM, Wade MS, Hysi P, Scuirba J, Richards TJ, Juan-Guardela BM, Vij R, Han MK, Martinez FJ, Kossen K, Seiwert SD, Christie JD, Nicolae D, Kaminski N, Garcia JG. Genetic variants associated with idiopathic pulmonary fibrosis susceptibility and mortality: a genome-wide association study. Lancet Respir Med. 2013;1:309–17.
22. Davies BH, Tuddenham EG. Familial pulmonary fibrosis associated with oculocutaneous albinism and platelet function defect. A new syndrome. Q J Med. 1976;45:219–32.
23. Terry RD, Sperry WM, Brodoff B. Adult lipidosis resembling Niemann-Pick's disease. Am J Pathol. 1954;30:263–85.
24. Schneider EL, Epstein CJ, Kaback MJ, Brandes D. Severe pulmonary involvement in adult Gaucher's disease. Report of three cases and review of the literature. Am J Med. 1977;63:475–80.
25. DePinho RA, Kaplan KL. The Hermansky-Pudlak syndrome. Report of three cases and review of pathophysiology and management considerations. Medicine (Baltimore). 1985;64:192–202.
26. Gahl WA, Brantly M, Kaiser-Kupfer MI, Iwata F, Hazelwood S, Shotelersuk V, Duffy LF, Kuehl EM, Troendle J, Bernardini I. Genetic defects and clinical characteristics of patients with a form of oculocutaneous albinism (Hermansky-Pudlak syndrome). N Engl J Med. 1998;338:1258–64.
27. Cullinane AR, Curry JA, Carmona-Rivera C, Summers CG, Ciccone C, Cardillo ND, Dorward H, Hess RA, White JG, Adams D, Huizing M, Gahl WAA. BLOC-1 mutation screen reveals that PLDN is mutated in Hermansky-Pudlak Syndrome type 9. Am J Hum Genet. 2011;88:778–87.
28. Ammann S, Schulz A, Krageloh-Mann I, Dieckmann NM, Niethammer K, Fuchs S, Eckl KM, Plank R, Werner R, Altmuller J, Thiele H, Nurnberg P, Bank J, Strauss A, von Bernuth H, Zur Stadt U, Grieve S, Griffiths GM, Lehmberg K, Hennies HC, Ehl S. Mutations in AP3D1 associated with immunodeficiency and seizures define a new type of Hermansky-Pudlak syndrome. Blood. 2016;127:997–1006.
29. Assoum M, Philippe C, Isidor B, Perrin L, Makrythanasis P, Sondheimer N, Paris C, Douglas J, Lesca G, Antonarakis S, Hamamy H, Jouan T, Duffourd Y, Auvin S, Saunier A, Begtrup A, Nowak C, Chatron N, Ville D, Mireskandari K, Milani P, Jonveaux P, Lemeur G, Milh M, Amamoto M, Kato M, Nakashima M, Miyake N, Matsumoto N, Masri A, Thauvin-Robinet C, Riviere JB, Faivre L, Thevenon J. Autosomal-recessive mutations in AP3B2, adaptor-related protein complex 3 beta 2 subunit, cause an early-onset epileptic encephalopathy with optic atrophy. Am J Hum Genet. 2016;99:1368–76.
30. Huizing M, Helip-Wooley A, Westbroek W, Gunay-Aygun M, Gahl WA. Disorders of lysosome-related organelle biogenesis: clinical and molecular genetics. Annu Rev Genomics Hum Genet. 2008;9:359–86.
31. Rouhani FN, Brantly ML, Markello TC, Helip-Wooley A, O'Brien K, Hess R, Huizing M, Gahl WA, Gochuico BR. Alveolar macrophage dysregulation in Hermansky-Pudlak syndrome type 1. Am J Respir Crit Care Med. 2009;180:1114–21.
32. Cullinane AR, Yeager C, Dorward H, Carmona-Rivera C, Wu HP, Moss J, O'Brien KJ, Nathan SD, Meyer KC, Rosas IO, Helip-Wooley A, Huizing M, Gahl WA, Gochuico

BR. Dysregulation of galectin-3. Implications for Hermansky-Pudlak syndrome pulmonary fibrosis. Am J Respir Cell Mol Biol. 2014;50:605–13.
33. Trimble A, Gochuico BR, Markello TC, Fischer R, Gahl WA, Lee JK, Kim Y, Burdick MD, Strieter RM, Mehrad B. Circulating fibrocytes as biomarker of prognosis in Hermansky-Pudlak syndrome. Am J Respir Crit Care Med. 2014;190:1395–401.
34. Gahl WA, Brantly M, Troendle J, Avila NA, Padua A, Montalvo C, Cardona H, Calis KA, Gochuico B. Effect of pirfenidone on the pulmonary fibrosis of Hermansky-Pudlak syndrome. Mol Genet Metab. 2002;76:234–42.
35. O'Brien K, Troendle J, Gochuico BR, Markello TC, Salas J, Cardona H, Yao J, Bernardini I, Hess R, Gahl WA. Pirfenidone for the treatment of Hermansky-Pudlak syndrome pulmonary fibrosis. Mol Genet Metab. 2011;103:128–34.
36. Dokal I. Dyskeratosis congenita in all its forms. Br J Haematol. 2000;110:768–79.
37. Heiss NS, Knight SW, Vulliamy TJ, Klauck SM, Wiemann S, Mason PJ, Poustka A, Dokal I. X-linked dyskeratosis congenita is caused by mutations in a highly conserved gene with putative nucleolar functions. Nat Genet. 1998;19:32–8.
38. Savage SA. Dyskeratosis congenita. In: Pagon RA, Adam MP, Ardinger HH, Wallace SE, Amemiya A, LJH B, Bird TD, Ledbetter N, Mefford HC, RJH S, Stephens K, editors. GeneReviews. Seattle, WA: University of Washington; 1993.
39. Savage SA, Giri N, Baerlocher GM, Orr N, Lansdorp PM, Alter BP. TINF2, a component of the shelterin telomere protection complex, is mutated in dyskeratosis congenita. Am J Hum Genet. 2008;82:501–9.
40. Walne AJ, Vulliamy T, Beswick R, Kirwan M, Dokal I. TINF2 mutations result in very short telomeres: analysis of a large cohort of patients with dyskeratosis congenita and related bone marrow failure syndromes. Blood. 2008;112:3594–600.
41. Armanios M, Chen JL, Chang YP, Brodsky RA, Hawkins A, Griffin CA, Eshleman JR, Cohen AR, Chakravarti A, Hamosh A, Greider CW. Haploinsufficiency of telomerase reverse transcriptase leads to anticipation in autosomal dominant dyskeratosis congenita. Proc Natl Acad Sci U S A. 2005;102:15960–4.
42. Vulliamy T, Marrone A, Goldman F, Dearlove A, Bessler M, Mason PJ, Dokal I. The RNA component of telomerase is mutated in autosomal dominant dyskeratosis congenita. Nature. 2001;413:432–5.
43. Fernandez BA, Fox G, Bhatia R, Sala E, Noble B, Denic N, Fernandez D, Duguid N, Dohey A, Kamel F, Edwards L, Mahoney K, Stuckless S, Parfrey PS, Woods MO. A Newfoundland cohort of familial and sporadic idiopathic pulmonary fibrosis patients: clinical and genetic features. Respir Res. 2012;13:64.
44. Talbert JL, Schwartz DA. Pulmonary fibrosis, familial. In: Pagon RA, Adam MP, Ardinger HH, Wallace SE, Amemiya A, LJH B, Bird TD, Ledbetter N, Mefford HC, RJH S, Stephens K, editors. GeneReviews. Seattle, WA: University of Washington; 1993.
45. Alder JK, Parry EM, Yegnasubramanian S, Wagner CL, Lieblich LM, Auerbach R, Auerbach AD, Wheelan SJ, Armanios M. Telomere phenotypes in females with heterozygous mutations in the dyskeratosis congenita 1 (DKC1) gene. Hum Mutat. 2013;34:1481–5.
46. Kropski JA, Mitchell DB, Markin C, Polosukhin VV, Choi L, Johnson JE, Lawson WE, Phillips JA III, Cogan JD, Blackwell TS, Loyd JE. A novel dyskerin (DKC1) mutation is associated with familial interstitial pneumonia. Chest. 2014;146:e1-e7.
47. Steele MP, Speer MC, Loyd JE, Brown KK, Herron A, Slifer SH, Burch LH, Wahidi MM, Phillips JA III, Sporn TA, McAdams HP, Schwarz MI, Schwartz DA. Clinical and pathologic features of familial interstitial pneumonia. Am J Respir Crit Care Med. 2005;172:1146–52.
48. Hamvas A, Cole FS, Nogee LM. Genetic disorders of surfactant proteins. Neonatology. 2007;91:311–7.
49. Mulugeta S, Nguyen V, Russo SJ, Muniswamy M, Beers MF. A surfactant protein C precursor protein BRICHOS domain mutation causes endoplasmic reticulum stress, proteasome dysfunction, and caspase 3 activation. Am J Respir Cell Mol Biol. 2005;32:521–30.

50. Mulugeta S, Maguire JA, Newitt JL, Russo SJ, Kotorashvili A, Beers MF. Misfolded BRICHOS SP-C mutant proteins induce apoptosis via caspase-4- and cytochrome c-related mechanisms. Am J Physiol Lung Cell Mol Physiol. 2007;293:L720–9.
51. Lawson WE, Crossno PF, Polosukhin VV, Roldan J, Cheng DS, Lane KB, Blackwell TR, Xu C, Markin C, Ware LB, Miller GG, Loyd JE, Blackwell TS. Endoplasmic reticulum stress in alveolar epithelial cells is prominent in IPF: association with altered surfactant protein processing and herpesvirus infection. Am J Physiol Lung Cell Mol Physiol. 2008;294:L1119–26.
52. Bridges JP, Wert SE, Nogee LM, Weaver TE. Expression of a human surfactant protein C mutation associated with interstitial lung disease disrupts lung development in transgenic mice. J Biol Chem. 2003;278:52739–46.
53. Wang WJ, Mulugeta S, Russo SJ, Beers MF. Deletion of exon 4 from human surfactant protein C results in aggresome formation and generation of a dominant negative. J Cell Sci. 2003;116:683–92.
54. Lawson WE, Cheng DS, Degryse AL, Tanjore H, Polosukhin VV, Xu XC, Newcomb DC, Jones BR, Roldan J, Lane KB, Morrisey EE, Beers MF, Yull FE, Blackwell TS. Endoplasmic reticulum stress enhances fibrotic remodeling in the lungs. Proc Natl Acad Sci U S A. 2011;108:10562–7.
55. Zhong Q, Zhou B, Ann DK, Minoo P, Liu Y, Banfalvi A, Krishnaveni MS, Dubourd M, Demaio L, Willis BC, Kim KJ, duBois RM, Crandall ED, Beers MF, Borok Z. Role of endoplasmic reticulum stress in epithelial-mesenchymal transition of alveolar epithelial cells: effects of misfolded surfactant protein. Am J Respir Cell Mol Biol. 2011;45:498–509.
56. Korfei M, Ruppert C, Mahavadi P, Henneke I, Markart P, Koch M, Lang G, Fink L, Bohle RM, Seeger W, Weaver TE, Guenther A. Epithelial endoplasmic reticulum stress and apoptosis in sporadic idiopathic pulmonary fibrosis. Am J Respir Crit Care Med. 2008;178:838–46.
57. Maitra M, Wang Y, Gerard RD, Mendelson CR, Garcia CK. Surfactant protein A2 mutations associated with pulmonary fibrosis lead to protein instability and endoplasmic reticulum stress. J Biol Chem. 2010;285:22103–13.
58. Shulenin S, Nogee LM, Annilo T, Wert SE, Whitsett JA, Dean M. ABCA3 gene mutations in newborns with fatal surfactant deficiency. N Engl J Med. 2004;350:1296–303.
59. Tryka AF, Wert SE, Mazursky JE, Arrington RW, Nogee LM. Absence of lamellar bodies with accumulation of dense bodies characterizes a novel form of congenital surfactant defect. Pediatr Dev Pathol. 2000;3:335–45.
60. Young LR, Nogee LM, Barnett B, Panos RJ, Colby TV, Deutsch GH. Usual interstitial pneumonia in an adolescent with ABCA3 mutations. Chest. 2008;134:192–5.
61. Ota C, Kimura M, Kure S. ABCA3 mutations led to pulmonary fibrosis and emphysema with pulmonary hypertension in an 8-year-old girl. Pediatr Pulmonol. 2016;51:E21–3.
62. Bullard JE, Nogee LM. Heterozygosity for ABCA3 mutations modifies the severity of lung disease associated with a surfactant protein C gene (SFTPC) mutation. Pediatr Res. 2007;62:176–9.
63. Petrovski S, Todd JL, Durheim MT, Wang Q, Chien JW, Kelly FL, Frankel C, Mebane CM, Ren Z, Bridgers J, Urban TJ, Malone CD, Finlen Copeland A, Brinkley C, Allen AS, O'Riordan T, McHutchison JG, Palmer SM, Goldstein DB. An Exome Sequencing Study to Assess the Role of Rare Genetic Variation in Pulmonary Fibrosis. Am J Respir Crit Care Med. 2017;196:82.
64. Juge PA, Borie R, Kannengiesser C, Gazal S, Revy P, Wemeau-Stervinou L, Debray MP, Ottaviani S, Marchand-Adam S, Nathan N, Thabut G, Richez C, Nunes H, Callebaut I, Justet A, Leulliot N, Bonnefond A, Salgado D, Richette P, Desvignes JP, Liote H, Froguel P, Allanore Y, Sand O, Dromer C, Flipo RM, Clement A, Beroud C, Sibilia J, Coustet B, Cottin V, Boissier MC, Wallaert B, Schaeverbeke T, Dastot le Moal F, Frazier A, Menard C, Soubrier M, Saidenberg N, Valeyre D, Amselem S, FREX consortium, Boileau C, Crestani B, Dieude P. Shared genetic predisposition in rheumatoid arthritis-interstitial lung disease and familial pulmonary fibrosis. Eur Respir J. 2017;49(5)

65. Alder JK, Chen JJ, Lancaster L, Danoff S, Su SC, Cogan JD, Vulto I, Xie M, Qi X, Tuder RM, Phillips JA III, Lansdorp PM, Loyd JE, Armanios MY. Short telomeres are a risk factor for idiopathic pulmonary fibrosis. Proc Natl Acad Sci U S A. 2008;105:13051–6.
66. Cronkhite JT, Xing C, Raghu G, Chin KM, Torres F, Rosenblatt RL, Garcia CK. Telomere shortening in familial and sporadic pulmonary fibrosis. Am J Respir Crit Care Med. 2008;178:729–37.
67. Stuart BD, Lee JS, Kozlitina J, Noth I, Devine MS, Glazer CS, Torres F, Kaza V, Girod CE, Jones KD, Elicker BM, Ma SF, Vij R, Collard HR, Wolters PJ, Garcia CK. Effect of telomere length on survival in patients with idiopathic pulmonary fibrosis: an observational cohort study with independent validation. Lancet Respir Med. 2014;2:557–65.
68. Dai J, Cai H, Li H, Zhuang Y, Min H, Wen Y, Yang J, Gao Q, Shi Y, Yi L. Association between telomere length and survival in patients with idiopathic pulmonary fibrosis. Respirology. 2015;20:947–52.
69. Mushiroda T, Wattanapokayakit S, Takahashi A, Nukiwa T, Kudoh S, Ogura T, Taniguchi H, Kubo M, Kamatani N, Nakamura Y, Pirfenidone Clinical Study Group. A genome-wide association study identifies an association of a common variant in TERT with susceptibility to idiopathic pulmonary fibrosis. J Med Genet. 2008;45:654–6.
70. Codd V, Nelson CP, Albrecht E, Mangino M, Deelen J, Buxton JL, Hottenga JJ, Fischer K, Esko T, Surakka I, Broer L, Nyholt DR, Mateo Leach I, Salo P, Hagg S, Matthews MK, Palmen J, Norata GD, O'Reilly PF, Saleheen D, Amin N, Balmforth AJ, Beekman M, de Boer RA, Bohringer S, Braund PS, Burton PR, de Craen AJ, Denniff M, Dong Y, Douroudis K, Dubinina E, Eriksson JG, Garlaschelli K, Guo D, Hartikainen AL, Henders AK, Houwing-Duistermaat JJ, Kananen L, Karssen LC, Kettunen J, Klopp N, Lagou V, van Leeuwen EM, Madden PA, Magi R, Magnusson PK, Mannisto S, MI MC, Medland SE, Mihailov E, Montgomery GW, Oostra BA, Palotie A, Peters A, Pollard H, Pouta A, Prokopenko I, Ripatti S, Salomaa V, Suchiman HE, Valdes AM, Verweij N, Vinuela A, Wang X, Wichmann HE, Widen E, Willemsen G, Wright MJ, Xia K, Xiao X, van Veldhuisen DJ, Catapano AL, Tobin MD, Hall AS, Blakemore AI, van Gilst WH, Zhu H, CARDIoGRAM consortium, Erdmann J, Reilly MP, Kathiresan S, Schunkert H, Talmud PJ, Pedersen NL, Perola M, Ouwehand W, Kaprio J, Martin NG, van Duijn CM, Hovatta I, Gieger C, Metspalu A, Boomsma DI, Jarvelin MR, Slagboom PE, Thompson JR, Spector TD, van der Harst P, Samani NJ. Identification of seven loci affecting mean telomere length and their association with disease. Nat Genet. 2013;45:422–7. 7e1-2.
71. Ballew BJ, Yeager M, Jacobs K, Giri N, Boland J, Burdett L, Alter BP, Savage SA. Germline mutations of regulator of telomere elongation helicase 1, RTEL1, in Dyskeratosis congenita. Hum Genet. 2013;132:473–80.
72. Kannengiesser C, Borie R, Menard C, Reocreux M, Nitschke P, Gazal S, Mal H, Taille C, Cadranel J, Nunes H, Valeyre D, Cordier JF, Callebaut I, Boileau C, Cottin V, Grandchamp B, Revy P, Crestani B. Heterozygous RTEL1 mutations are associated with familial pulmonary fibrosis. Eur Respir J. 2015;46:474–85.
73. Tummala H, Walne A, Collopy L, Cardoso S, de la Fuente J, Lawson S, Powell J, Cooper N, Foster A, Mohammed S, Plagnol V, Vulliamy T, Dokal I. Poly(A)-specific ribonuclease deficiency impacts telomere biology and causes dyskeratosis congenita. J Clin Invest. 2015;125:2151–60.
74. Seibold MA, Wise AL, Speer MC, Steele MP, Brown KK, Loyd JE, Fingerlin TE, Zhang W, Gudmundsson G, Groshong SD, Evans CM, Garantziotis S, Adler KB, Dickey BF, du Bois RM, Yang IV, Herron A, Kervitsky D, Talbert JL, Markin C, Park J, Crews AL, Slifer SH, Auerbach S, Roy MG, Lin J, Hennessy CE, Schwarz MI, Schwartz DAA. common MUC5B promoter polymorphism and pulmonary fibrosis. N Engl J Med. 2011;364:1503–12.
75. Peljto AL, Steele MP, Fingerlin TE, Hinchcliff ME, Murphy E, Podlusky S, Carns M, Schwarz M, Varga J, Schwartz DA. The pulmonary fibrosis-associated MUC5B promoter polymorphism does not influence the development of interstitial pneumonia in systemic sclerosis. Chest. 2012;142:1584–8.

76. Borie R, Crestani B, Dieude P, Nunes H, Allanore Y, Kannengiesser C, Airo P, Matucci-Cerinic M, Wallaert B, Israel-Biet D, Cadranel J, Cottin V, Gazal S, Peljto AL, Varga J, Schwartz DA, Valeyre D, Grandchamp B. The MUC5B variant is associated with idiopathic pulmonary fibrosis but not with systemic sclerosis interstitial lung disease in the European Caucasian population. PLoS One. 2013;8:e70621.
77. Stock CJ, Sato H, Fonseca C, Banya WA, Molyneaux PL, Adamali H, Russell AM, Denton CP, Abraham DJ, Hansell DM, Nicholson AG, Maher TM, Wells AU, Lindahl GE, Renzoni EA. Mucin 5B promoter polymorphism is associated with idiopathic pulmonary fibrosis but not with development of lung fibrosis in systemic sclerosis or sarcoidosis. Thorax. 2013;68:436–41.
78. Zhang Y, Noth I, Garcia JG, Kaminski N. A variant in the promoter of MUC5B and idiopathic pulmonary fibrosis. N Engl J Med. 2011;364:1576–7.
79. Peljto AL, Selman M, Kim DS, Murphy E, Tucker L, Pardo A, Lee JS, Ji W, Schwarz MI, Yang IV, Schwartz DA, Fingerlin TE. The MUC5B promoter polymorphism is associated with idiopathic pulmonary fibrosis in a Mexican cohort but is rare among Asian ancestries. Chest. 2015;147:460–4.
80. Wang C, Zhuang Y, Guo W, Cao L, Zhang H, Xu L, Fan Y, Zhang D, Wang Y. Mucin 5B promoter polymorphism is associated with susceptibility to interstitial lung diseases in Chinese males. PLoS One. 2014;9:e104919.
81. Horimasu Y, Ohshimo S, Bonella F, Tanaka S, Ishikawa N, Hattori N, Kohno N, Guzman J, Costabel U. MUC5B promoter polymorphism in Japanese patients with idiopathic pulmonary fibrosis. Respirology. 2015;20:439–44.
82. Jin GY, Lynch D, Chawla A, Garg K, Tammemagi MC, Sahin H, Misumi S, Kwon KS. Interstitial lung abnormalities in a CT lung cancer screening population: prevalence and progression rate. Radiology. 2013;268:563–71.
83. Hunninghake GM, Hatabu H, Okajima Y, Gao W, Dupuis J, Latourelle JC, Nishino M, Araki T, Zazueta OE, Kurugol S, Ross JC, San Jose Estepar R, Murphy E, Steele MP, Loyd JE, Schwarz MI, Fingerlin TE, Rosas IO, Washko GR, O'Connor GT, Schwartz DA. MUC5B promoter polymorphism and interstitial lung abnormalities. N Engl J Med. 2013;368:2192–200.
84. Araki T, Putman RK, Hatabu H, Gao W, Dupuis J, Latourelle JC, Nishino M, Zazueta OE, Kurugol S, Ross JC, San Jose Estepar R, Schwartz DA, Rosas IO, Washko GR, O'Connor GT, Hunninghake GM. Development and Progression of Interstitial Lung Abnormalities in the Framingham Heart Study. Am J Respir Crit Care Med. 2016;194:1514–22.
85. Fahy JV, Dickey BF. Airway mucus function and dysfunction. N Engl J Med. 2010;363:2233–47.
86. Nakano Y, Yang IV, Walts AD, Watson AM, Helling BA, Fletcher AA, Lara AR, Schwarz MI, Evans CM, Schwartz DA. MUC5B promoter variant rs35705950 affects MUC5B expression in the distal airways in idiopathic pulmonary fibrosis. Am J Respir Crit Care Med. 2016;193:464–6.
87. Plantier L, Crestani B, Wert SE, Dehoux M, Zweytick B, Guenther A, Whitsett JA. Ectopic respiratory epithelial cell differentiation in bronchiolised distal airspaces in idiopathic pulmonary fibrosis. Thorax. 2011;66:651–7.
88. Peljto AL, Zhang Y, Fingerlin TE, Ma SF, Garcia JG, Richards TJ, Silveira LJ, Lindell KO, Steele MP, Loyd JE, Gibson KF, Seibold MA, Brown KK, Talbert JL, Markin C, Kossen K, Seiwert SD, Murphy E, Noth I, Schwarz MI, Kaminski N, Schwartz DA. Association between the MUC5B promoter polymorphism and survival in patients with idiopathic pulmonary fibrosis. JAMA. 2013;309:2232–9.
89. Yang HZ, Cui B, Liu HZ, Chen ZR, Yan HM, Hua F, Hu ZW. Targeting TLR2 attenuates pulmonary inflammation and fibrosis by reversion of suppressive immune microenvironment. J Immunol. 2009;182:692–702.
90. Meneghin A, Choi ES, Evanoff HL, Kunkel SL, Martinez FJ, Flaherty KR, Toews GB, Hogaboam CM. TLR9 is expressed in idiopathic interstitial pneumonia and its activation promotes in vitro myofibroblast differentiation. Histochem Cell Biol. 2008;130:979–92.

91. Kirillov V, Siler JT, Ramadass M, Ge L, Davis J, Grant G, Nathan SD, Jarai G, Trujillo G. Sustained activation of toll-like receptor 9 induces an invasive phenotype in lung fibroblasts: possible implications in idiopathic pulmonary fibrosis. Am J Pathol. 2015;185:943–57.
92. O'Dwyer DN, Armstrong ME, Trujillo G, Cooke G, Keane MP, Fallon PG, Simpson AJ, Millar AB, McGrath EE, Whyte MK, Hirani N, Hogaboam CM, Donnelly SC. The Toll-like receptor 3 L412F polymorphism and disease progression in idiopathic pulmonary fibrosis. Am J Respir Crit Care Med. 2013;188:1442–50.
93. Yang HZ, Wang JP, Mi S, Liu HZ, Cui B, Yan HM, Yan J, Li Z, Liu H, Hua F, Lu W, Hu ZW. TLR4 activity is required in the resolution of pulmonary inflammation and fibrosis after acute and chronic lung injury. Am J Pathol. 2012;180:275–92.
94. Hams E, Armstrong ME, Barlow JL, Saunders SP, Schwartz C, Cooke G, Fahy RJ, Crotty TB, Hirani N, Flynn RJ, Voehringer D, McKenzie AN, Donnelly SC, Fallon PG. IL-25 and type 2 innate lymphoid cells induce pulmonary fibrosis. Proc Natl Acad Sci U S A. 2014;111:367–72.
95. Pulkkinen V, Bruce S, Rintahaka J, Hodgson U, Laitinen T, Alenius H, Kinnula VL, Myllarniemi M, Matikainen S, Kere J. ELMOD2, a candidate gene for idiopathic pulmonary fibrosis, regulates antiviral responses. FASEB J. 2010;24:1167–77.
96. Ranjith-Kumar CT, Miller W, Sun J, Xiong J, Santos J, Yarbrough I, Lamb RJ, Mills J, Duffy KE, Hoose S, Cunningham M, Holzenburg A, Mbow ML, Sarisky RT, Kao CC. Effects of single nucleotide polymorphisms on Toll-like receptor 3 activity and expression in cultured cells. J Biol Chem. 2007;282:17696–705.
97. Hodgson U, Pulkkinen V, Dixon M, Peyrard-Janvid M, Rehn M, Lahermo P, Ollikainen V, Salmenkivi K, Kinnula V, Kere J, Tukiainen P, Laitinen T. ELMOD2 is a candidate gene for familial idiopathic pulmonary fibrosis. Am J Hum Genet. 2006;79:149–54.
98. Oldham JM, Ma SF, Martinez FJ, Anstrom KJ, Raghu G, Schwartz DA, Valenzi E, Witt L, Lee C, Vij R, Huang Y, Strek ME, Noth I, Investigators IP. TOLLIP, MUC5B, and the response to N-acetylcysteine among individuals with idiopathic pulmonary fibrosis. Am J Respir Crit Care Med. 2015;192:1475–82.
99. Crystal RG, Bitterman PB, Rennard SI, Hance AJ, Keogh BA. Interstitial lung diseases of unknown cause. Disorders characterized by chronic inflammation of the lower respiratory tract (first of two parts). N Engl J Med. 1984;310:154–66.
100. Whyte M, Hubbard R, Meliconi R, Whidborne M, Eaton V, Bingle C, Timms J, Duff G, Facchini A, Pacilli A, Fabbri M, Hall I, Britton J, Johnston I, Di Giovine F. Increased risk of fibrosing alveolitis associated with interleukin-1 receptor antagonist and tumor necrosis factor-alpha gene polymorphisms. Am J Respir Crit Care Med. 2000;162:755–8.
101. Hutyrova B, Pantelidis P, Drabek J, Zurkova M, Kolek V, Lenhart K, Welsh KI, Du Bois RM, Petrek M. Interleukin-1 gene cluster polymorphisms in sarcoidosis and idiopathic pulmonary fibrosis. Am J Respir Crit Care Med. 2002;165:148–51.
102. Pantelidis P, Fanning GC, Wells AU, Welsh KI, Du Bois RM. Analysis of tumor necrosis factor-alpha, lymphotoxin-alpha, tumor necrosis factor receptor II, and interleukin-6 polymorphisms in patients with idiopathic pulmonary fibrosis. Am J Respir Crit Care Med. 2001;163(6):1432.
103. Barlo NP, van Moorsel CH, Korthagen NM, Heron M, Rijkers GT, Ruven HJ, van den Bosch JM, Grutters JC. Genetic variability in the IL1RN gene and the balance between interleukin (IL)-1 receptor agonist and IL-1beta in idiopathic pulmonary fibrosis. Clin Exp Immunol. 2011;166:346–51.
104. Korthagen NM, van Moorsel CH, Kazemier KM, Ruven HJ, Grutters JC. IL1RN genetic variations and risk of IPF: a meta-analysis and mRNA expression study. Immunogenetics. 2012;64:371–7.
105. Kolahian S, Fernandez IE, Eickelberg O, Hartl D. Immune mechanisms in pulmonary fibrosis. Am J Respir Cell Mol Biol. 2016;55:309–22.
106. Vasakova M, Striz I, Slavcev A, Jandova S, Kolesar L, Sulc J. Th1/Th2 cytokine gene polymorphisms in patients with idiopathic pulmonary fibrosis. Tissue Antigens. 2006;67:229–32.

107. Xaubet A, Marin-Arguedas A, Lario S, Ancochea J, Morell F, Ruiz-Manzano J, Rodriguez-Becerra E, Rodriguez-Arias JM, Inigo P, Sanz S, Campistol JM, Mullol J, Picado C. Transforming growth factor-beta1 gene polymorphisms are associated with disease progression in idiopathic pulmonary fibrosis. Am J Respir Crit Care Med. 2003;168:431–5.
108. Son JY, Kim SY, Cho SH, Shim HS, Jung JY, Kim EY, Lim JE, Park BH, Kang YA, Kim YS, Kim SK, Chang J, Park MS. TGF-beta1 T869C polymorphism may affect susceptibility to idiopathic pulmonary fibrosis and disease severity. Lung. 2013;191:199–205.
109. Carre PC, Mortenson RL, King TE Jr, Noble PW, Sable CL, Riches DW. Increased expression of the interleukin-8 gene by alveolar macrophages in idiopathic pulmonary fibrosis. A potential mechanism for the recruitment and activation of neutrophils in lung fibrosis. J Clin Invest. 1991;88:1802–10.
110. Lynch JP III, Standiford TJ, Rolfe MW, Kunkel SL, Strieter RM. Neutrophilic alveolitis in idiopathic pulmonary fibrosis. The role of interleukin-8. Am Rev Respir Dis. 1992;145:1433–9.
111. Southcott AM, Jones KP, Li D, Majumdar S, Cambrey AD, Pantelidis P, Black CM, Laurent GJ, Davies BH, Jeffery PK, et al. Interleukin-8. Differential expression in lone fibrosing alveolitis and systemic sclerosis. Am J Respir Crit Care Med. 1995;151:1604–12.
112. Ahn MH, Park BL, Lee SH, Park SW, Park JS, Kim DJ, Jang AS, Park JS, Shin HK, Uh ST, Kim YK, Kim YW, Han SK, Jung KS, Lee KY, Jeong SH, Park JW, Choi BW, Park IW, Chung MP, Shin HD, Song JW, Kim DS, Park CS, Shim YS. A promoter SNP rs4073T>A in the common allele of the interleukin 8 gene is associated with the development of idiopathic pulmonary fibrosis via the IL-8 protein enhancing mode. Respir Res. 2011;12:73.
113. Nakagome K, Dohi M, Okunishi K, Tanaka R, Miyazaki J, Yamamoto K. In vivo IL-10 gene delivery attenuates bleomycin induced pulmonary fibrosis by inhibiting the production and activation of TGF-beta in the lung. Thorax. 2006;61:886–94.
114. Sun L, Louie MC, Vannella KM, Wilke CA, LeVine AM, Moore BB, Shanley TP. New concepts of IL-10-induced lung fibrosis: fibrocyte recruitment and M2 activation in a CCL2/CCR2 axis. Am J Physiol Lung Cell Mol Physiol. 2011;300:L341–53.
115. Whittington HA, Freeburn RW, Godinho SI, Egan J, Haider Y, Millar AB. Analysis of an IL-10 polymorphism in idiopathic pulmonary fibrosis. Genes Immun. 2003;4:258–64.
116. Zorzetto M, Ferrarotti I, Trisolini R, Lazzari Agli L, Scabini R, Novo M, De Silvestri A, Patelli M, Martinetti M, Cuccia M, Poletti V, Pozzi E, Luisetti M. Complement receptor 1 gene polymorphisms are associated with idiopathic pulmonary fibrosis. Am J Respir Crit Care Med. 2003;168:330–4.
117. Hodgson U, Tukiainen P, Laitinen T. The polymorphism C5507G of complement receptor 1 does not explain idiopathic pulmonary fibrosis among the Finns. Respir Med. 2005;99:265–7.
118. Kubistova Z, Mrazek F, Lympany PA, Lagan AL, Arakelyan A, Kriegova E, Welsh KI, Kolek V, Zatloukal J, Hutyrova B, du Bois RM, Petrek M. The CR1 C5507G polymorphism is not involved in susceptibility to idiopathic pulmonary fibrosis in two European populations. Tissue Antigens. 2008;72:483–6.
119. Bournazos S, Grinfeld J, Alexander KM, Murchison JT, Wallace WA, McFarlane P, Hirani N, Simpson AJ, Dransfield I, Hart SP. Association of FcgammaRIIa R131H polymorphism with idiopathic pulmonary fibrosis severity and progression. BMC Pulm Med. 2010;10:51.
120. Bournazos S, Bournazou I, Murchison JT, Wallace WA, McFarlane P, Hirani N, Simpson AJ, Dransfield I, Fcgamma HSP. receptor IIIb (CD16b) polymorphisms are associated with susceptibility to idiopathic pulmonary fibrosis. Lung. 2010;188:475–81.
121. Bournazos S, Bournazou I, Murchison JT, Wallace WA, McFarlane P, Hirani N, Simpson AJ, Dransfield I, Hart SP. Copy number variation of FCGR3B is associated with susceptibility to idiopathic pulmonary fibrosis. Respiration. 2011;81:142–9.
122. Swiderski RE, Dencoff JE, Floerchinger CS, Shapiro SD, Hunninghake GW. Differential expression of extracellular matrix remodeling genes in a murine model of bleomycin-induced pulmonary fibrosis. Am J Pathol. 1998;152:821–8.
123. Rutter JL, Mitchell TI, Buttice G, Meyers J, Gusella JF, Ozelius LJ, Brinckerhoff CE. A single nucleotide polymorphism in the matrix metalloproteinase-1 promoter creates an Ets binding site and augments transcription. Cancer Res. 1998;58:5321–5.

124. Checa M, Ruiz V, Montano M, Velazquez-Cruz R, Selman M, Pardo A. MMP-1 polymorphisms and the risk of idiopathic pulmonary fibrosis. Hum Genet. 2008;124:465–72.
125. Xu L, Bian W, Gu XH, Shen C. Genetic polymorphism in matrix metalloproteinase-9 and transforming growth factor-beta1 and susceptibility to combined pulmonary fibrosis and emphysema in a Chinese population. Kaohsiung J Med Sci. 2017;33:124–9.
126. Turton CW, Morris LM, Lawler SD, Turner-Warwick M. HLA in cryptogenic fibrosing alveolitis. Lancet. 1978;1:507–8.
127. Varpela E, Tiilikainen A, Varpela M, Tukiainen P. High prevalences of HLA-B15 and HLA-Dw6 in patients with cryptogenic fibrosing alveolitis. Tissue Antigens. 1979;14:68–71.
128. Falfan-Valencia R, Camarena A, Juarez A, Becerril C, Montano M, Cisneros J, Mendoza F, Granados J, Pardo A, Selman M. Major histocompatibility complex and alveolar epithelial apoptosis in idiopathic pulmonary fibrosis. Hum Genet. 2005;118:235–44.
129. Xue J, Gochuico BR, Alawad AS, Feghali-Bostwick CA, Noth I, Nathan SD, Rosen GD, Rosas IO, Dacic S, Ocak I, Fuhrman CR, Cuenco KT, Smith MA, Jacobs SS, Zeevi A, Morel PA, Pilewski JM, Valentine VG, Gibson KF, Kaminski N, Sciurba FC, Zhang Y, Duncan SR. The HLA class II Allele DRB1*1501 is over-represented in patients with idiopathic pulmonary fibrosis. PLoS One. 2011;6:e14715.
130. Markart P, Ruppert C, Wygrecka M, Schmidt R, Korfei M, Harbach H, Theruvath I, Pison U, Seeger W, Guenther A, Witt H. Surfactant protein C mutations in sporadic forms of idiopathic interstitial pneumonias. Eur Respir J. 2007;29:134–7.

Chapter 8
Other Diffuse Lung Diseases: Diffuse Cystic Lung Diseases (LAM, TSC, BHD), Sarcoidosis, Pulmonary Alveolar Proteinosis, and Pulmonary Alveolar Microlithiasis—What Are the Roles of Genetic Factors in the Pathogenesis of These Diseases?

Haruhiko Furusawa, Masahiro Masuo, Yoshihisa Nukui, Yasunari Miyazaki, and Naohiko Inase

Abstract Lymphangioleiomyomatosis (LAM) is a rare multisystem disorder that mostly affects women in their reproductive years and predominantly affects the lungs. LAM occurs in patients with tuberous sclerosis complex (TSC-LAM) and as a sporadic form in patients who do not have tuberous sclerosis (S-LAM). Patients with TSC-LAM have germline mutations either in TSC1 located on chromosome 9q34 or TSC2 located on chromosome 16p13.3, and the majority have a germline mutation in TCS2.

Birt-Hogg-Dubé (BHD) syndrome is a rare autosomal dominant disorder that is characterized by the development of cutaneous fibrofolliculomas, renal tumors, and pulmonary cysts, causing spontaneous pneumothorax. BHD is caused by germline mutations in the folliculin (FLCN) gene on chromosome 17 (17p12q11.2), which encodes the protein FLCN.

Sarcoidosis is a systemic granulomatous disease that affects young and middle-aged adults. It frequently presents with bilateral hilar lymphadenopathy, pulmonary

H. Furusawa · M. Masuo · Y. Nukui · N. Inase
Department of Respiratory Medicine, Graduate School of Medical and Dental Sciences, TMDU, Tokyo, Japan

Y. Miyazaki (✉)
Student Support and Health Administration Organization, Tokyo Medical and Dental University (TMDU), Tokyo, Japan

Department of Respiratory Medicine, Graduate School of Medical and Dental Sciences, TMDU, Tokyo, Japan
e-mail: miyazaki.pilm@tmd.ac.jp

T. Kaneko (ed.), *Clinical Relevance of Genetic Factors in Pulmonary Diseases*, Respiratory Disease Series: Diagnostic Tools and Disease Managements,
https://doi.org/10.1007/978-981-10-8144-6_8

infiltration, and ocular and skin lesions. Granuloma formation is caused by T-cell activation by antigen presentation; therefore, the most prominent finding was a linkage to a section within human leukocyte antigens (HLA), a linkage to HLA-DRB1-alleles, and variants of these alleles are associated with the disease course and specific organ involvement.

Pulmonary alveolar proteinosis (PAP) is a rare disease in which surfactants mainly accumulate in the alveolar space due to the dysregulation of surfactant clearance by AMs. GM-CSF receptor gene mutations, surfactant-related genes SFTPB and SFTPC, gene mutations in ATP-binding cassette 3 (ABCA3), which is essential for the intracellular transport of surfactant, and NK2 homeobox 1 (NKX2-1), which is essential for the development of alveolar epithelial cells, have been reported in PAP patients.

Pulmonary alveolar microlithiasis (PAM) is an extremely rare disease and an autosomal recessive genetic disorder. Inactivating mutations are present in the solute carrier family 34 member 2 (SLC34A2) gene, which encodes the IIb type sodium-dependent phosphoryl transport protein.

Keywords Lymphangioleiomyomatosis · TSC · Birt-Hogg-Dubé syndrome FLCN · Sarcoidosis · HLA-DRB1 · Pulmonary alveolar proteinosis GM-CSF receptor · SFTPB · SFTPC · ABCA3 · NKX2-1 Pulmonary alveolar microlithiasis · SLC34A2

8.1 Diffuse Cystic Lung Diseases (LAM, TSC, BHD)

8.1.1 Lymphangioleiomyomatosis, Sporadic and Tuberous Sclerosis Complex

8.1.1.1 Introduction

Lymphangioleiomyomatosis (LAM) is a rare multisystem disorder that mostly affects women in their reproductive years and predominantly affects the lungs [1, 2]. LAM occurs in patients with tuberous sclerosis complex (TSC-LAM) and as a sporadic form in patients who do not have tuberous sclerosis (S-LAM) [3]. Both TSC-LAM and S-LAM are characterized by the proliferation of abnormal smooth muscle-like cells (LAM cells) in the lungs, lymphatics, and kidney, leading to cystic destruction in the lungs, chylous effusion, and abdominal tumors, such as angiomyolipoma (AML), respectively.

The prevalence of LAM is 4.9 cases/million for females (range 3.35–7.76), and the average age at diagnosis of LAM is approximately 35 years [4]. TSC is an autosomal dominant genetic disorder that is characterized by seizures, mental retardation, and hamartoma of the brain, retina, skin, heart, lungs, and kidneys [3]. TSC occurs in 30–40% of women and 10% of men [5]. S-LAM appears to be limited to women, with the exception of one case report [6].

Clinical Manifestations

The clinical course of LAM is characterized by worsening dyspnea on effort, recurrent pneumothorax, and accumulation of chylous effusions in the chest and abdomen [1]. Ten years after diagnosis, approximately 55% of patients with LAM experience shortness of breath with walking, 20% require supplemental oxygen, and 10% die [7]. Airflow obstruction and hyperinflation are the most common physiologic features. Pulmonary function tests show a decline in forced expiratory volume in 1 s (FEV_1) and diffusing capacity for carbon monoxide (DL_{CO}) [8, 9]. The progression of lung disease in patients with LAM is best estimated by serial measurements of lung function [10].

Although S-LAM and TSC-LAM are associated with the same genetic mutation, there are differences in their clinical presentation. Ryu JH et al. reported that normal lung function was observed in approximately 31% of patients with S-LAM and in approximately 53% of patients with TSC-LAM [11]. In a study that compared CT findings, patients with S-LAM often had a higher frequency of pulmonary nodules than those with TSC-LAM, whereas patients with TSC-LAM had a higher frequency of pneumothorax and AMLs [12].

8.1.1.2 Diagnosis

Radiological HRCT images show multiple thin-walled round well-defined cysts distributed evenly throughout the lungs. The cysts vary, typically ranging from 2 to 5 mm in diameter, and their wall thickness varies from 0.1 to 2 mm (Fig. 8.1) [13, 14].

Histologically, LAM cells are found in the walls of the cysts and along bronchioles, lymphatics, and blood vessels in the lung. LAM cells consist of two types: smaller spindle-shaped cells and larger epithelioid cells (Fig. 8.2). LAM cells are positive for smooth muscle action, vimentin, desmin, and estrogen and progesterone receptors. While cells positive for human melanoma black-45 (HMB-45) are classically associated with the diagnosis LAM, they are not detectable in all LAM cells, and HMB-45 expression may vary from case to case [15–17]. LAM cells also stain positively for vascular endothelial growth factor (VEGF)-C and VEGF-D [18].

The definitive diagnosis is made by tissue biopsy (usually from the lung). However, surgical lung biopsy is associated with a risk of developing pneumothorax, which must be considered. The European Respiratory Society Guidelines indicate that the diagnosis of LAM can be made with reasonable certainty on the basis of characteristic cystic changes on HRCT in patients with tuberous sclerosis, AML, chylous effusion, or lymphadenopathy [14]. The exclusion of an alternative cause of cystic lung disease should be carefully conducted. Recently, a serum VEGF-D level >800 pg/ml in a patient with typical HRCT findings has been proposed as a diagnostic marker [19].

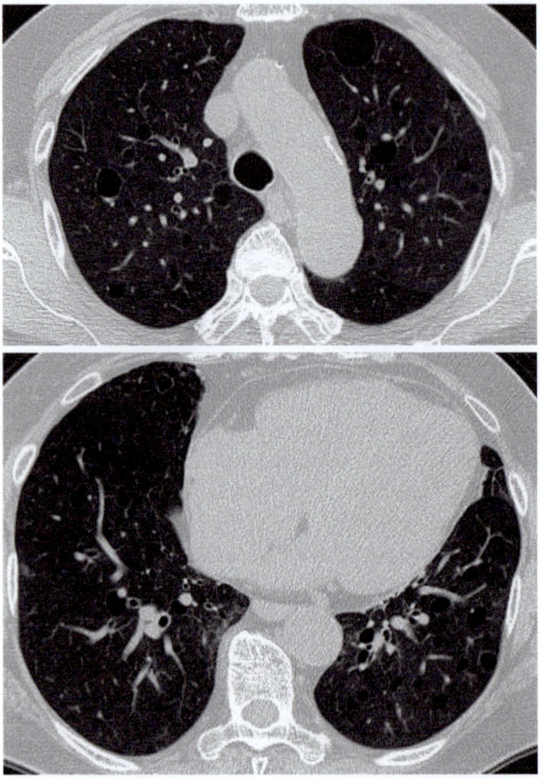

Fig. 8.1 Computed tomography scan of the lung. Multiple round thin-walled cysts are diffusely distributed without any zonal predominance (Provided by the authors)

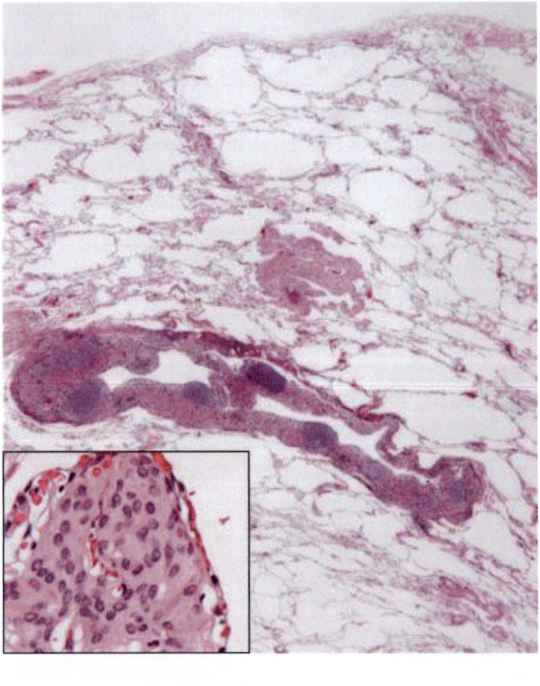

Fig. 8.2 Pathological findings of the surgically biopsied lung specimen (hematoxylin and eosin stain). A cystic lesion and nodular lesions are observed. Focal proliferation of short spindle-shaped cells is present (inset) (Provided by Dr. Hiroshi Ishii et al. Respir Investig. 2014;52:261–4)

8.1.1.3 Genetic Aspects and Relevance

TSC1, located on chromosome 9q34, and TSC2, located on chromosome 16p13.3, were identified as the genes responsible for TSC in 1997 and 1993, respectively [20, 21]. Patients with TSC-LAM have germline mutations either in *TSC1* or *TSC2*, and the majority has a germline mutation in *TCS2* [22]. Patients with S-LAM have no *TSC2* germline mutation [23]. Loss of the heterozygosity (LOH) of *TSC2* was found in LAM lesions from patients with TSC-LAM and S-LAM patients and not in surrounding normal tissue [24, 25]. In addition, an inactivating somatic mutation was present in the lungs and kidneys of the same patients with S-LAM [26]. These results indicate that inactivation of both alleles of *TSC1* or *TSC2* is the cause of LAM in both TSC-LAM and S-LAM and that LAM cells have metastatic properties.

The microdissection of LAM nodules from patients with S-LAM revealed that inactivating *TSC2* mutations were found in 8/10 cases, with mutant allele frequencies of 4–60% in microdissected cells, which were positive for both SMA and HMB45 [27]. This result suggests that a high degree of heterogeneity is present in LAM nodule cell populations, including both *TSC2*-mutant cells and wild-type cells. The relationship between these cells and their role in the development of LAM remains to be resolved. Moreover, this study demonstrated that two cases without a *TSC1* or *TSC2* mutation were identified, which suggests that another genetic mechanism may be involved in the pathogenesis of LAM.

TSC1 and *TSC2* encode the proteins hamartin and tuberin, respectively, and these proteins form a heterodimeric complex that inhibits the mammalian target of rapamycin (mTOR) signaling pathway [28, 29]. Dysregulation of the mTOR signaling pathway is the cause of abnormal LAM cell proliferation. The large serine/threonine protein kinase mTOR belongs to the phosphatidylinositol kinase-related kinase family and regulates cell growth as well as cell proliferation, migration, survival, and metabolism [30].

8.1.1.4 Treatment and Management

The Multicenter International LAM Efficacy of Sirolimus (MILES) trial was a double-blind, randomized, placebo-controlled study of 1 year of treatment with the mTOR inhibitor sirolimus versus placebo followed by 1 year of off-treatment observation. This study showed that sirolimus stabilized the forced expiratory volume in 1 s, improved the forced vital capacity, and improved quality of life. However, during the 1 year of off-treatment observation, lung function declined in both groups, which indicates the need for continuous treatment for the stability of lung function [31]. For patients with LAM with a decline in lung function or with persistent chylous effusion, treatment with mTOR inhibitors should be considered [32]. Bronchodilators are prescribed to patients with airway reversibility and to patients with obstructive ventilatory impairment for symptom relief. Due to the high recurrence rate of pneumothorax (70%), pleurodesis is recommended at the time of the initial pneumothorax [33]. Lung transplantation is an important option for patients with progressive respiratory failure [34].

8.1.2 Birt-Hogg-Dubé Syndrome

8.1.2.1 Introduction and Clinical Aspects

Birt-Hogg-Dubé (BHD) syndrome was initially described in 1977 as kindred; 15 of 70 family members developed multiple, small, white, or skin-colored papules on the face, neck, and upper trunk after the age of 25 years [35]. BHD syndrome is a rare autosomal dominant disorder that is characterized by the development of cutaneous fibrofolliculomas, renal tumors, and pulmonary cysts, causing spontaneous pneumothorax [36]. However, it does not necessarily present all of these characteristics, and patients with different phenotypes have been shown to exhibit various combinations or single lesions.

Regarding clinical manifestations, lung cysts have been described in most (77–89%) patients with BHD syndrome, and the estimated incidence of pneumothorax in these patients is 33–38%. No evidence of neoplasia, inflammation, or fibrosis has been found in association with these lung cysts. Classically described skin findings consist of a triad of hamartomas of the hair follicles (fibrofolliculomas), tumors of the hair disk (trichodiscomas), and skin tags (acrochordons). Renal tumors, when present, are often multiple and bilateral [36]. There was no significant difference in the diagnosis of colorectal polyps or colon cancer compared to the non-BHD syndrome group.

8.1.2.2 Clinical Manifestations

Pulmonary Lesions

Pulmonary cysts and spontaneous pneumothorax are the important symptoms of BHD syndrome. A family history of pneumothorax is present in 35% of patients with BHD syndrome [37]. The risk of pneumothorax in BHD patients is 50-fold higher than that in the general population. Toro et al. evaluated 198 patients from 89 families with BHD syndrome and focused on lung cysts and spontaneous pneumothorax. They reported that 89% (177/198) of patients with BHD syndrome had lung cysts, which were detected with CT scans of the chest, and approximately 24% (48/198) of patients and 35% (31/89) of BHDS families screened for lung cysts had a history of spontaneous pneumothorax [38]. There was no gender difference for the onset of pneumothorax. The median age of occurrence was 38 years (range, 22–71 years), and 75% (36/48) of patients had a second pneumothorax.

In CT scans of the chest, lung cysts have a tendency to exhibit thin/smooth walls and no fusion, and relatively large cysts can be present in the basal or subpleural lungs (Fig. 8.3). Tobino et al. analyzed thin-section CT images of the chest in 12 patients and showed that the number (range, 29–407/person) and size (from a few mm to 2 cm or more) of the cysts varied. Most cysts were irregular-shaped, and

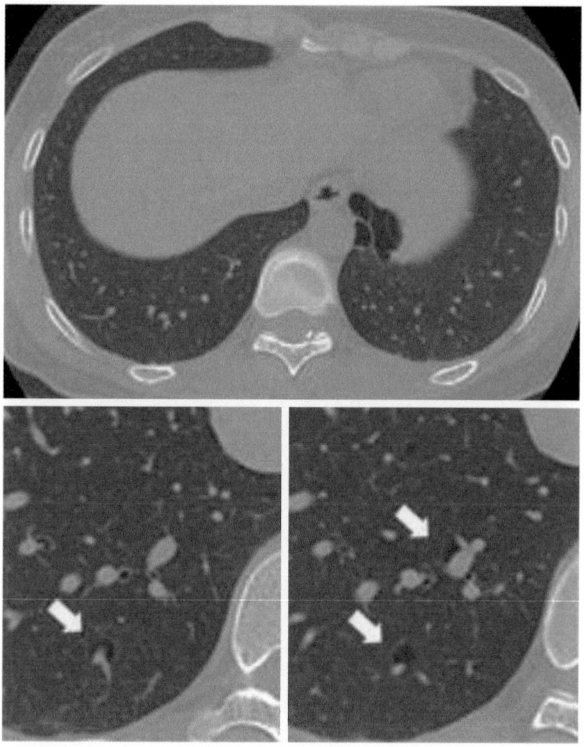

Fig. 8.3 CT scan of the lung. Upper row, multiple cysts are observed in left S10; lower row: cysts in contact with blood vessels are observed in the lower right lobe (white arrows) (Provided by the authors)

approximately 40% of cysts were located along the pleura, predominantly in the lower medial zone. Furthermore, they found cysts located in, and abutting on, the proximal portions of lower pulmonary arteries or veins.

Furuya et al. used histology to investigate the lungs of 11 patients from nine families and found that the cysts had walls that were partially incorporated with the interstitial stroma of the interlobular septum, visceral pleura, or bronchovascular bundle and that the inner surface was lined by epithelial cells, sometimes with a predominance of type II pneumocyte-like cuboidal cells, and occasionally contained internal septa consisting of alveolar walls or showed an "alveoli within an alveolus" pattern (Fig. 8.4) [39].

Kumasaka et al. hypothesized that the cysts possibly expanded in size as the alveolar walls disappeared at the alveolar-septal junction and grew even larger when several cysts fused [40].

Cutaneous Lesions

Fibrofolliculomas, trichodiscomas, and acrochordons are the triad of skin lesions that characterize BHD syndrome [35]. Fibrofolliculomas are the most common phenotypic features of BHD syndrome, occurring in more than 85% of BHD patients

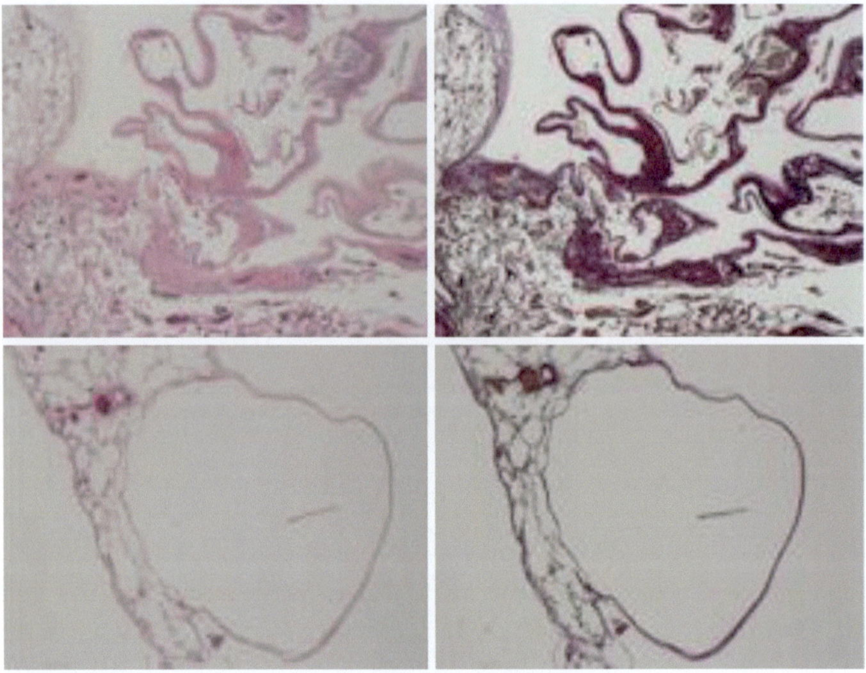

Fig. 8.4 Pathological findings of the left lower lobe. Upper row: In the left S10 tissue, ruptured cysts, bullae, and emphysematous cystic cavities are observed in part of the subpleura. Bottom: In the left S8 tissue, a bleb is observed adjacent to the pleura (left, HE staining; right, EVG staining) (Provided by the authors)

over the age of 25 on the face, neck, and upper trunk and less frequently on ear lobes or oral mucosa [41].

Renal Lesions

The incidence of renal tumors is 6–34% and increases after the age of 40. Renal tumors are usually bilateral and multiple. Unlike pulmonary lesions and skin lesions, in addition to the germline mutation of the FLCN gene, a somatic mutation of an allele or a "second hit," such as LOH, is considered to be to be the cause of onset [42].

8.1.3 Diagnostic Criteria for BHD Syndrome

Schmidt et al. proposed the following diagnostic criteria to be suggestive of BHD syndrome: (1) at least two cutaneous papules that are clinically consistent with fibrofolliculoma/trichodiscoma and at least one histologically confirmed fibrofolliculoma; (2) multiple bilateral pulmonary cysts located mainly in the basilar regions of the lung with or without a history of spontaneous pneumothorax that develops prior to age 40, but especially with a family history of these pulmonary manifestations; (3) bilateral, multifocal chromophobe renal carcinomas or hybrid oncocytic tumors, especially with a family history of renal tumors or an early age (<50 years) of onset; and (4) a combination of these cutaneous, pulmonary or renal manifestations in a patient or members of his family. A definitive diagnosis of BHD syndrome is confirmed with a diagnostic genetic test that is positive for a germline FLCN mutation [41].

8.1.4 Genetic Aspects and Relevance

BHD is caused by germline mutations in the folliculin (*FLCN*) gene, which encodes the protein FLCN [37]. In 2001, Khoo et al. (Sweden) and Schmidt et al. (USA) identified the responsible gene on chromosome 17 (17p12q11.2) almost simultaneously via mapping analysis [43, 44]. The *FLCN* gene sequence was identified and named in 2002 by Nickerson. FLCN consists of 14 exons that span approximately 20 kb of genomic DNA, 11 kb of which encode transcript mRNA and a 579-amino acid protein [45].

More than 150 unique *FLCN* germline mutations have been reported, as updated by the European Birt-Hogg-Dubé Consortium (https://grenada.lumc.nl/LOVD2/shared1/home.php?select_db=FLCN). They are predominantly mutations (base substitution, deletion, duplication, indel, insertion) that result in premature protein truncation and a presumed loss of FLCN function. In addition, nine large intragenic deletions or duplications are expected to severely disrupt protein structure or, at a minimum, to delete the last exon, and seven missense mutations that result in amino acid substitutions have been documented [41]. The most frequent mutation is a "hot spot" mutation that occurs in almost half of patients within a polycytosine C8 tract of exon 11.

The primary functions of the folliculin protein include roles in mTOR and AMPK signaling via the interaction of FLCN with FNIP1/2 and cell-cell adhesion via the physical interaction of FLCN with plakophilin 4 (PKP4), an armadillo-repeat-containing protein that interacts with E-cadherin and is a component of adherent junctions. However, the mechanism through which the loss of a single *FLCN* allele leads to pathogenesis is unclear. In renal lesions in BHD patients, the *FLCN* gene functions as a tumor suppressor gene, which fits the Knudson "two-hit" tumor suppressor gene model; a germline event inactivates one allele; and a somatic event, often the loss of heterozygosity, inactivates the second allele in renal cell carcinoma. On the other hand, it is unknown if a second hit event is required for the initiation of pulmonary cyst formation in BHD. Kennedy et al. described a "stretch hypothesis," which proposes that cysts arise because of fundamental defects in cell-cell adhesion due to FLCN deficiency, leading to repeated respiration-induced physical stretch-induced stress and, over time, the expansion of alveolar spaces, particularly in regions of the lung with larger changes in alveolar volume and at weaker "anchor points" to the pleura, including the interlobular septa and attachments to the visceral pleura in the secondary lobule [46].

Currently, although there is no clear correlation between the type or location of the *FLCN* gene mutation and organs with phenotype:genotype-phenotype correlations, several trends have been noted [41]. In a Japanese cohort of 36 BHD patients with multiple lung cysts, mutations that were most frequently identified in the 3′-end of the *FLCN* gene, including exons 12 and 13 (13/25.52.0%), and mutations that were related to a history of pneumothorax were the predominant phenotypic features [47].

In analyses of genotype-phenotype correlations, Toro et al. reported that among patients with mutations in exon 9, the number of lung cysts was higher, and the cysts were larger, and among the patients with mutations in exon 12, the cysts were larger. Particularly in exon 9 mutant cases, there were more patients with renal tumors. These results suggested that exon 9 is a functionally important site [38]. Another report by Schmidt et al. noted that BHD-affected individuals with the c.1285delC mutation in the exon 11 mutation "hot spot" had fewer renal tumors (1/26) compared to BHD-affected individuals with the c.1285dupC mutation (13/56), although the sample size was too small for significance to be reached [48].

8.1.5 *Treatment and Management*

To date, there is no treatment for the disease; however, the advantage of an early diagnosis is in the initiation of screening for renal tumors. If the syndrome is suspected, full family and genetic histories should be taken because of the autosomal dominant nature of its transmission and the fact that cutaneous symptoms are often absent or subtle or exhibit a late onset.

For pulmonary involvement, therapy is largely focused on the treatment and prevention of pneumothorax. Because of its high recurrence rate, surgical intervention with resection and pleurodesis is an acceptable option, even in patients with a first episode of pneumothorax. Patients should be cautioned about the increased risk of pneumothorax in association with scuba diving and air travel [36].

8.2 Sarcoidosis

8.2.1 *Introduction and Clinical Aspects*

Sarcoidosis is a systemic granulomatous disease that affects young and middle-aged adults. It frequently presents with bilateral hilar lymphadenopathy, pulmonary infiltration, and ocular and skin lesions. The liver, spleen, kidney, heart, nervous system, muscles, and other organs may also be involved. A diagnosis of the disorder usually requires the demonstration of typical lesions in more than one organ system and

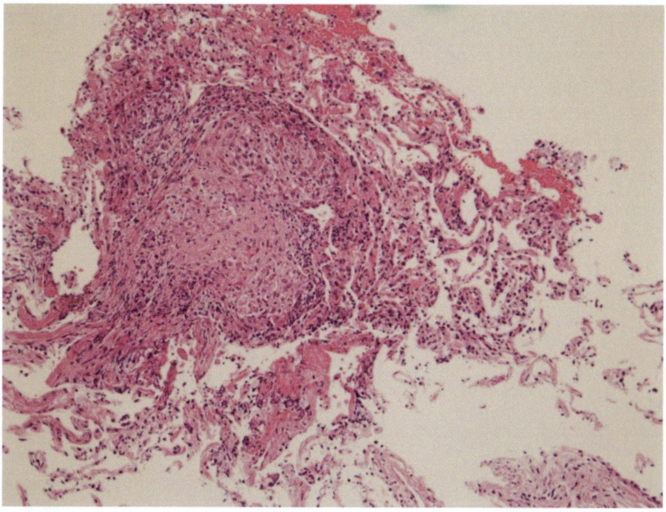

Fig. 8.5 A well-circumscribed, non-necrotizing granuloma in the lung showing central epithelioid histiocytes surrounded by lymphocytes

exclusion of other disorders that are known to cause granulomatous disease [49] (Fig. 8.5).

The clinical expression, natural history, and prognosis of sarcoidosis are highly variable and depend on the pattern of onset, race, and development organ. This disease occurs more often in women; the peak incidence in men occurs at 20–29 years old, while women displayed two peak incidences at 25–29 and 65–69 years old in a Northern European country and Japan. The incidence risk of sarcoidosis in US blacks is approximately three times higher than in US whites. Sarcoidosis is relatively rare in Japan, while Northern European countries reported the highest prevalence rates in the world.

A Case Control Etiologic Study of Sarcoidosis (ACCESS) enrolled 736 patients with sarcoidosis in the United States. In this study, women were more likely to have eye and neurologic involvement and to have erythema nodosum, whereas men were more likely to be hypercalcemic. Blacks were more likely to have eye, liver, bone marrow, skin, and extrathoracic lymph node involvement other than erythema nodosum [50].

8.2.2 Clinical Manifestations

Patients with sarcoidosis exhibit specific organ disorders and nonspecific systemic constitutional symptoms, such as fever, fatigue, malaise, pain, and weight loss. The most frequently involved organ is the lung, which is affected in more than 90% of patients. Two-thirds of sarcoidosis patients can expect to achieve remission; however, approximately 20% of patients evolve toward pulmonary fibrosis. Common symptoms include cough, dyspnea, and chest pain. Lung parenchymal manifestation is predominant in the upper to middle lung field, and four stages of intrathoracic findings have been identified on chest X-ray images: stage I is bilateral hilar adenopathy (Fig. 8.6a, b), stage II is bilateral hilar adenopathy with parenchymal infiltration, stage III is parenchymal infiltration without hilar adenopathy, and stage IV is pulmonary fibrosis (Fig. 8.7). Stage IV sarcoidosis is generally associated with poor pulmonary function and a poor prognosis.

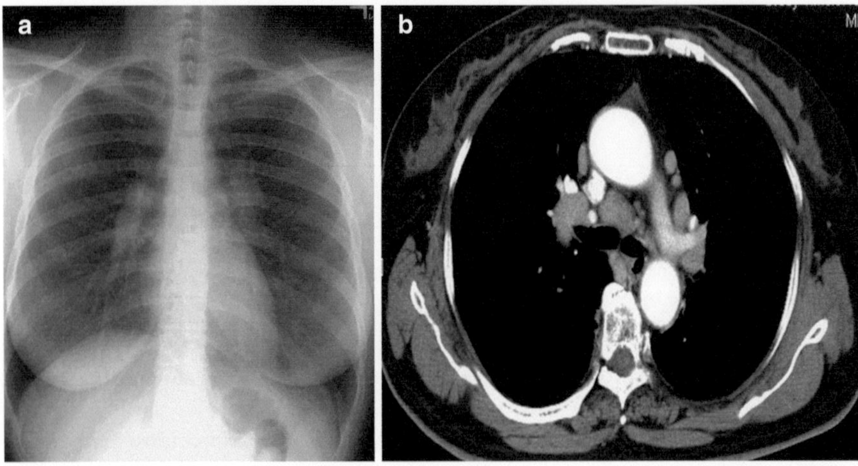

Fig. 8.6 Bilateral hilar lymphadenopathy on a chest X-ray (**a**) and extensive mediastinal and hilar lymph node enlargement on a chest CT (**b**)

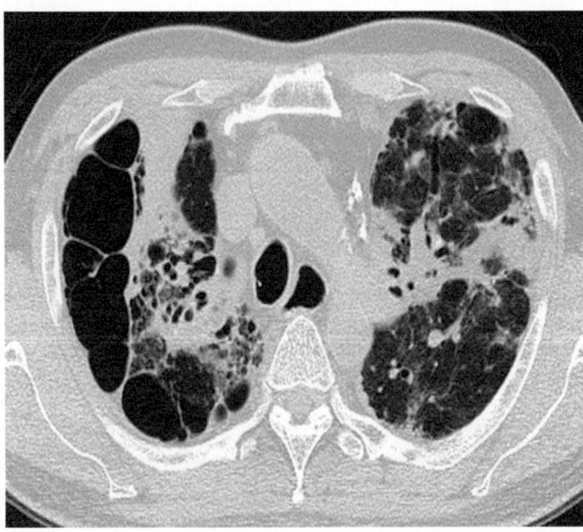

Fig. 8.7 Extensive pulmonary fibrosis

Ocular lesions frequently occur in Japanese patients (38%). Uveitis is the most common and can cause glaucoma or cataracts. Local therapy with corticosteroids may spontaneously resolve the inflammation.

Myocardial involvement occurs in approximately 5% of sarcoidosis patients; however, it is found at autopsy in up to 25% of patients in the United States and more than 50% of patients in Japan. Cardiac sarcoidosis can affect any part of the heart and the conduction system. The symptoms and clinical course vary from asymptomatic to syncope, heart failure, or sudden death. Electrocardiogram, echocardiogram, and myocardial imaging with thallium-201 are used for diagnosis. The presence of granulomas in an endomyocardial biopsy can confirm the diagnosis of cardiac sarcoidosis; however, the low positive rate of this procedure makes diagnosis difficult to obtain [51].

8.2.3 Diagnosis

Diagnosis of sarcoidosis is made via identification of noncaseating granulomas with the exclusion of other diseases (e.g., tuberculosis, lymphoma, and lung cancer) and compatible clinical and radiographic manifestations. Biopsies should be performed on the most accessible lesion, such as cutaneous lesions or superficial lymph node swellings. If there is no involvement, flexible bronchoscopy with transbronchial lung biopsies (TBLB) or endobronchial ultrasound-guided transbronchial needle aspiration (EBUS-TBNA) is recommended. There are several reports that EBUS-TBNA yields a higher positivity rate of granulomas compared to TBLB [52].

8.2.4 Genetic Aspects and Relevance

The pathogenesis of sarcoidosis is unknown; however, both environmental and hereditary etiologies have been considered. The existence of hereditary etiologies, supported by many reports of familial clustering, has been observed worldwide; monozygotic twins are more often concordant for disease than dizygotic twins, and blacks are more frequently affected by this disease and show more severe and chronic clinical courses than individuals of other ethnicities. However, this disease is not caused by a single major gene, and there are many candidate causes due to immunological or genetic aspects. Granuloma formation is caused by T-cell activation by antigen presentation; therefore, the most prominent finding was a linkage to a section within human leukocyte antigens (HLA). Several specific HLA alleles are thought to influence the incident rate and clinical course of this disease. The most prominent finding is a linkage to HLA-DRB1 alleles, and variants of these alleles are associated with the disease course and specific organ involvement.

HLA-DRB1*03 is strongly associated with Lofgren's syndrome, and Grunewald et al. demonstrated that *03-positivity was strongly correlated with a good prognosis in Swedish patients with Lofgren's syndrome [53]. This allele is common in Europeans and very rare in Japanese, and there are few patients with Lofgren's syndrome. HLA-DRB1*1101, DRB1*1201, DRB1*1501, and DRB1*0402 are also correlated with the incidence risk of sarcoidosis [54], and DRB1*08 is a candidate allele that only appears in Japanese patients [55].

Non-HLA genes that influence antigen processing, antigen presentation, granuloma formation, or autophagy may also be considered sarcoidosis candidate genes. BTNL2 (butyrophilin-like 2), located on chromosome 6p at the junction of HLA class II and class III regions, is a member of the immunoglobulin superfamily and has been implicated as a costimulatory molecule that is involved in T-cell activation on the basis of its homology to B7-1. The G→A transition that constitutes rs2076530 leads to a premature truncation of the protein and may result in insufficient T-cell regulation [56]. The A allele frequency of rs2076530 was significantly increased in sarcoidosis patients compared with controls, and this allele correlated with a chronic and severe clinical course [57]. On the other hand, the annexin A11 (ANXA11) gene, which may affect the apoptosis pathway, was also identified as a susceptibility locus for sarcoidosis [58], but the T allele of rs1049550 leads to a mild form of the disease that resolves spontaneously in the majority of cases [59].

The CARD15 gene, known as the nucleotide-binding oligomerization domain 2 gene (NOD2), is involved in innate immunity through recognition of bacterial pathogens. This gene is a causative gene of Blau syndrome and early onset sarcoidosis (EOS) [60]. Sato et al. reported that the NOD2 genotype did not differ between adult sarcoidosis patients and controls; however, the 2104T polymorphism was associated with worse lung function, and the 1761G polymorphism was associated with better lung function [61].

8.2.5 Treatment and Management

Sarcoidosis shows spontaneous remission in more than half of patients without any systemic treatment or with local corticosteroid treatment (such as ointment or eye drops) only, but this disease persists as a chronic disease in approximately one-third of those affected. Therefore, the use of systemic steroids must be considered carefully. Severe lung involvement and myocardial and nervous lesions require systemic therapy. The most commonly used agent is a corticosteroid. Generally, 20–40 mg of prednisolone is initially started and continued with gradual tapering for 1 month. If the patient has a recurrence of symptoms and the involvement is remitted after 6–12 months, systemic therapy may be finished. Methotrexate and azathioprine or infliximab might be considered when patients show an insufficient response in spite of adequate corticosteroid treatment.

8.3 Pulmonary Alveolar Proteinosis

8.3.1 Introduction and Clinical Aspects

Pulmonary surfactant is composed of protein and phospholipid; its surfactant action prevents the collapse of the lung by reducing surface tension and plays an important role in respiratory function. Pulmonary surfactant is synthesized and secreted by type II alveolar epithelial cells. Alveolar macrophages (AMs) play a critical role in surfactant uptake and degradation in a process that depends on signaling by granulocyte macrophage colony-stimulating factor (GM-CSF). Pulmonary alveolar proteinosis (PAP) is a rare disease in which surfactants mainly accumulate in the alveolar space due to the dysregulation of surfactant clearance by AMs.

GM-CSF is an important cytokine in the pathology of PAP. In 1994, PAP-like lung lesions were observed in GM-CSF knockout mice [62]. In GM-CSF knockout mice, a lung-specific transgenic system for GM-CSF and the inhalation of GM-CSF improve the pathology of PAP. In addition, GM-CSF was required when alveolar macrophages were treated with pulmonary surfactant, and GM-CSF could be an option for treatment [63]. In addition, it was reported that a high level of autoantibodies against GM-CSF (anti-GM-CSF antibodies) was present in the sera of patients with idiopathic PAP, but not in the sera of S-PAP patients. The dysfunction of AMs due to the neutralization of GM-CSF bioactivity by an autoantibody was indicated to be the pathogenesis of human idiopathic PAP [64].

Other genetic abnormalities associated with PAP, including mutations in the GM-CSF receptor α chain gene (*CSF 2 RA*) on the X chromosome pseudoautosomal region 1 and in the β chain gene (*CSF 2 RB*) on chromosome 22, inhibit GM-CSF signaling and have been detected in patients with congenital PAP [65, 66]. The four main surfactant proteins are SP-A, SP-B, SP-C, and SP-D, and the corresponding genes are *SFTPA*, *SFTPB*, *SFTPC*, and *SFTPD*, respectively. Mutations of surfactant protein genes are responsible for quantitative and qualitative alterations in secreted surfactant, consequently leading to ineffective surfactant and abnormal clearance. These are known to be the causes of PAP due to the mutations as well.

PAP is classified depending on the etiology: (1) autoimmune PAP (previously named primary or idiopathic), (2) genetic PAP, and (3) secondary PAP. Autoimmune PAP represents ~90% of all PAP cases and is rarely associated with another autoimmune disease; indeed, in the study by Seymour et al., only 7 (1.7%) out of 410 patients had another autoimmune disease [67]. GM-CSF receptor gene mutations were found in PAP patients who were anti-GM-CSF antibody negative. In addition to the surfactant-related genes *SFTPB* and *SFTPC*, gene mutations in ATP-binding cassette 3 (*ABCA3*), which is essential for the intracellular transport of surfactant, and NK2 homeobox 1 (*NKX2-1*), which is essential for the development of alveolar epithelial cells, have been reported. Secondary PAP is recognized as a PAP that develops with some underlying disease, such as malignant tumors (especially a blood malignancy, such as myelodysplastic syndromes, MDS), and inhalation of toxins, such as dust [68].

8.3.2 Diagnosis

In autoimmune PAP patients, symptoms are not specific, and almost one-third of patients are asymptomatic. Dyspnea is present in 39% of cases, and cough, productive or not, is present in 21% of patients. Chest pain, loss of weight, fatigue, and fever are rare. The clinical examination results are often normal. Cyanosis or digital clubbing may be present in up to 30% of cases, and auscultation may reveal crackles [68]. On the other hand, in secondary PAP with MDS, it is reported that 45% of patients had fever. Genetic PAP is similar to autoimmune PAP in clinical presentation except that patients have no anti-GM-CSF antibody and the age of onset is young. PAP with surfactant-related gene mutations, although dependent on the causative gene, shows respiratory failure during the neonatal period, possibly leading to death.

Bronchoalveolar lavage is useful for the diagnosis. It has a milky appearance and has precipitation when standing still (Fig. 8.8). Cytological examination and periodic acid-Schiff (PAS) staining reveal large, foamy macrophages that contain eosinophilic granules, with extracellular globular hyaline material found homogeneously positive on PAS.

In radiological findings, chest radiography reveals symmetric, bilateral alveolar opacities, without air bronchogram, that exhibit a perihilar and basal distribution. The levels of opacities and symptoms are often discrepant. A chest CT scan is a major tool in the diagnosis of PAP. Major abnormalities are ground-glass opacities, septal reticulations, and parenchymal consolidation. Reticulations are frequently superimposed on ground-glass opacities, forming a "crazy-paving" pattern that is characteristic of PAP. Opacities have a typically geographic distribution, with a juxtaposition of healthy and sick zones.

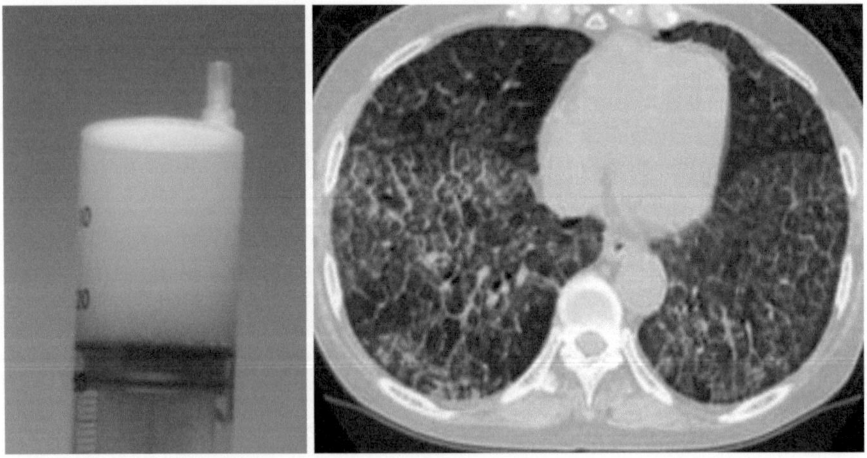

Fig. 8.8 Bronchial lavage fluid and CT scans of the lungs of patients with PAP (Provided by the authors)

8.3.3 Genetic Aspects and Relevance

Genetic PAP includes mutations in the GM-CSF receptor α (CD116) or β (CD131) chains, *SFTPB*, *SFTPC*, *ABCA3*, *NKX2-1*, and lysinuric protein intolerance.

The GM-CSF receptor is composed of the binding α chain, encoded by *CSF2RA*, and the common β chain (CD131), encoded by *CSF2RB*, which is also used by IL-3 and IL-5 receptors. Transmission in both mutations is autosomal recessive. Mutations in the *CSF2RA* gene have only been reported in children, not in neonates, corresponding to 6% of all PAP cases. A mutation in *CSF2RB* has been reported in children, but there are reports of individuals who are diagnosed in their 30s.

The term PAP has been widely used in patients with surfactant mutation-associated disorders. Historically, these disorders are referred to as congenital PAP, which is mainly seen in the neonatal period. Mutations of SP-B (*SFTPB*), SP-C (*SFTPC*), and ABCA3 (*ABCA3*), which are necessary for the intracellular transport of surfactant, and NKX2-N (or TTF-1), which is necessary for lung development, have been reported in patients with congenital PAP. Most cases of congenital PAP are transmitted in an autosomal recessive manner. The surfactant protein SP-B is encoded by *SFTPB* on human chromosome 2p11.2, which produces a 381-amino acid preproprotein that is expressed and processed by type II epithelial cells. Congenital PAP is most often caused by homozygosity for a frameshift mutation (121ins2) in the *SP-B* gene, which has a lethal course in the neonatal period. *SFTPC* is located on chromosome 8p21.3 and encodes the preprotein pro-SP-C, which is selectively expressed in alveolar type II epithelial cells in the lung. Mutations of SP-C are transmitted in a dominant or point mutation (de novo) manner. The most frequent mutation is a point mutation that causes substitution of threonine by isoleucine at the position 73 codon, I73T. Compared with the PAP of the *SFTPB* mutation, the age of onset varies, and there are cases of insidious onset and relatively long-term survival. *SFTPC* mutations are associated with interstitial lung diseases in neonates, children, and adults. While ABCA3 is expressed in various tissues, abnormalities are only found in the lung. Mutations in *ABCA3* (chromosome 16p13.3) are the most common cause of hereditary respiratory failure in newborns, are inherited in an autosomal recessive manner, and have a fatal course at the neonatal stage or lead to chronic respiratory failure during childhood. The most common genetic mutation is a missense point mutation, which causes the substitution of glutamic acid at the 292th codon by valine, E292V. NKX2-1 (TTF-1) is a protein that is specifically expressed in the thyroid gland, lung, and mesencephalon and regulates the expression of *SFTPA*, *SFTPB*, *SFFTPC*, Clara cell secretory protein, and *ABCA3*.

The NKX2-1 gene mutation is characterized by a disease that is similar to PAP of *SPTPB*, *SPTPC*, and *ABCA3* mutation and repeated infection. In addition, PAP due to lysinuric protein intolerance caused by an *SLC7A7* mutation has also been reported.

8.3.4 Treatment and Management

Clinical courses of PAP vary from natural remission to death. Among the 39 asymptomatic, untreated patients with autoimmune PAP from the Japanese cohort (17%), 11 (28%) showed spontaneous improvement, 3 (7%) had worsened disease and symptoms, and 25 (64%) had stable disease [69].

Treatment via lung lavage has recently become common, and the 5-year survival rate of autoimmune PAP in patients who receive this treatment is reported to be 95%. On the other hand, the median survival time of secondary PAP is 16 months, and the prognosis is relatively worse.

Because autoimmune PAP has spontaneous remission, no therapy is required in asymptomatic cases or in cases with mild respiratory failure. However, treatments such as lung lavage are selected for patients with progressive respiratory failure. The improvement of survival rate, symptoms, images, and pulmonary function has been reported, although the observations are retrospective [67].

GM-CSF replacement therapies with inhalation or subcutaneous injection are other options for treatment. These treatments are often administered to patients in whom total lung lavage has been ineffective and for patients who are not eligible to receive lung lavage because of poor cardiopulmonary function. In a retrospective study of 12 patients with autoimmune PAP, the improvement rate of GM-CSF inhalation therapy is reported to be 91%. GM-CSF subcutaneous injection therapy has been conducted in Europe and the United States, and it is reported that the effective rate is 40–50%. GM-CSF therapy has few serious side effects; however, there is no fixed predictor for the effect, which is a future task. Rituximab, also known as an anti-CD20 monoclonal antibody, can treat autoimmune PAP by lowering the concentration of the anti-GM-CSF antibody. There are a few reports that rituximab has been effective for all ineffective lung lavage cases [70]. Immunosuppressants and corticosteroid are considered to be ineffective for autoimmune PAP. In secondary PAP, pulmonary lesions may improve due to the treatment of the underlying disease. Total lung lavage can be used in combination. In the case of secondary PAP caused by inhalation exposure, avoidance of inhalation exposure is important.

8.4 Pulmonary Alveolar Microlithiasis

8.4.1 Introduction and Clinical Aspects

Pulmonary alveolar microlithiasis (PAM) is an extremely rare disease and an autosomal recessive genetic disorder in which the responsible gene was unidentified until recently. Familial cases of PAM occur at frequencies ranging from 36% to 61%; the disorder has been reported to occur among siblings and cousins in a horizontal pattern and less frequently between parents and children in a vertical pattern of familial inheritance [71]. In patients with PAM, microliths made of calcium phosphate arise in the alveolar space, slowly grow and occupy the space, and cause chronic inflammation or fibrosis in the alveolar wall. Ultimately, these lesions lead to a state of chronic respiratory failure.

An Italian scientist, Malpighi, was the first to provide a concise and detailed macroscopic description of the disease in 1686: "In vesciculis pulmonum innumeri lapilli sunt." Centuries later, the second case was reported by Harbitz in 1918 and was named PAM by Puhr in 1933 [72–74]. More than 1000 cases have been reported worldwide, and the most reports come from Japan; approximately 120 cases have been reported in the past 60 years [74].

8.4.2 Diagnosis

PAM may affect people of any age, ranging from early childhood to advanced age. However, affected individuals usually become symptomatic in the third or fourth decade of life.

Radiologically, a remarkable diffuse fine granular shade as a composite image of shadows by many microliths is observed in the chest X-ray, namely, exhibiting a snowstorm or sandstorm appearance (Fig. 8.9a). Chest CT images show characteristic image findings, such as calcification along the pleura, intralobular septum, and bronchovascular bundle, which sometimes develops partially fusible calcification (Fig. 8.9b).

Generally, the clinical symptoms are milder than indicated by the appearance of chest X-rays and CT images. Most of the reported cases are found during health

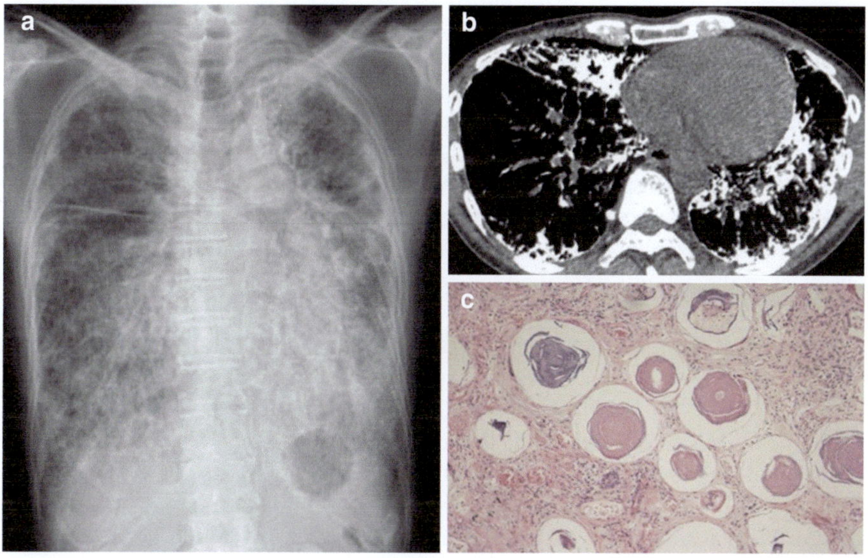

Fig. 8.9 Chest X-ray, CT scan of the lung, and autopsy in a patient with PAM (Provided by Dr. Torahiko Jinta, St. Luku Hospital, Nihon Kokyuuki Gakkaishi 2012;1:267–272)

checkups or checkups of family members of affected patients and are diagnosed by radiology and family history.

Histologically, PAM is characterized by the presence of microliths and alveolitis with a layered structure inside the alveoli (Fig. 8.9c) in samples from transbronchial lung biopsy, surgical biopsy, necropsy, bronchoalveolar lavage, and so on.

8.4.3 Extrapulmonary Manifestations

The *SLC34A2* gene is also expressed in the mammary glands, small intestine, kidneys, pancreas, ovaries, liver, testes, placenta, and prostate [71]. As a consequence, extrapulmonary calcifications can occur, including medullary nephrocalcinosis, nephrolithiasis, cholelithiasis, calcification of the lumbar sympathetic chain, and testicular involvement. A total of 34 cardiac complications, such as aortic and mitral valve and pericardial calcifications, have been reported.

8.4.4 Genetic Aspects and Relevance

In patients with PAM, there are findings consistent with autosomal recessive inheritance, such as a high frequency of consanguineous marriage, high-rate horizontal transfer, accumulation in marriage between relatives, and identical occurrence between men and women.

In recent years, two groups, Hagiwara et al. (Japan) and Corut et al. (Turkey), reported that inactivating mutations are present in the solute carrier family 34 member 2 (*SLC34A2*) gene, which encodes the Ilb-type sodium-dependent phosphoryl transport protein [75–76]. Alveolar type II cells produce pulmonary surfactant, of which phospholipids are essential constituents. Outdated surfactant is taken up by type II cells for recycling and degradation and by alveolar macrophages for degradation. Degraded phospholipids release phosphate that should be cleared from the alveolar space [77]. Huqun et al. showed that SLC34A2 was highly expressed in type II cells, and treatment with the proteins that had the mutations observed in the patients abolished the normal transporter function, as observed in the results of the microinjection assay in *Xenopus* oocytes [76]. Therefore, the dysfunction of SLC34A2 in type II cells may reduce the clearance of phosphorus ions from the alveolar space and lead to microlith formation in the extracellular fluids [71].

The *SLC34A2* gene is located on the short arm of chromosome 4 (4p15). It has 13 exons; the first exon is noncoding and encodes a 2280-nt mRNA and a 690-amino acid protein [71]. Many researchers have described homozygous mutation in this gene in PAM patients. A total of 18 mutant alleles have currently been identified (Table 8.1). Huqun et al. calculated that the frequency of a mutant allele in the general population is <0.008. Regarding mutations, exon 8 and exon 12 are more commonly

Table 8.1 SLC34A2 mutations reported in the patients with PAM

Location	Mutation	Effect of translation	Predicted consequence on protein	References
Promoter exon 1	c.[-6773_-6588del]	–	Not synthesized	Corut et al. [75]
Exon 2	insT (not specified)	Frameshift	Truncation	Dogan (2010) [78]
Exon 2–6	5.5 Kb deletion	Intragenetic deletion	Truncation	Ishihara (2008) [79]
Exon 3	c.212-224delACCTACCCACTCT	p.A71IfsX25	Truncation	Vismara (2015) [80]
Exon 3	c.114delA	Frameshift	Truncation	Corut et al. [75]
Exon 3	c.226C→T	p.Q76X	Truncation	Corut et al. [75]
Exon 4	c.316G→C	p.G106R	Substitution	Corut et al. [75], Özbudak et al. [81]
Exon 6	c.575C>A	p.T192K	Substitution	Ma (2014) [82]
Exon 7	insdel857-871	Splicing failure	Truncation	Huqun et al. [76]
Exon 8	c.910A>T	Premature stop codon	Truncation	Wang (2014) [83]
Intron 9	c.1048+1G>A	Splicing failure	Truncation	Huqun et al. [76]
Exon 11	c.1328delT	Frameshift	Truncation	Corut et al. [75]
Exon 12	c.1342delG	p.V448X	Truncation	Corut et al. [75]
Exon 12	c.1363T>C	p.Y455H	Substitution	Wang (2014) [83]
Exon 12	c.1390G>C	p.G464R	Substitution	Izumi (2017) [84]
Exon 12	c.1393-1404delACC	Threonine deletion	Aberrant	Jönsson (2012) [85]
Exon 12	c.1402-1404delACC	Threonine deletion	Aberrant	Jönsson (2012) [85]
Exon 12	c.1456C>T	G46Term	Truncation	Proesmans (2012) [86]

involved. In particular, the c. 910A>T exon 8 mutation appears to be common and might be the screening target for Chinese patients. There appears to be a high prevalence of PAM disease in some populations, including Turks and Italians [74].

8.4.5 *Treatment and Management*

PAM has been diagnosed in patients at various stages of life, and the disease has a long and progressive course that results in the deterioration of lung function [87]. However, to date, there is no medical or gene therapy for the management of patients with PAM. Systemic corticosteroids, calcium-chelating agents, and serial bronchopulmonary lavage have been shown to be ineffective. Based on the analyses of case series and experiences, lung transplantation remains the only possible treatment for patients with end-stage disease. Since PAM involves the dysregulation of phosphorus metabolism, a treatment strategy may target the reduction of the phosphorus ion concentration in the alveolar space [74, 76, 88, 89].

References

1. McCormack FX. Lymphangioleiomyomatosis: a clinical update. Chest. 2008;133(2):507–16. https://doi.org/10.1378/chest.07-0898.
2. Gupta N, Vassallo R, Wikenheiser-Brokamp KA, McCormack FX. Diffuse Cystic Lung Disease. Part I. Am J Respir Crit Care Med. 2015;191(12):1354–66. https://doi.org/10.1164/rccm.201411-2094CI.
3. Crino PB, Nathanson KL, Henske EP. The tuberous sclerosis complex. N Engl J Med. 2006;355(13):1345–56. https://doi.org/10.1056/NEJMra055323.
4. Harknett EC, Chang WY, Byrnes S, Johnson J, Lazor R, Cohen MM, et al. Use of variability in national and regional data to estimate the prevalence of lymphangioleiomyomatosis. QJM. 2011;104(11):971–9. https://doi.org/10.1093/qjmed/hcr116.
5. Adriaensen ME, Schaefer-Prokop CM, Duyndam DA, Zonnenberg BA, Prokop M. Radiological evidence of lymphangioleiomyomatosis in female and male patients with tuberous sclerosis complex. Clin Radiol. 2011;66(7):625–8. https://doi.org/10.1016/j.crad.2011.02.009.
6. Schiavina M, Di Scioscio V, Contini P, Cavazza A, Fabiani A, Barberis M, et al. Pulmonary lymphangioleiomyomatosis in a karyotypically normal man without tuberous sclerosis complex. Am J Respir Crit Care Med. 2007;176(1):96–8. https://doi.org/10.1164/rccm.200610-1408CR.
7. Johnson SR, Whale CI, Hubbard RB, Lewis SA, Tattersfield AE. Survival and disease progression in UK patients with lymphangioleiomyomatosis. Thorax. 2004;59(9):800–3. https://doi.org/10.1136/thx.2004.023283.
8. Hayashida M, Yasuo M, Hanaoka M, Seyama K, Inoue Y, Tatsumi K, et al. Reductions in pulmonary function detected in patients with lymphangioleiomyomatosis: an analysis of the Japanese National Research Project on Intractable Diseases database. Respir Investig. 2016;54(3):193–200. https://doi.org/10.1016/j.resinv.2015.11.003.
9. Taveira-DaSilva AM, Hedin C, Stylianou MP, Travis WD, Matsui K, Ferrans VJ, et al. Reversible airflow obstruction, proliferation of abnormal smooth muscle cells, and impairment of gas exchange as predictors of outcome in lymphangioleiomyomatosis. Am J Respir Crit Care Med. 2001;164(6):1072–6. https://doi.org/10.1164/ajrccm.164.6.2102125.
10. Taveira-DaSilva AM, Pacheco-Rodriguez G, Moss J. The natural history of lymphangioleiomyomatosis: markers of severity, rate of progression and prognosis. Lymphat Res Biol. 2010;8(1):9–19. https://doi.org/10.1089/lrb.2009.0024.
11. Ryu JH, Moss J, Beck GJ, Lee JC, Brown KK, Chapman JT, et al. The NHLBI lymphangioleiomyomatosis registry: characteristics of 230 patients at enrollment. Am J Respir Crit Care Med. 2006;173(1):105–11. https://doi.org/10.1164/rccm.200409-1298OC.
12. Tobino K, Johkoh T, Fujimoto K, Sakai F, Arakawa H, Kurihara M, et al. Computed tomographic features of lymphangioleiomyomatosis: evaluation in 138 patients. Eur J Radiol. 2015;84(3):534–41. https://doi.org/10.1016/j.ejrad.2014.12.008.
13. Lenoir S, Grenier P, Brauner MW, Frija J, Remy-Jardin M, Revel D, et al. Pulmonary lymphangiomyomatosis and tuberous sclerosis: comparison of radiographic and thin-section CT findings. Radiology. 1990;175(2):329–34. https://doi.org/10.1148/radiology.175.2.2326456.
14. Johnson SR, Cordier JF, Lazor R, Cottin V, Costabel U, Harari S, et al. European Respiratory Society guidelines for the diagnosis and management of lymphangioleiomyomatosis. Eur Respir J. 2010;35(1):14–26. https://doi.org/10.1183/09031936.00076209.

15. Ferrans VJ, Yu ZX, Nelson WK, Valencia JC, Tatsuguchi A, Avila NA, et al. Lymphangioleiomyomatosis (LAM): a review of clinical and morphological features. J Nippon Med Sch. 2000;67(5):311–29.
16. Matsumoto Y, Horiba K, Usuki J, Chu SC, Ferrans VJ, Moss J. Markers of cell proliferation and expression of melanosomal antigen in lymphangioleiomyomatosis. Am J Respir Cell Mol Biol. 1999;21(3):327–36. https://doi.org/10.1165/ajrcmb.21.3.3693.
17. Gao L, Yue MM, Davis J, Hyjek E, Schuger L. In pulmonary lymphangioleiomyomatosis expression of progesterone receptor is frequently higher than that of estrogen receptor. Virchows Arch. 2014;464(4):495–503. https://doi.org/10.1007/s00428-014-1559-9.
18. Kumasaka T, Seyama K, Mitani K, Sato T, Souma S, Kondo T, et al. Lymphangiogenesis in lymphangioleiomyomatosis: its implication in the progression of lymphangioleiomyomatosis. Am J Surg Pathol. 2004;28(8):1007–16.
19. Young LR, Vandyke R, Gulleman PM, Inoue Y, Brown KK, Schmidt LS, et al. Serum vascular endothelial growth factor-D prospectively distinguishes lymphangioleiomyomatosis from other diseases. Chest. 2010;138(3):674–81. https://doi.org/10.1378/chest.10-0573.
20. van Slegtenhorst M, de Hoogt R, Hermans C, Nellist M, Janssen B, Verhoef S, et al. Identification of the tuberous sclerosis gene TSC1 on chromosome 9q34. Science. 1997;277(5327):805–8.
21. European Chromosome 16 Tuberous Sclerosis C. Identification and characterization of the tuberous sclerosis gene on chromosome 16. Cell. 1993;75(7):1305–15.
22. Strizheva GD, Carsillo T, Kruger WD, Sullivan EJ, Ryu JH, Henske EP. The spectrum of mutations in TSC1 and TSC2 in women with tuberous sclerosis and lymphangiomyomatosis. Am J Respir Crit Care Med. 2001;163(1):253–8. https://doi.org/10.1164/ajrccm.163.1.2005004.
23. Astrinidis A, Khare L, Carsillo T, Smolarek T, Au KS, Northrup H, et al. Mutational analysis of the tuberous sclerosis gene TSC2 in patients with pulmonary lymphangioleiomyomatosis. J Med Genet. 2000;37(1):55–7.
24. Smolarek TA, Wessner LL, McCormack FX, Mylet JC, Menon AG, Henske EP. Evidence that lymphangiomyomatosis is caused by TSC2 mutations: chromosome 16p13 loss of heterozygosity in angiomyolipomas and lymph nodes from women with lymphangiomyomatosis. Am J Hum Genet. 1998;62(4):810–5. https://doi.org/10.1086/301804.
25. Yu J, Astrinidis A, Henske EP. Chromosome 16 loss of heterozygosity in tuberous sclerosis and sporadic lymphangiomyomatosis. Am J Respir Crit Care Med. 2001;164(8 Pt 1):1537–40. https://doi.org/10.1164/ajrccm.164.8.2104095.
26. Carsillo T, Astrinidis A, Henske EP. Mutations in the tuberous sclerosis complex gene TSC2 are a cause of sporadic pulmonary lymphangioleiomyomatosis. Proc Natl Acad Sci U S A. 2000;97(11):6085–90.
27. Badri KR, Gao L, Hyjek E, Schuger N, Schuger L, Qin W, et al. Exonic mutations of TSC2/TSC1 are common but not seen in all sporadic pulmonary lymphangioleiomyomatosis. Am J Respir Crit Care Med. 2013;187(6):663–5. https://doi.org/10.1164/ajrccm.187.6.663.
28. Ito N, Rubin GM. gigas, a Drosophila homolog of tuberous sclerosis gene product-2, regulates the cell cycle. Cell. 1999;96(4):529–39.
29. Tapon N, Ito N, Dickson BJ, Treisman JE, Hariharan IK. The Drosophila tuberous sclerosis complex gene homologs restrict cell growth and cell proliferation. Cell. 2001;105(3):345–55.
30. Sengupta S, Peterson TR, Sabatini DM. Regulation of the mTOR complex 1 pathway by nutrients, growth factors, and stress. Mol Cell. 2010;40(2):310–22. https://doi.org/10.1016/j.molcel.2010.09.026.
31. McCormack FX, Inoue Y, Moss J, Singer LG, Strange C, Nakata K, et al. Efficacy and safety of sirolimus in lymphangioleiomyomatosis. N Engl J Med. 2011;364(17):1595–606. https://doi.org/10.1056/NEJMoa1100391.
32. McCormack FX, Gupta N, Finlay GR, Young LR, Taveira-DaSilva AM, Glasgow CG, et al. Official American Thoracic Society/Japanese Respiratory Society clinical practice guidelines: lymphangioleiomyomatosis diagnosis and management. Am J Respir Crit Care Med. 2016;194(6):748–61. https://doi.org/10.1164/rccm.201607-1384ST.

33. Almoosa KF, Ryu JH, Mendez J, Huggins JT, Young LR, Sullivan EJ, et al. Management of pneumothorax in lymphangioleiomyomatosis: effects on recurrence and lung transplantation complications. Chest. 2006;129(5):1274–81. https://doi.org/10.1378/chest.129.5.1274.
34. Boehler A, Speich R, Russi EW, Weder W. Lung transplantation for lymphangioleiomyomatosis. N Engl J Med. 1996;335(17):1275–80. https://doi.org/10.1056/nejm199610243351704.
35. Birt AR, Hogg GR, Dube WJ. Hereditary multiple fibrofolliculomas with trichodiscomas and acrochordons. Arch Dermatol. 1977;113(12):1674–7.
36. Dal Sasso AA, Belem LC, Zanetti G, Souza CA, Escuissato DL, Irion KL, et al. Birt-Hogg-Dube syndrome. State-of-the-art review with emphasis on pulmonary involvement. Respir Med. 2015;109(3):289–96. https://doi.org/10.1016/j.rmed.2014.11.008.
37. Gupta N, Seyama K, McCormack FX. Pulmonary manifestations of Birt-Hogg-Dube syndrome. Fam Cancer. 2013;12(3):387–96. https://doi.org/10.1007/s10689-013-9660-9.
38. Toro JR, Pautler SE, Stewart L, Glenn GM, Weinreich M, Toure O, et al. Lung cysts, spontaneous pneumothorax, and genetic associations in 89 families with Birt-Hogg-Dube syndrome. Am J Respir Crit Care Med. 2007;175(10):1044–53. https://doi.org/10.1164/rccm.200610-1483OC.
39. Furuya M, Tanaka R, Koga S, Yatabe Y, Gotoda H, Takagi S, et al. Pulmonary cysts of Birt-Hogg-Dube syndrome: a clinicopathologic and immunohistochemical study of 9 families. Am J Surg Pathol. 2012;36(4):589–600. https://doi.org/10.1097/PAS.0b013e3182475240.
40. Kumasaka T, Hayashi T, Mitani K, Kataoka H, Kikkawa M, Tobino K, et al. Characterization of pulmonary cysts in Birt-Hogg-Dube syndrome: histopathological and morphometric analysis of 229 pulmonary cysts from 50 unrelated patients. Histopathology. 2014;65(1):100–10. https://doi.org/10.1111/his.12368.
41. Schmidt LS, Linehan WM. Molecular genetics and clinical features of Birt-Hogg-Dube syndrome. Nat Rev Urol. 2015;12(10):558–69. https://doi.org/10.1038/nrurol.2015.206.
42. Vocke CD, Yang Y, Pavlovich CP, Schmidt LS, Nickerson ML, Torres-Cabala CA, et al. High frequency of somatic frameshift BHD gene mutations in Birt-Hogg-Dube-associated renal tumors. J Natl Cancer Inst. 2005;97(12):931–5. https://doi.org/10.1093/jnci/dji154.
43. Khoo SK, Bradley M, Wong FK, Hedblad MA, Nordenskjold M, Teh BT. Birt-Hogg-Dube syndrome: mapping of a novel hereditary neoplasia gene to chromosome 17p12-q11.2. Oncogene. 2001;20(37):5239–42. https://doi.org/10.1038/sj.onc.1204703.
44. Schmidt LS, Warren MB, Nickerson ML, Weirich G, Matrosova V, Toro JR, et al. Birt-Hogg-Dube syndrome, a genodermatosis associated with spontaneous pneumothorax and kidney neoplasia, maps to chromosome 17p11.2. Am J Hum Genet. 2001;69(4):876–82. https://doi.org/10.1086/323744.
45. Nickerson ML, Warren MB, Toro JR, Matrosova V, Glenn G, Turner ML, et al. Mutations in a novel gene lead to kidney tumors, lung wall defects, and benign tumors of the hair follicle in patients with the Birt-Hogg-Dube syndrome. Cancer Cell. 2002;2(2):157–64.
46. Kennedy JC, Khabibullin D, Henske EP. Mechanisms of pulmonary cyst pathogenesis in Birt-Hogg-Dube syndrome: the stretch hypothesis. Semin Cell Dev Biol. 2016;52:47–52. https://doi.org/10.1016/j.semcdb.2016.02.014.
47. Kunogi M, Kurihara M, Ikegami TS, Kobayashi T, Shindo N, Kumasaka T, et al. Clinical and genetic spectrum of Birt-Hogg-Dube syndrome patients in whom pneumothorax and/or multiple lung cysts are the presenting feature. J Med Genet. 2010;47(4):281–7. https://doi.org/10.1136/jmg.2009.070565.
48. Schmidt LS, Nickerson ML, Warren MB, Glenn GM, Toro JR, Merino MJ, et al. Germline BHD-mutation spectrum and phenotype analysis of a large cohort of families with Birt-Hogg-Dube syndrome. Am J Hum Genet. 2005;76(6):1023–33. https://doi.org/10.1086/430842.
49. Hunninghake GW, Costabel U, Ando M, Baughman R, Cordier JF, du Bois R, et al. ATS/ERS/WASOG statement on sarcoidosis. American Thoracic Society/European Respiratory Society/World Association of Sarcoidosis and other Granulomatous Disorders. Sarcoidosis Vasc Diffuse Lung Dis. 1999;16(2):149–73.
50. Baughman RP, Teirstein AS, Judson MA, Rossman MD, Yeager H Jr, Bresnitz EA, et al. Clinical characteristics of patients in a case control study of sarcoidosis. Am J Respir Crit Care Med. 2001;164(10 Pt 1):1885–9.

51. Iannuzzi MC, Fontana JR. Sarcoidosis: clinical presentation, immunopathogenesis, and therapeutics. JAMA. 2011;305(4):391–9. https://doi.org/10.1001/jama.2011.10.
52. von Bartheld MB, Dekkers OM, Szlubowski A, Eberhardt R, Herth FJ, in't Veen JC, et al. Endosonography vs conventional bronchoscopy for the diagnosis of sarcoidosis: the GRANULOMA randomized clinical trial. JAMA. 2013;309(23):2457–64. https://doi.org/10.1001/jama.2013.5823.
53. Grunewald J, Eklund A. Lofgren's syndrome: human leukocyte antigen strongly influences the disease course. Am J Respir Crit Care Med. 2009;179(4):307–12. https://doi.org/10.1164/rccm.200807-1082OC.
54. Rossman MD, Thompson B, Frederick M, Maliarik M, Iannuzzi MC, Rybicki BA, et al. HLA-DRB1*1101: a significant risk factor for sarcoidosis in blacks and whites. Am J Hum Genet. 2003;73(4):720–35. https://doi.org/10.1086/378097.
55. Suzuki H, Ota M, Meguro A, Katsuyama Y, Kawagoe T, Ishihara M, et al. Genetic characterization and susceptibility for sarcoidosis in Japanese patients: risk factors of BTNL2 gene polymorphisms and HLA class II alleles. Invest Ophthalmol Vis Sci. 2012;53(11):7109–15. https://doi.org/10.1167/iovs.12-10491.
56. Valentonyte R, Hampe J, Huse K, Rosenstiel P, Albrecht M, Stenzel A, et al. Sarcoidosis is associated with a truncating splice site mutation in BTNL2. Nat Genet. 2005;37(4):357–64. https://doi.org/10.1038/ng1519.
57. Li Y, Wollnik B, Pabst S, Lennarz M, Rohmann E, Gillissen A, et al. BTNL2 gene variant and sarcoidosis. Thorax. 2006;61(3):273–4. https://doi.org/10.1136/thx.2005.056564.
58. Hofmann S, Franke A, Fischer A, Jacobs G, Nothnagel M, Gaede KI, et al. Genome-wide association study identifies ANXA11 as a new susceptibility locus for sarcoidosis. Nat Genet. 2008;40(9):1103–6. https://doi.org/10.1038/ng.198.
59. Feng X, Zang S, Yang Y, Zhao S, Li Y, Gao X, et al. Annexin A11 (ANXA11) gene polymorphisms are associated with sarcoidosis in a Han Chinese population: a case-control study. BMJ Open. 2014;4(7):e004466. https://doi.org/10.1136/bmjopen-2013-004466.
60. Miceli-Richard C, Lesage S, Rybojad M, Prieur AM, Manouvrier-Hanu S, Hafner R, et al. CARD15 mutations in Blau syndrome. Nat Genet. 2001;29(1):19–20. https://doi.org/10.1038/ng720.
61. Sato H, Williams HR, Spagnolo P, Abdallah A, Ahmad T, Orchard TR, et al. CARD15/NOD2 polymorphisms are associated with severe pulmonary sarcoidosis. Eur Respir J. 2010;35(2):324–30. https://doi.org/10.1183/09031936.00010209.
62. Stanley E, Lieschke GJ, Grail D, Metcalf D, Hodgson G, Gall JA, et al. Granulocyte/macrophage colony-stimulating factor-deficient mice show no major perturbation of hematopoiesis but develop a characteristic pulmonary pathology. Proc Natl Acad Sci U S A. 1994;91(12):5592–6.
63. Whitsett JA, Wert SE, Weaver TE. Diseases of pulmonary surfactant homeostasis. Annu Rev Pathol. 2015;10:371–93. https://doi.org/10.1146/annurev-pathol-012513-104644.
64. Kitamura T, Tanaka N, Watanabe J, Uchida, Kanegasaki S, Yamada Y, et al. Idiopathic pulmonary alveolar proteinosis as an autoimmune disease with neutralizing antibody against granulocyte/macrophage colony-stimulating factor. J Exp Med. 1999;190(6):875–80.
65. Suzuki T, Sakagami T, Rubin BK, Nogee LM, Wood RE, Zimmerman SL, et al. Familial pulmonary alveolar proteinosis caused by mutations in CSF2RA. J Exp Med. 2008;205(12):2703–10. https://doi.org/10.1084/jem.20080990.
66. Tanaka T, Motoi N, Tsuchihashi Y, Tazawa R, Kaneko C, Nei T, et al. Adult-onset hereditary pulmonary alveolar proteinosis caused by a single-base deletion in CSF2RB. J Med Genet. 2011;48(3):205–9. https://doi.org/10.1136/jmg.2010.082586.
67. Seymour JF, Presneill JJ. Pulmonary alveolar proteinosis: progress in the first 44 years. Am J Respir Crit Care Med. 2002;166(2):215–35. https://doi.org/10.1164/rccm.2109105.
68. Borie R, Danel C, Debray MP, Taille C, Dombret MC, Aubier M, et al. Pulmonary alveolar proteinosis. Eur Respir Rev. 2011;20(120):98–107. https://doi.org/10.1183/09059180.00001311.
69. Inoue Y, Trapnell BC, Tazawa R, Arai T, Takada T, Hizawa N, et al. Characteristics of a large cohort of patients with autoimmune pulmonary alveolar proteinosis in Japan. Am J Respir Crit Care Med. 2008;177(7):752–62. https://doi.org/10.1164/rccm.200708-1271OC.
70. Amital A, Dux S, Shitrit D, Shpilberg O, Kramer MR. Therapeutic effectiveness of rituximab in a patient with unresponsive autoimmune pulmonary alveolar proteinosis. Thorax. 2010;65(11):1025–6. https://doi.org/10.1136/thx.2010.140673.

71. Ferreira Francisco FA, Pereira e Silva JL, Hochhegger B, Zanetti G, Marchiori E. Pulmonary alveolar microlithiasis. State-of-the-art review. Respir Med. 2013;107(1):1–9. https://doi.org/10.1016/j.rmed.2012.10.014.
72. Harbitz F. Extensive calcification of the lungs as a distinct disease. Arch Intern Med. 1918;21:139–46.
73. Puhr L. Mikrolithiasis alveolaris pulmonum. Virchows Arch. 1933;290:156–60.
74. Castellana G, Castellana G, Gentile M, Castellana R, Resta O. Pulmonary alveolar microlithiasis: review of the 1022 cases reported worldwide. Eur Respir Rev. 2015;24(138):607–20. https://doi.org/10.1183/16000617.0036-2015.
75. Corut A, Senyigit A, Ugur SA, Altin S, Ozcelik U, Calisir H, et al. Mutations in SLC34A2 cause pulmonary alveolar microlithiasis and are possibly associated with testicular microlithiasis. Am J Hum Genet. 2006;79(4):650–6. https://doi.org/10.1086/508263.
76. Huqun, Izumi S, Miyazawa H, Ishii K, Uchiyama B, Ishida T, et al. Mutations in the SLC34A2 gene are associated with pulmonary alveolar microlithiasis. Am J Respir Crit Care Med. 2007;175(3):263–8. https://doi.org/10.1164/rccm.200609-1274OC.
77. Poelma DL, Ju MR, Bakker SC, Zimmermann LJ, Lachmann BF, van Iwaarden JF. A common pathway for the uptake of surfactant lipids by alveolar cells. Am J Respir Cell Mol Biol. 2004;30(5):751–8. https://doi.org/10.1165/rcmb.2003-0127OC.
78. Dogan OT, Ozsahin SL, Gul E, Arslan S, Koksal B, Berk S, Ozdemir O, Akkurt I. A frameshift mutation in the SLC34A2 gene in three patients with pulmonary alveolar microlithiasis in an inbred family. Intern Med. 2010;49(1):45–9.
79. Ishihara Y, Hagiwara K, Zen K, Huqun HY, Natsuhara A. A case of pulmonary alveolar microlithiasis with an intragenetic deletion in SLC34A2 detected by a genome-wide SNP study. Thorax. 2009;64(4):365–7.
80. Vismara MF, Colao E, Fabiani F, Bombardiere F, Tamburrini O, Alessio C, Manti F, Pelaia G, Romeo P, Iuliano R, Perrotti N. The sodium-phosphate co-transporter SLC34A2, and pulmonary alveolar microlithiasis: Presentation of an inbred family and a novel truncating mutation in exon 3. Respir Med Case Rep. 2015;16:77–80.
81. Özbudak IH, Başsorgun CI, Ozbılım G, Lülecı G, Sarper A, Erdoğan A, Taylan F, Altiok E. Pulmonary alveolar microlithiasis with homozygous c.316G > C (p.G106R) mutation: a case report. Turk Patoloji Derg. 2012;28(3):282–5. https://doi.org/10.5146/tjpath.2012.01138. https://www.ncbi.nlm.nih.gov/pubmed/23011834
82. Ma T, Ren J, Yin J, Ma Z. A pedigree with pulmonary alveolar microlithiasis: a clinical case report and literature review. Cell Biochem Biophys. 2014;70(1):565–72.
83. Wang H, Yin X, Wu D, Jiang X. SLC34A2 gene compound heterozygous mutation identification in a patient with pulmonary alveolar microlithiasis and computational 3D protein structure prediction. Meta Gene. 2014;2:557–64.
84. Izumi H, Kurai J, Kodani M, Watanabe M, Yamamoto A, Nanba E, Adachi K, Igishi T, Shimizu E. A novel SLC34A2 mutation in a patient with pulmonary alveolar microlithiasis. Hum Genome Var. 2017 Jan 26;4:16047.
85. Jönsson ÅL, Hilberg O, Bendstrup EM, Mogensen S, Simonsen U. SLC34A2 gene mutation may explain comorbidity of pulmonary alveolar microlithiasis and aortic valve sclerosis. Am J Respir Crit Care Med. 2012;185(4):464.
86. Proesmans M, Boon M, Verbeken E, Ozcelik U, Kiper N, Van de Casseye W, De Boeck K. Pulmonary alveolar microlithiasis: a case report and review of the literature. Eur J Pediatr. 2012;171(7):1069–72.
87. Mariotta S, Ricci A, Papale M, De Clementi F, Sposato B, Guidi L, et al. Pulmonary alveolar microlithiasis: report on 576 cases published in the literature. Sarcoidosis Vasc Diffuse Lung Dis. 2004;21(3):173–81.
88. Stamatis G, Zerkowski HR, Doetsch N, Greschuchna D, Konietzko N, Reidemeister JC. Sequential bilateral lung transplantation for pulmonary alveolar microlithiasis. Ann Thorac Surg. 1993;56(4):972–5.
89. Edelman JD, Bavaria J, Kaiser LR, Litzky LA, Palevsky HI, Kotloff RM. Bilateral sequential lung transplantation for pulmonary alveolar microlithiasis. Chest. 1997;112(4):1140–4.

Chapter 9
Pulmonary Vascular Diseases: Pulmonary Hypertension and HHT—What Are the Roles of Genetic Factors in the Pathogenesis of Pulmonary Vascular Diseases?

Toshihiko Sugiura and Koichiro Tatsumi

Abstract Heritable pulmonary arterial hypertension (HPAH) and hereditary hemorrhagic telangiectasia (HHT) are rare diseases with autosomal dominant inheritance. HHT is often found to be the underlying cause of pulmonary arteriovenous malformations (PAVMs). Mutations in *BMPR2*, *ACVRLK1*, *ENG*, *SMAD9*, *CAV1*, and *KCNK3* have been identified in cases of HPAH. Mutations in *ACVRLK1*, *ENG*, and *SMAD4* have been identified in cases of HHT. The average penetrance of *BMPR2* mutations is only 30% in HPAH. In contrast, the average penetrance of *ACVRLK1* and *ENG* mutations is almost 100% in HHT, but the affected organs often differ within the family. It is likely that there are additional genes and genetic/epigenetic or environmental modifiers such as hormones, inflammation, hypoxia, medications/drugs, or infections that play important roles to form phenotypes in HPAH and HHT. Further research is required to fully elucidate these potential mechanisms.

Keywords Heritable pulmonary arterial hypertension · Hereditary hemorrhagic telangiectasia · *BMPR2* · *ACVRLK1* · *ENG*

T. Sugiura (✉) · K. Tatsumi
Department of Respirology, Graduate School of Medicine, Chiba University, Chiba, Japan
e-mail: sugiura-respi@chiba-u.jp

T. Kaneko (ed.), *Clinical Relevance of Genetic Factors in Pulmonary Diseases*, Respiratory Disease Series: Diagnostic Tools and Disease Managements,
https://doi.org/10.1007/978-981-10-8144-6_9

9.1 Introduction

9.1.1 Pulmonary Hypertension (PH)

Pulmonary hypertension (PH) is defined by a mean pulmonary artery pressure of ≥25 mmHg at rest, as measured by right heart catheterization [1]. Recently, PH has been classified into five groups according to its cause: pulmonary arterial hypertension (PAH) (Group 1), PH due to left heart disease (Group 2), PH due to chronic lung disease and/or hypoxia (Group 3), chronic thromboembolic PH (Group 4), and PH due to unclear multifactorial mechanisms (Group 5) [2].

9.1.2 Pulmonary Arterial Hypertension (PAH)

PAH is an uncommon condition characterized by excessive pulmonary vasoconstriction, abnormal vascular remodeling (including medial hypertrophy, intimal fibrosis, and adventitial proliferation), and obliteration of small pulmonary arterioles. PAH has a poor prognosis and leads to right ventricular overload associated with severe right-sided heart failure [3]. The male-to-female ratio of PAH is 1:1.7, and it commonly occurs at the relatively young people with mean age of 36 years. PAH has a prevalence of 1–2 cases per million persons. In the past, PAH had a poor prognosis; however, advances in treatment, mainly novel pulmonary vasodilators, have improved the prognosis dramatically [4].

9.1.3 Heritable Pulmonary Arterial Hypertension (HPAH)

Familial cases of PAH were recognized in 1954 [5]. Before the availability of modern genetic tools, examination of family trees showed that heritable PAH is an autosomal dominant disease with incomplete penetrance. Previous studies reported that 6–8% of all PAH cases were familial [6].

In 2000, linkage analysis of PAH families and analysis of candidate genes identified mutations in the bone morphogenetic protein receptor type II gene (*BMPR2*) as a predisposition of heritable PAH [7]. Subsequently, other culprit genes such as *ACVRLK1* [8], *ENG* [9], and *SMAD9* [10] were also identified. Furthermore, beginning in 2010, whole exome sequencing using next-generation sequencing techniques led to the identification of more genes, such as *CAV1* [11] and *KCNK3* [12]. All identified genes exhibit an autosomal dominant inheritance pattern. Based on the results of these studies, PAH cases with the expression of culprit genes and a clear pattern of familial onset are now diagnosed as heritable PAH (HPAH). Mutations in *BMPR2* are detected in 75% of HPAH cases, whereas other genes are detected in <1% of all cases [13, 14].

9.1.4 Hereditary Hemorrhagic Telangiectasia (HHT)

Hereditary hemorrhagic telangiectasia (HHT) is a genetic systemic vascular disease characterized by recurrent epistaxis, cutaneous telangiectasia, and arteriovenous malformations (AVMs) that affect many organs including the lungs. According to the Curaçao criteria, a definitive diagnosis of this disease requires at least three of the four following features: spontaneous and recurrent epistaxis, telangiectasia, visceral AVMs, and a positive family history. HHT shows primarily dominant autosomal hereditary transmission with an estimated prevalence of 1 in 6000 [15].

For respirologists, HHT is often found to be the underlying cause of pulmonary arteriovenous malformations (PAVMs). PAVMs affect no more than 50% of all HHT patients. PAVMs provide direct capillary-free communications between the pulmonary and systemic circulations, which causes a right-to-left shunt in the lungs. The major consequences of PAVMs are paradoxical emboli and hypoxemia. Furthermore, a ruptured fistula can lead to expectoration of the blood and hemothorax [16].

About 8% of HHT patients develop PH. It is usually secondary to high cardiac output caused by visceral AVMs and to portal hypertension in association with liver vascular malformations. PAH is rarely observed in HHT patients [17].

The culprit genes for HHT have been identified as *ACVRLK1* [18], *ENG* [9], and *SMAD4* [19]; all of these show an autosomal dominant inheritance pattern.

9.2 Genetics of HPAH and HHT

9.2.1 BMPR2

BMPR-II, which is encoded by *BMPR2*, is a receptor of the bone morphogenetic protein (BMP) family, which performs an important function in angiogenesis [7]. This receptor is a member of the transforming growth factor (TGF)-β superfamily. After ligand binding, BMPR-II binds to and phosphorylates a type I receptor. The activated type I receptor then transmits the BMP signal to cells by phosphorylating downstream SMAD1/5/8, which is involved in regulating the expression of target genes.

The BMP signal plays an important role in the formation and maintenance of blood vessels and can suppress differentiation, proliferation, and apoptosis of vascular endothelial cells; it can also restrict the proliferation of vascular smooth muscle cells. Consequently, its action is directly opposite to that of the TGF-β signal. As a result, when the action of BMPR-II is attenuated due to mutations in *BMPR2*, the TGF-β signal is activated due to a reduction in the BMP signal, resulting in the apoptosis of vascular endothelial cells. Some remaining apoptosis-resistant cells become highly proliferative due to phenotypic transformation, and these can cause occlusion of the lumen if they proliferate in a disorderly manner. Furthermore, as the inhibitory effect on vascular smooth muscle cells is lost, the vascular intima thickens. These mechanisms result in stenotic and plexiform lesions in the pulmonary artery [20, 21].

To date, 390 different *BMPR2* mutations have been identified. These are all loss-of-function mutations and include nonsense, missense, splicing, and frameshift mutations and deletions or rearrangements affecting one or more exons or the entire *BMPR2* gene [22].

9.2.2 ACVRLK1 and ENG

ALK-I, which is encoded by *ACVRLK1*, is a TGF-β signal receptor. In the presence of endoglin, which is encoded by *ENG*, ALK-I undergoes phosphorylation, and the activated ALK-I transmits the BMP signal to cells by phosphorylating downstream SMAD1/5, which is involved in the regulation of target gene expression. All genetic abnormalities cause reductions in the TGF-β signal leading to functional disorders of vascular endothelial cells and weakening of the vascular structure, although the mechanisms involved remain unknown. This suggests that such genetic abnormalities can result in a variety of vascular lesions throughout the body. Interestingly, when ALK-I converts BMPR-II to a type II receptor through the BMP9 ligand, the downstream signal is SMAD1/5/8, which transmits the BMP signal. This may be the reason why mutations in *ACVRLK1* and *ENG* cause HPAH [23].

SMAD9, which is encoded by *SMAD9*, functions to positively regulate the signal transmission of BMP. However, as only a few cases of PAH have been reported to have mutations in *SMAD9*, the relationship between such mutations and patient symptoms remains unclear at the present time [10].

9.2.3 CAV1

CAV1 encodes the caveolon1 branch, which functions as a lipid raft on cell membranes. In the lungs, this is expressed in alveolar epithelial cells and pulmonary vascular endothelial cells. PAH patients experience reduced expression of *CAV1* in pulmonary arterial endothelial cells [24], and *CAV1*-deficient rat models have long been known to suffer from PAH-related complications [25]. However, as only a few cases of PAH have been reported to possess *CAV1* mutations, the relationship between this mutation and clinical symptoms remains unclear at the present time.

9.2.4 KCNK3

KCNK3 is a gene that encodes TASK-1, which is a pH-sensitive potassium channel. TASK-1 forms a variety of cellular resting membrane potentials, including those of pulmonary arterial smooth muscle cells. TASK-1 is also involved in the regulation of pulmonary vascular tone via the regulation of membrane resistance. TASK-1 has also been suggested to be involved in the regulation of pulmonary vascular remodeling and apoptosis [12].

9.3 Genetic Mutations and Clinical Disease Type

9.3.1 HPAH

PAH is usually diagnosed at a younger age and is associated with more serious hemodynamic compromise at the time of diagnosis in patients with than without *BMPR2* mutations. Moreover, the incidence of serious events such as death and lung transplantation in PAH patients <50 years old is higher in those patients with than without *BMPR2* mutations [26]. However, treatment with recently developed drugs has improved the prognosis of PAH patients with *BMPR2* mutations [27].

PAH patients with *ACVRLK1* mutations are younger at the time of diagnosis than patients with *BMPR2* mutations and noncarriers of a PAH-causing mutation. In the majority of patients with *ACVRLK1* mutations, the diagnosis of PAH precedes clinical manifestations of HHT. Despite more normal pulmonary hemodynamics at the time of presentation, *ACVRLK1* mutation carriers have a worse survival, suggesting either a poor response to PAH therapy or more rapid disease progression [28].

9.3.2 HHT

Cases of HHT with *ENG* mutations are known as HHT1, whereas those with *ACVRLK1* mutations are known as HHT2. HHT1 is more commonly complicated by lung and brain AVMs, whereas liver AVMs are more common in HHT2. Telangiectasia of the mucosa of the nose and mouth commonly accompanies HHT1 in younger patients [29].

9.4 Conclusion

The average penetrance of *BMPR2* mutations is only 30% in HPAH [7]. In contrast, the average penetrance of *ACVRLK1* and *ENG* mutations is almost 100% in HHT [17]. However, the affected organs often differ in the family, so that identical genes must be involved. Collectively, there are probably additional genes and genetic and environmental modifiers such as hormones, inflammation, hypoxia, medications/drugs, or infections that play important roles in HPAH and HHT. Further research is required to fully elucidate these potential mechanisms. Understanding the genetic etiology of PAH and HHT should facilitate better diagnosis and the development of novel therapies in the future.

References

1. Hoeper MM, Bogaard HJ, Condliffe R, et al. Definitions and diagnosis of pulmonary hypertension. J Am Coll Cardiol. 2013;62(Suppl):D42–50.
2. Simonneau G, Gatzoulis MA, Adatia I, et al. Updated clinical classification of pulmonary hypertension. J Am Coll Cardiol. 2013;62(Suppl):D34–41.
3. Tuder RM, Marecki JC, Richter A, et al. Pathology of pulmonary hypertension. Clin Chest Med. 2007;28:23–42.
4. Tamura Y, Kumamaru H, Satoh T, et al. Effectiveness and outcome of pulmonary arterial hypertension-specific therapy in Japanese patients with pulmonary arterial hypertension. Circ J. 2017;82(1):275–82.
5. Dresdale DT, Michtom RJ, Schultz M. Recent studies in primary pulmonary hypertension, including pharmacodynamic observations on pulmonary vascular resistance. Bull N Y Acad Med. 1954;30:195–207.
6. Lane KB, Machado RD, Pauciulo MW, et al. Heterozygous germline mutations in BMPR2, encoding a TGF-beta receptor, cause familial primary pulmonary hypertension. The International PPH Consortium. Nat Genet. 2000;26:81–4.
7. Deng Z, Morse JH, Slager SL, et al. Familial primary pulmonary hypertension (gene PPH1) is caused by mutations in the bone morphogenetic protein receptor-II gene. Am J Hum Genet. 2000;67:737–44.
8. Harrison RE, Flanagan JA, Sankelo M, et al. Molecular and functional analysis identifies ALK-1 as the predominant cause of pulmonary hypertension related to hereditary haemorrhagic telangiectasia. J Med Genet. 2003;40:865–71.
9. McAllister KA, Grogg KM, Johnson DW, et al. Endoglin, a TGF-beta binding protein of endothelial cells, is the gene for hereditary haemorrhagic telangiectasia type 1. Nat Genet. 1994;8:345–51.
10. Shintani M, Yagi H, Nakayama T, et al. A new nonsense mutation of SMAD8 associated with pulmonary arterial hypertension. J Med Genet. 2009;46:331–7.
11. Austin ED, Ma L, LeDuc C, et al. Whole exome sequencing to identify a novel gene (caveolin-1) associated with human pulmonary arterial hypertension. Circ Cardiovasc Genet. 2012;5:336–43.
12. Ma L, Roman-Campos D, Austin ED, et al. A novel channelopathy in pulmonary arterial hypertension. N Engl J Med. 2013;369:351–61.
13. Cogan JD, Pauciulo MW, Batchman AP, et al. High frequency of BMPR2 exonic deletions/duplications in familial pulmonary arterial hypertension. Am J Respir Crit Care Med. 2006;174:590–8.
14. Aldred MA, Vijayakrishnan J, James V, et al. BMPR2 gene rearrangements account for a significant proportion of mutations in familial and idiopathic pulmonary arterial hypertension. Hum Mutat. 2006;27:212–3.
15. Shovlin CL, Guttmacher AE, Buscarini E, et al. Diagnostic criteria for hereditary hemorrhagic telangiectasia (Rendu-Osler-Weber syndrome). Am J Med Genet. 2000;91(1):66–7.
16. Cottin V, Chinet T, Lavole A, et al. Pulmonary arteriovenous malformations in hereditary hemorrhagic telangiectasia: a series of 126 patients. Medicine (Baltimore). 2007;86:1–17.
17. Vorselaars VM, Velthuis S, Snijder RJ, et al. Pulmonary hypertension in hereditary haemorrhagic telangiectasia. World J Cardiol. 2015;7:230–7.
18. Johnson DW, Berg JN, Baldwin MA, et al. Mutations in the activin receptor-like kinase 1 gene in hereditary haemorrhagic telangiectasia type 2. Nat Genet. 1996;13:189–95.
19. Gallione CJ, Repetto GM, Legius E, et al. A combined syndrome of juvenile polyposis and hereditary haemorrhagic telangiectasia associated with mutations in MADH4 (SMAD4). Lancet. 2004;363:852–9.
20. Gore B, Izikki M, Mercier O, et al. Key role of the endothelial TGF-β/ALK1/endoglin signaling pathway in humans and rodents pulmonary hypertension. PLoS One. 2014;9:e100310.

21. Aschner Y, Downey GP. Transforming growth factor-β: master regulator of the respiratory system in health and disease. Am J Respir Cell Mol Biol. 2016;54:647–55.
22. Ma L, Chung WK. The genetic basis of pulmonary arterial hypertension. Hum Genet. 2014;133:471–9.
23. Upton PD, Davies RJ, Trembath RC, et al. Bone morphogenetic protein (BMP) and activine type 2 receptors balance BMP9 signals mediated by activing receptor-like kinase-1 in human pulmonary artery endothelial cells. J Biol Chem. 2009;284:15794–804.
24. Quest AF, Leyton L, Parraga M. Caveolins, caveolae, and lipid rafts in cellular transport, signaling, and disease. Biochem Cell Biol. 2004;82:129–44.
25. Drab M, Verkade P, Elger M, et al. Loss of caveolae, vascular dysfunction, and pulmonary defects in caveolin-1 gene-disrupted mice. Science. 2001;293:2449–52.
26. Evans JD, Girerd B, Montani D, et al. BMPR2 mutations and survival in pulmonary arterial hypertension: an individual participant data meta-analysis. Lancet Respir Med. 2016;4:129–37.
27. Isobe S, Kataoka M, Aimi Y, et al. Improved survival of patients with pulmonary arterial hypertension with BMPR2 mutations in the last decade. Am J Respir Crit Care Med. 2016;193:1310–4.
28. Girerd B, Montani D, Coulet F, et al. Clinical outcomes of pulmonary arterial hypertension in patients carrying an ACVRL1 (ALK1) mutation. Am J Respir Crit Care Med. 2010;181:851–61.
29. Letteboer TG, Mager JJ, Snijder RJ, et al. Genotype-phenotype relationship in hereditary haemorrhagic telangiectasia. J Med Genet. 2006;43:371–7.

Chapter 10
Mycobacterial Infection: TB and NTM—What Are the Roles of Genetic Factors in the Pathogenesis of Mycobacterial Infection?

Kazuko Yamamoto and Hiroshi Mukae

Abstract Human lung infections due to *Mycobacterium tuberculosis* have had a major impact on society. Nontuberculous mycobacterial infections have recently increased especially in developed countries and now being more prevalent than tuberculosis. Severe mycobacterial disease is mostly confined to patients who are immunocompromised either by acquired or inherited causes. Genetic aberrations in pathways critical for host defense against mycobacteria—which involve functional interleukin 12/interferon γ and the integrity of macrophages that modulate T lymphocytes—can lead to disseminated and fatal mycobacterial disease ranging from early-onset systemic infection to adult-onset localized disease, with clinical outcome dependent on the extent to which host genes are depleted and the pattern of inheritance. In addition, polymorphisms in genes encoding receptors and cytokines involved in innate immunity and host defense against mycobacteria are linked to mycobacterial disease susceptibility. The elucidation of genetic factors underlying mycobacterial disease can reveal the contribution of specific genes to immunological processes essential for the pathogenesis and control of mycobacterial infections in humans.

Keywords Mycobacteria · Tuberculosis · Gene · MSMD · Polymorphism

10.1 Introduction

Studies published over 50 years indicate that host genetic factors play an important role in determining susceptibility to and severity of infectious diseases. Tuberculosis (TB), which is caused by *Mycobacterium tuberculosis* (*Mtb*) infection, remains a

K. Yamamoto (✉) · H. Mukae
Department of Respiratory Medicine, Nagasaki University Hospital, Nagasaki, Japan
e-mail: kazukomd@nagasaki-u.ac.jp

T. Kaneko (ed.), *Clinical Relevance of Genetic Factors in Pulmonary Diseases*, Respiratory Disease Series: Diagnostic Tools and Disease Managements, https://doi.org/10.1007/978-981-10-8144-6_10

major cause of morbidity and mortality worldwide [1]. Approximately one-third of the world's population is infected with *Mtb*, with 10% developing clinical disease. Nontuberculous mycobacteria (NTM) are ubiquitous in soil, water, and man-made environments. Infectious diseases caused by NTM are increasing worldwide and are now more prevalent than TB in developed countries [2, 3].

Widespread mycobacterial infection of the human population over a long period of time creates evolutionary pressure in interactions between host and pathogen genomes. Mycobacterial diseases have been extensively analyzed from a human genetics point of view using various approaches such as case-control studies, candidate gene approaches, and family-based, genome-wide linkage analyses. Natural immunity to mycobacteria depends on the interleukin (IL)12/interferon (IFN)γ signaling pathway, which links myeloid cells (monocytes, macrophages, and dendritic cells [DCs]) to lymphoid cells (T cells and natural killer [NK] cells). Deficiencies and/or mutations in genes encoding components of this pathway are the major causes of genetic mycobacterial diseases, especially those caused by inherited inborn or childhood errors of immunity. Polymorphisms in host innate immunity genes have also been investigated, especially macrophage receptors involved in TB pathogenesis. This chapter describes recent findings on human genetic susceptibility to *Mtb* and/or NTM.

10.2 Mendelian Susceptibility to Mycobacterial Disease (MSMD)

MSMD is a rare congenital syndrome caused by genetic defects in the mononuclear phagocyte/T helper cell type 1 (Th1) pathway. MSMD patients have increased susceptibility to systemic infections by weakly virulent mycobacteria such as Bacillus Calmette-Guerin (BCG) vaccine strain and NTM. Mycobacterial disease generally begins in childhood and has diverse phenotypes ranging from localized to disseminated infection by single or multiple mycobacterial species that may or may not recur. Affected individuals are also vulnerable to the more virulent *Mtb*, and about half of patients also experience systemic salmonellosis, which is typically non-typhoidal and caused by *Salmonella* spp. Other severe infections can also occur—usually in single patients—that are caused by intracellular bacteria such as *Nocardia* and *Listeria* spp., intracellular fungi such as *Histoplasma* and *Coccidioides* spp., intracellular parasites such as *Leishmania* spp., and certain viruses. MSMD-causing mutations have been identified in seven autosomal genes (IFNγ ligand-binding chain [*IFNGR1*], IFNγ receptor signal-transducing chain [*IFNGR2*], Signal transducer and activator of transcription [*STAT*]*1*, *IL12B*, IL12 receptor subunit beta [*IL12RB*]*1*, Interferon regulatory factor [*IRF*]*8*, and Interferon-stimulated gene [*ISG*]*15*) and two X-linked MSMD genes (Nuclear factor kappa B essential modulator [*NEMO*] and Cytochrome B-245 beta chain [*CYBB*]) that are expressed in recessive, dominant, and haploinsufficient forms (Table 10.1 and Fig. 10.1). Three

Table 10.1 Characteristics of mycobacterial infection in MSMD

Gene	Inheritance	Disease onset	BCG infection	Systemic salmonella infection	TB	Other infections	Granuloma formation	Response to antimicrobial therapy	Indication for immunotherapy	Prognosis
IFGR1/R2										
Complete	AR	Infancy/early childhood	Yes	Yes	Yes	Listeriosis, herpes virus, respiratory syncytial virus, parainfluenza virus	No	Poor	No	Poor
Partial	AR	Late childhood	Yes	Yes	Yes	Bacteria, viruses, parasites	No	Favorable	Variable	Good
	AD	Late childhood/ adolescence	Yes	Yes	Yes	Histoplasmosis, Coccidiodes, VZV	Yes	Favorable	Yes	Good
IL12RB1	AR	Early childhood	Yes	Yes	Yes	CMC, *Klebsiella* spp. infection	Yes	Favorable	Yes	Fair
IL12p40	AR	Infancy/early childhood	Yes	Yes	Yes	CMC, Nocardia, *Klebsiella* spp. infection	Yes	Favorable	Yes	Fair
STAT1 LOF										
Complete	AR	Infancy	Yes	No	Yes	Fulminant viral infection	Yes	Poor	No	Poor
Partial	AR	Infancy/early childhood/ adolescence	Yes	Yes		Severe viral infection	No	Favorable	Yes	Fair

(continued)

Table 10.1 (continued)

Gene	Inheritance	Disease onset	BCG infection	Systemic salmonella infection	TB	Other infections	Granuloma formation	Response to antimicrobial therapy	Indication for immunotherapy	Prognosis
	AD	Infancy/early childhood/ adolescence	Yes	No	Yes	CMC	Yes	Favorable	Yes	Good
IRF8	AR	Infancy	Yes	No		CMC	Poorly formed	Poor	No	Poor
	AD	Late infancy	Yes	No	No	No	Yes	Favorable	No	Good
ISG15	AR	Infancy	Yes	Yes			No	Favorable	Yes	Good
NEMO	XR	Infancy/early childhood	Yes	No	Yes	Invasive pneumococcal disease	Yes	Variable	Yes	Fair
CYBB	XR	Infancy/early childhood	Yes	No	Yes		Yes	Fair	No	Fair
GATA2	AD	Late childhood/ adulthood	No	No		HPV, CMV, EBV, *Clostridium difficile*, histoplasmosis, aspergillosis	Yes	Poor	Yes	Poor

LOF = loss of function, AR = autosomal recessive, AD = autosomal dominant, XR = X-linked recessive, VZV = varicella zoster virus
CMC = chronic mucocutaneous candidasis, HPV = human papilloma sirus, CMV = cytomegalovirus, EBV = Epstein-Barr virus

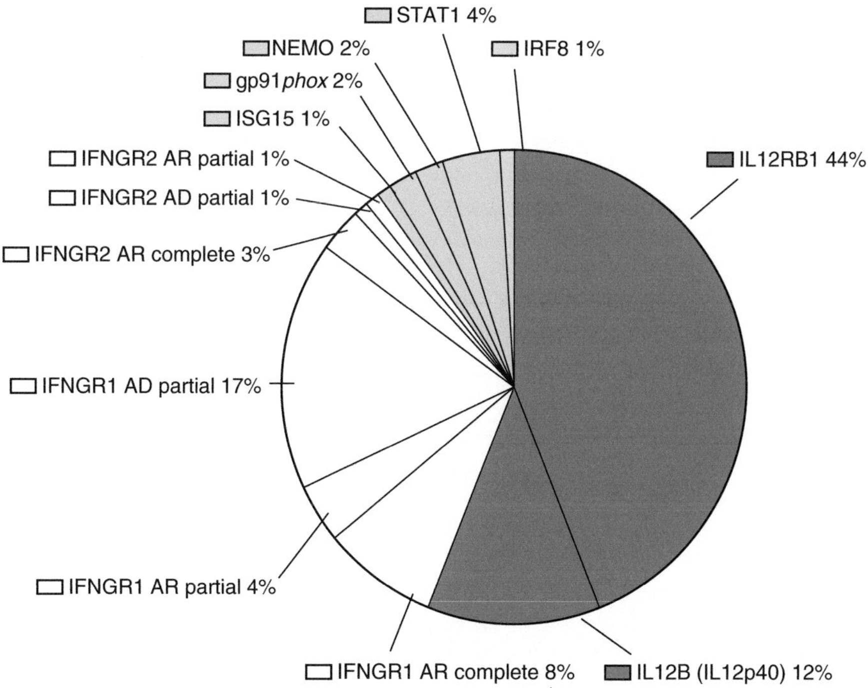

Fig. 10.1 Distribution of genetic disorders among MSMD patients with known etiologies. Genetic defects observed in MSMD patients with known mutations are shown. The proportions of AR (autosomal recessive) and AD (autosomal dominant) defects in autosomal genes (*IFNGR1*, *IFNGR2*, *STAT1*, *IRF8*, *IL12B*, *IL12RB1* and *ISG15*) and X-linked recessive (XR) genes (*NEMO* and *CYBB*) are indicated

of the autosomal genes (*IL12B*, *IL12RB1*, and *ISG15*) are implicated in the control of IFNγ production, while four (*IFNGR1*, *IFNGR2*, *STAT1*, and *IRF8*) are associated with IFNγ responsiveness. *IFNGR1* or *IL12RB1* deficiency is the most common cause of MSMD, accounting for almost 80% of all genetically diagnosed cases (Fig. 10.1). Immune deficiency is more severe in patients who completely lack *IFNGR1* as compared to those with partial *IFNGR1* or other gene deficiencies.

10.2.1 IFNGR Deficiency

IFNγ is critical for the immune response to mycobacterial infections, and defects in IFNγ production and response are associated with severe NTM infections. Mutations in *IFNGR1* and *IFNGR2* encoding IFNGR subunits can manifest as autosomal recessive (AR), or autosomal dominant (AD) mutations that can be subdivided into complete or partial forms. The first genetic cause of MSMD was discovered in 1996 as bi-allelic null mutations in the *IFNGR1* gene underlying AR complete *IFNGR1* deficiency [4, 5]. A total of 142 patients have been reported to harbor *IFNGR1* mutation and 27 have *IFNGR2* mutation worldwide (https:grenada.lumc.nl/LOVD2/mendelian_genes/status, Sep 2017).

AR complete *IFNGR1* or *IFNGR2* deficiency is typically associated with severe disseminated mycobacterial disease in infancy or early childhood (before 3 years of age) and is caused by BCG and/or weakly virulent environmental NTM such as *M. chelonae*, *M. fortuitum*, *M. mageritense*, *M. peregrinum*, *M. smegmatis*, and *M. scrofulaceum* [6] [7–9]. To date, 36 patients with 25 different variant mutations of AR complete *IFNGR1* deficiency and 13 patients with AR complete *IFNGR2* deficiency have been described [10, 11]. Compared to AD disease, AR complete *IFNGR1* deficiency is associated with more frequent mycobacterial disease episodes (a mean of 19 per person-years), greater dissemination (a mean of 4 affected organs per infection), and shorter disease-free intervals (a mean of 1.6 years) [6]. A typical histopathological feature in patients with AR complete *IFNGR2* deficiency is loss of granuloma formation [6]. Salmonellosis is less frequent (around 15%) compared to the IL12 receptor or ligand deficiency; however, the phenotype also includes increased susceptibility to cytomegalovirus, respiratory syncytial virus (RSV), varicella-zoster virus (VZV), and *Listeria monocytogenes* [12–14]. AR defects in *IFNGR1* or *IFNGR2* lead to complete loss of IFNGR protein expression [5, 15]. Over 50% of children with AR complete *IFNGR1* or *IFNGR2* deficiency die before 10 years of age as a result of severe and disseminated NTM infection and/or life-threatening infection by BCG [6, 16]. Cytokine replacement therapy has limited efficacy due to the lack of receptors, and the only curative treatment is hematopoietic stem cell transplantation (HSCT). However, it has a fairly low success rate because of fatal graft-versus-host disease and severe complications and generalized granulomatous response and bacterial sepsis [16]. Thus, patients with AR complete *IFNGR1* or *IFNGR2* deficiency have poor prognosis (58% and 33%, respectively, including deaths after HSCT) [16–19].

Rare AR partial defects in both *IFNGR1* and *IFNGR2*—in which IFNγ transduction is impaired but not abolished—have also been identified. In these patients, IFNGR is expressed on the cell surface but the response to IFNγ is diminished. A total of 15 cases of AR partial *IFNGR1* deficiency have been recorded in the Canary Islands, Portugal, Poland, and Chile, and 6 patients with AR partial *IFNGR2* deficiency were identified in Saudi Arabia, Israel, Mexico, Turkey, and France. Three of these 21 patients (14.2%) have died [11]. The disease typically presents in late childhood or even early adulthood and is usually less severe than AR complete disease but is nonetheless associated with disseminated mycobacterial infections. HSCT is not indicated, but treatment with antibiotics and IFNγ is necessary to control the infection [20].

AD partial *IFNGR1* deficiency has been described in 68 patients and is thus more common than AR complete deficiency [11]. The clinical presentation of this form is usually in late childhood or in adolescence, with a mean age of disease onset of 13.4 years. The typical presentation is mild, with fewer organs involved, good treatment response, less recurrence, and better survival; indeed, only 1.5% of cases result in death [6]. Patients are susceptible to BCG and NTM, which can in most cases be controlled by prolonged treatment with antibiotics with or without recombinant IFNγ. Histologically, more mature-looking granulomas similar to those seen in patients with AR partial *IFNGR1* deficiency are observed. Approximately 80% of patients with AD partial *IFNGR1* deficiency develop multifocal NTM osteomyelitis with almost no other sites of mycobacterial disease [6], which has become the hallmark of this genotype. *Salmonella* infection is rare (5%) [6]; other associated pathogens include *Coccidioides* spp. [21], *Histoplasma capsulatum* [22], and VZV [23]. The clinical penetrance of AD *IFNGR2* deficiency is very low, being confined to two affected siblings in a single family. The only treatment for symptomatic individuals is curative antibiotic administration [11].

10.2.2 IL12RB1 *and* IL12p40 *Deficiency*

IL12RB1 and *IL12B* encode the β1 chain and the p40 subunit, respectively, of the IL12 and IL23 receptors. Mutations in *IL12RB1*, which have been reported in over 220 patients worldwide (https:grenada.lumc.nl/LOVD2/mendelian_genes/status, Sep 2017), are the most common genetic cause of MSMD [24]. The combination of IL12RB1 and IL12RB2 is required for high-affinity IL12 binding and signaling. Patients with *IL12RB1* mutations present disseminated non-typhoidal salmonellosis and NTM infections or disseminated BCG infection following inoculation with the vaccine. In these patients, IFNγ secretion by otherwise healthy T cells and NK cells is impaired as a result of defective IL12R signaling. Clinical symptoms of patients with *IL12RB1* deficiency typically manifest in early childhood (around 2.4 years of age) and are most frequently caused by BCG (64%) [24]. The mortality associated with *IL12RB1* deficiency is around 30% and is largely due to severe NTM infection [24]. However, recurrent NTM infections are uncommon, possibly because of protection conferred by a previous BCG episode. Non-typhoidal, extraintestinal salmonellosis is the second most common infection in patients with *IL12RB1* deficiency (43%), and importantly, *Mtb* [25] and *Klebsiella pneumoniae* are also pathogenic in these patients [24]. Mild chronic mucocutaneous candidiasis (CMC) is commonly observed (27%), whereas invasive candidiasis is rare [26]. Patients must receive prolonged treatment with antibiotics against mycobacteria in addition to subcutaneous IFNγ administration [27]. HSCT is not indicated, although the overall mortality of 26% suggests that this option should be considered in select cases—for instance, when IFNγ treatment is not feasible or when a human leukocyte antigen (HLA)-compatible donor is available within the family [28]. Despite the large number of patients with AR *IL12RB1* deficiency, none with AR complete *IL12RB2* deficiency have yet been identified with MSMD.

The *IL12p40* gene mutation was the first inherited cytokine defect to be identified [29]; to date, 9 mutations in 50 patients from 5 countries (India, Iran, Pakistan, Saudi Arabia, and Tunisia) have been reported [11]. AR complete *IL12p40* deficiency appears to clinically phenocopy *IL12RB1* deficiency. BCG disease frequently occurs after vaccination, and infections caused by *Mtb* and NTM have also been reported

[30]. Salmonellosis occurred in 25% of patients and was often recurrent (36%) [31]. Other infections caused by various pathogens including fungi (*Candida* spp.) and bacteria (*Klebsiella* and *Nocardia* spp.) have been reported. The clinical penetrance of *IL12p40* deficiency can reach 50% before the age of 12 months. The mortality rate in the largest series was 32% in symptomatic patients, with a mean age at the time of death of 7 years [24]. HSCT is not indicated in most cases, and patients are treated with antibiotics and recombinant IFNγ over a prolonged period [11].

10.2.3 STAT1 *Deficiency*

STAT1 is a transcription factor downstream of the IFNγ receptor in the Janus kinase-STAT signaling pathway (Fig. 10.2) that plays a crucial role in the signal transduction of type I (IFNα/β), type II (IFNγ), and type III (IFNλ) IFNs. Following IFNγ stimulation, STAT1 is phospholylated and homodimerized to form γ-activating factor (GAF) (Fig. 10.2). *STAT1* deficiency varies in terms of severity and clinical presentation depending on whether the mutation is complete or partial and its effects on protein expression and function. Heterozygous loss-of-function (LOF) mutations in *STAT1* lead to impaired but not fully abolished responses to IFNγ, while

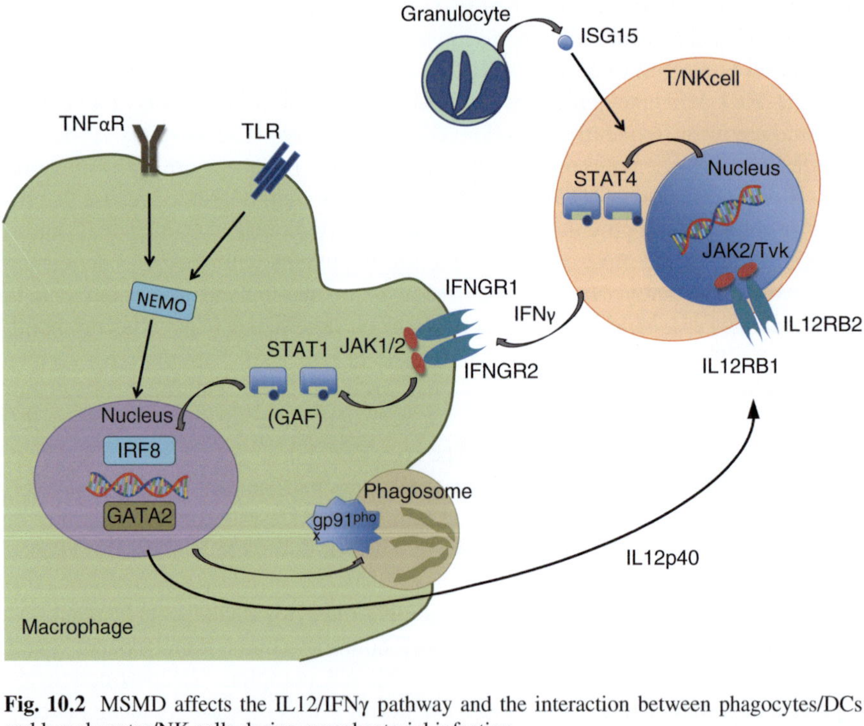

Fig. 10.2 MSMD affects the IL12/IFNγ pathway and the interaction between phagocytes/DCs and lymphocytes/NK cells during mycobacterial infection

homozygous mutations lead to partial or complete STAT1 deficiency. Gain-of-function (GOF) mutations can cause CMC [32], disseminated fungal infections [33], and NTM infections.

Patients with AR complete *STAT1* deficiency caused by bialleic *STAT1* LOF present a rare, life-threatening immunodeficiency that leads to increased susceptibility to both mycobacterial and viral infections [34]. Three unrelated patients with complete AR *STAT1* deficiency have been reported; all had disseminated BCG vaccine-related infection and died in infancy due to severe viral infection, including herpes simplex virus (HSV) and Epstein-Barr virus [34].

In contrast, AR partial *STAT1* deficiency has been associated with severe but curable intracellular bacterial and viral infections. This form is caused by a hypomorphic missense mutation that leads to impaired splicing of *STAT1* mRNA, which is not translated into a stable protein, resulting in low levels of functional STAT1 [35]. Two siblings identified with this defect both had recurrent and disseminated salmonellosis. Other reported manifestations include recurrent HSV and RSV infections and hepatosplenic mycobacterial disease [35].

AD *STAT1* deficiency, which has been described in two unrelated individuals, arises from a heterozygous point mutation in the *STAT1* gene [36]. *STAT1* LOF mutations predispose patients to mycobacterial infections due to selective impairment of the IFNγ-STAT1-GAF pathway, resulting in a mild clinical phenotype. Since the cellular response to IFNα/β in these patients is maintained, severe viral infections are rarely seen. Patients with AD partial *STAT1* GOF mutations predominantly exhibit CMC and have a much broader phenotype than those with LOF mutations that can range from recurrent infections by NTM, fungi, and John Cunningham virus (progressive multifocal leukoencephalopathy) [37]. Antibiotics and supplemental IFNγ are effective treatments.

10.2.4 IRF8 *Deficiency*

IRF8 is one of the nine members of the IRF family of transcription factors. Human IRF8 is present in mononuclear phagocytes that regulate the expression of IFNα and IFNβ response genes (Fig. 10.2) and is crucial for their ontogeny, maturation, and production of IL12 in response to IFNγ, which mediates protection against mycobacteria [38]. Two types of *IRF8* deficiency have been reported. AR complete *IRF8* deficiency leads to a total absence of circulating monocytes and DCs; one patient with a K108E mutation presented with disseminated BCG disease, oral candidiasis, severe respiratory infections in early infancy, and myeloproliferative syndrome necessitating HSCT [39]. The milder AD partial form of *IRF8* deficiency causes selective depletion of circulating DCs. This genotype was observed in two unrelated patients carrying the same mono-allelic mutation (T80A) of *IRF8* who had disseminated BCG disease in early childhood. IFNγ does not appear to be required and HSCT is not indicated [39].

10.2.5 ISG15 *Deficiency*

ISG15 is an intracellular ubiquitin-like molecule that stimulates the production of IFNγ by T and NK cells [40] (Fig. 10.2). Three patients from two consanguineous families and three unrelated patients have been reported with AR complete *ISG15* deficiency. The clinical phenotype is similar to that of *IL12p40* or *IL12RB1* deficiency and develops into disseminated mycobacterial diseases after BCG vaccination, but the infections are resolved by prolonged antimycobacterial therapy [41].

10.2.6 *X-Linked Mendelian Susceptibility to Mycobacterial Disease*

10.2.6.1 *NEMO* Deficiency

Outside of the IFNγ pathway, nuclear factor kappa (NFκ)B is a transcription factor that regulates a large number of genes with roles in immune and inflammatory responses. NFκB also regulates the development of tissues such as the skin, hair, and teeth. Its activity is partly controlled by NFκB inhibitor molecules including inhibitor (I)κB. NFκB is active when IκB is degraded upon phosphorylation by IκB kinase, which is an α/β/γ heterotrimer (also called NEMO) [42]. To date, six patients with hypomorphic mutations in *NEMO* have been reported as MSMD cases [43]. Complete deficiency in *NEMO* leads to incontinentia pigmenti in girls, which is usually prenatally lethal in males. Partial deficiency confers phenotypes ranging from anhidrotic ectodermal dysplasia with immunodeficiency to osteoporosis and lymphedema [44]. Increased susceptibility to a wide range of pathogens (NTM, encapsulated bacteria, some herpes viruses, and *Pneumocystis jirovecii*) has been observed, but most patients suffer from invasive pneumococcal disease [45]. Prognosis differs among patients, who may benefit from both antibiotics and IFNγ treatment [28].

10.2.6.2 *CYBB* Deficiency

CYBB (also known as gp91^{phox} or NADPH oxidase [NOX]2) is an essential IFNγ-inducible component of the NADPH oxidase complex that is strongly expressed in all phagocytic cells (Fig. 10.2). Seven males from two French families have been reported with two discrete mutations in *CYBB* (Q231P and T178P), which is the X-linked form of MSMD [46]. The normal respiratory burst by phagocytes, which produces reactive oxygen species that kill microorganisms, was impaired in patients due to a lack of NOX activity; these patients presented with recurrent or disseminated TB and BCG disease [46], and unlike those with *CYBB*-mutated chronic granulomatous disease (CGD), they more frequently experienced recurrent fungal and bacterial infections—especially of *Staphylococcus* spp. and *Aspergillus* spp.—as well as granuloma formation. The discrepancy in the infectious phenotype between *CYBB*-mutated MSMD and CGD patients may be explained by the impairment of the oxidative burst in macrophages but not in neutrophils and monocytes [47].

10.2.6.3 GATA-Binding Protein (*GATA*)*2* Deficiency

GATA2 is a hematopoietic transcription factor activated at the early stage of myeloid development. *GATA2* haploinsufficiency causes a wide range of clinical manifestations and is considered as a bone marrow failure/infection susceptibility defect. *GATA2* deficiency most often leads to monocytopenia and mycobacterial disease (MonoMAC), which is characterized by late-childhood or adult-onset disseminated NTM or fungal disease [48]. A decrease in or absence of circulating monocytes, DCs, NK cells, and B cells characterizes the hemograms of patients with *GATA2* mutation. Other infections observed in this syndrome include human papillomavirus infection, disseminated histoplasmosis, cryptococcal meningitis, invasive aspergillosis, and severe *Clostridium difficile* infection [49]. Noninfectious conditions including pulmonary alveolar proteinosis, erythema nodosum, and lymphedema also occur. Progression to aplastic anemia, hypoplastic myelodysplastic syndrome, or acute myeloid leukemia is a serious complication of *GATA2* deficiency [49]. HSCT has been successfully performed in several of these patients [50].

10.3 Genetic Polymorphisms and Mycobacterial Disease

Although mutations in these rare Mendelian susceptibility genes highlight the importance of IFNγ signaling in mycobacterial immunity, they cannot explain susceptibility to mycobacteria in the larger population. Polymorphisms—which are defined as genetic variations occurring in more than 1% of the population—are sufficiently common to contribute to the risk of mycobacterial infection at the population level. The immune response to mycobacteria is regulated by interactions between lymphocytes or antigen-presenting cells and the cytokines secreted by these cell types, and immunogenetics studies have revealed that polymorphisms in genes implicated in innate immunity increase susceptibility to mycobacterial infection. Although cytokines exhibit a low degree of genetic variation, an increasing number of association studies have shown that polymorphisms located in promoter regions of cytokine genes influence susceptibility to infectious diseases. Mutations in these genes may alter transcription factor recognition sites and thereby affect transcriptional activation and cytokine production. Representative polymorphisms in gene encoding cytokines and their receptors are presented in Table 10.2.

Table 10.2 Representative gane polymorphisms related to mycobacterial disease

Gene	Polymorphism(s)	Population(s)
MRC1	1186G/A(exon)	China
DC-SIGN	−336G/A (promoter), −871G/A (promoter)	South Africa, SSA, Gambia
TLR1	N248S, S602I (exon)	USA (African-American), Europe (Caucasian)
TLR2	R753Q (exon), R677W (exon), Insertion/deletion (promoter)	Turkey, Tunisia, Vietnam, Guinea-Bissau, USA (Caucasian)
TLR4	D299G	Tanzania, Spain
TLR8	rs3764879, rs3788935, rs3761624, rs3764880 (exon)	Indonesia, Russia
TLR9	rs352143, rs574386 (exon)	USA (Caucasian), USA (African-American)
TIRAP	S180L (exon)	Vietnam
CD14	−159C/T (promoter)	Mexico, Korea
VDR	ApaI (exon), BsmI (exon), FolkI (exon), TaqI (exon), FolkI-BsmI-ApaI-TaqI haplotype	Guinea-Bissau, China, Gambia, West Africa, South Africa
SP-A1	1416C/T (intron), 307G/A, 776C/T (exon)	India, Ethiopia
SP-A2	1382C/G (intron), 355C/G, 751A/C (exon)	India, Ethiopia
MBL	O allele, B allele, HYA/HYA, LYB/LYD haplotypes, G57E (exon)	India, USA (African-American), Italy, India, Ghana
TNF	−238G/A (promoter), −238GG genotype, −308G/A (promoter)	Colombia, Iran
IFNΥ	1616A/G, 874T/A, 3234C/T (promoter)	Gambia, Guinea-Bissau
IL10	−1082G/A (promoter), −1082G allele, −592A/C (promoter)	Cambodia, China, Turkey, Korea
IL12RB1	M365T, G278R, Q214R	Japan
MCP1 (*CCL2*)	−2518A/G (promoter), −2518GG genotype, −362G/C (promoter)	Zambia, Tunisia, Mexico, South Korea, Ghana

10.3.1 Pattern Recognition Receptors (PRRs)

One of the first lines of immune defense is the recognition and uptake of microorganisms by professional phagocytes—i.e., macrophages and DCs. Macrophage PRRs and phagocytic receptors include cell membrane-bound receptors such as the mannose receptor (MR)C1 (also known as cluster of differentiation [CD]206), DC-specific ICAM3-grabbing nonintegrin (DC-SIGN, also known as CD209), toll-like receptors (TLRs), and the vitamin D nuclear receptor (VDR); soluble C-type lectins (CTLs) such as surfactant protein (SP)-A, SP-D, and mannose-binding lectin (MBL); phagocyte cytokines such as tumor necrosis factor (TNF)α; and chemokines such as monocyte chemoattractant protein (MCP)1 (also known as chemokine [C-C motif] ligand [CCL]2). Polymorphisms in these genes have been linked to susceptibility to *Mtb* in different populations.

10.3.1.1 TLRs

TLRs are classified as members of the IL1R superfamily based on a shared cytoplasmic region known as the Toll/IL1 receptor (TIR) domain and are expressed by various cell types including host immune cells. TLRs stimulate the innate immune response to a variety of pathogens including *Mtb* [51]. Single nucleotide polymorphisms (SNPs) in TLR-encoding genes have been shown to influence interactions between ligands and receptors and determine susceptibility to infectious diseases including TB. TLRs are expressed either on the cell surface (e.g., TLR2 and TLR4) or intracellularly (e.g., TLR8 and TLR9) (Fig. 10.3). TLR1, TLR2, TLR4, TLR6, TLR9, and possibly TLR8 are involved in recognition of *Mtb* [52]. Evidence for genetic variants associated with TB is most abundant for TLR2, which functions

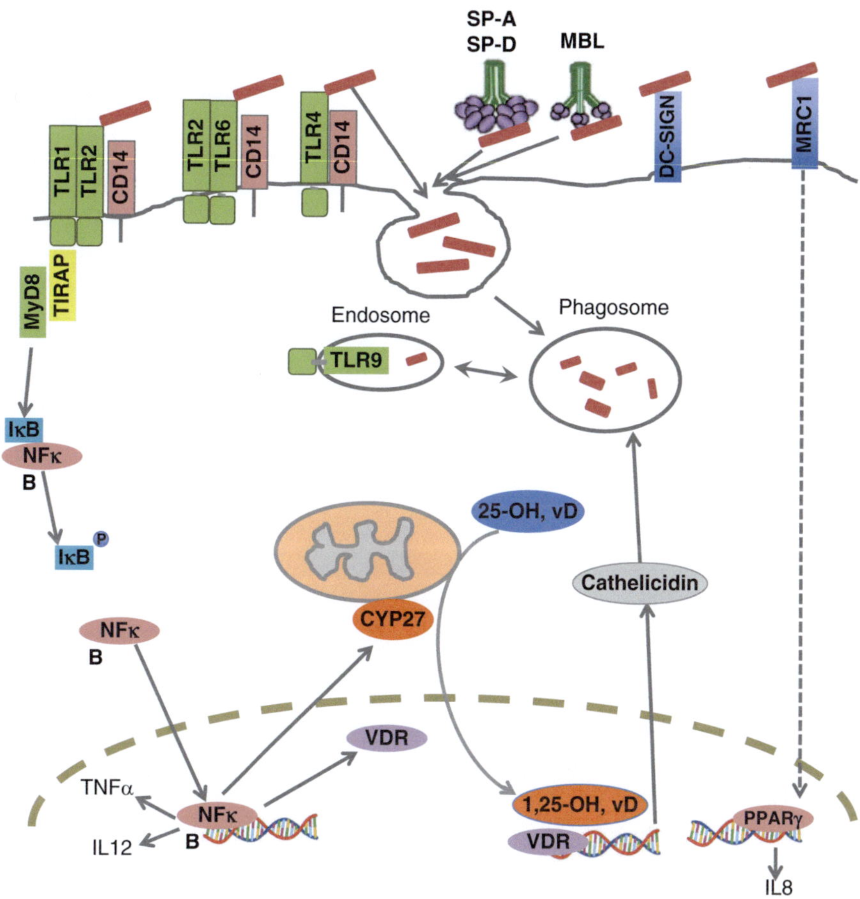

Fig. 10.3 Scheme of the macrophage innate immune network in response to mycobacterial infection

alone or as a heterodimer with either TLR1 or TLR6 (Fig. 10.3) [53]. The strong proinflammatory response to *Mtb* infection involving the TLR2 signaling pathway is mediated via its adaptor proteins myeloid differentiation primary response 88 and TIR domain-containing adaptor protein (TIRAP) [54]. This cascade leads to activation of NFκB, which induces the secretion of proinflammatory cytokines such as TNFα and IL12 by macrophages (Fig. 10.3).

Several polymorphisms associated with TB have been reported for different TLRs (Table 10.2). The *TLR2* R753Q [55] and R677W [56] variants are risk factors for TB in Turkish and Tunisian populations, respectively. Another SNP of *TLR2* (597T/C) was found to be strongly associated with TB meningitis and miliary TB in Vietnam [57]. Although there are no reports of an association between the *TLR4* D299G polymorphism and pulmonary TB, this variant was shown to be a risk factor for TB in human immunodeficiency virus-infected patients in Tanzania and Spain [58, 59]. In a diversified racial study evaluating 71 SNPs in 5 TLRs (TLR1, TLR2, TLR4, TLR6, and TLR9), significant associations with TB were observed for 2 variants each of *TLR2* (an insertion/deletion from −196 to −174) and *TLR9* in some, but not all, study populations [60]. In a large study of Indonesian and Russian populations, four sequence polymorphisms (rs3764879, rs3788935, rs3761624, and rs3764880) in the *TLR8* gene on chromosome X were associated with TB susceptibility in males [61]. A recent meta-analysis of 29 studies revealed an obvious increase in TB risk for *TLR2* R753Q, *TLR6* 745T/T, and *TLR8* rs3761624 GA genotypes [62]. The missense variant SNP S180L (975C/T) in TIRAP was found to contribute to TB susceptibility, and another polymorphic variant (558C/T) of TIRAP was associated with TB meningitis but not pulmonary TB in Vietnam [63]. These results provide evidence that TLRs and their signaling partners are true mycobacterial susceptibility genes; however, the functional significance of candidate mutations is unknown and varies according to the specific gene and allele, making it difficult to assess the clinical relevance of TLR-related genetic factors.

10.3.1.2 CD14

Efficient microbial recognition by TLR2 and TLR4 requires the activity of the co-receptor CD14, which is a 55-kDa glycosyl phosphatidylinositol-anchored glycoprotein expressed at the cell surface of monocytes, macrophages, and neutrophils [64]. A soluble form of CD14 (sCD14) produced during enzymatic cleavage of membrane-bound CD14 is an important acute-phase protein. CD14 interacts with various pathogen-associated molecular patterns, including lipopolysaccharide of Gram-negative bacteria and mycobacterial lipoarabinomannan (LAM). CD14 can also bind double-stranded RNA intracellularly and interact with TLR3 [65]. A study on the role of *CD14* gene polymorphisms in mycobacteria-associated infection identified the −159C/T SNP in the *CD14* gene promoter, which increased sCD14 production and decreased IFNγ secretion. The −159T/T genotype of the *CD14* gene reduced promoter binding and enhanced the transcriptional activity of CD14 [64]. A meta-analysis suggested that −159C/T polymorphism in *CD14* gene was associated with an increased risk of TB in Asians but not in Caucasians [66]. Additional studies in different populations are required to clarify the biological effects of the C/T SNP in the *CD14* gene and its relationship to TB development.

10.3.2 CTL Receptors (CTLRs)

CTLRs are a class of PRRs expressed in various immune cells that play an important role in *Mtb* recognition. This large protein family is divided into 17 groups that share a CTL domain. Among soluble CTLs, the main modulators of inflammation are MBL and SP-A and -D. Among transmembrane CTLs, DC-SIGN (CD209) and MR (CD207) are the most critical for the induction of an immune response against *Mtb*.

10.3.2.1 MBL

MBL is a collectin family member that recognizes pathogens via a carbohydrate-recognition domain and is an acute-phase serum protein secreted by the liver. Of the two human MBL genes, *MBL1* is a pseudogene, whereas the functional *MBL2* gene encodes MBL protein. By binding to *Mtb*, MBL acts as an opsonin, enhancing complement-dependent and complement-independent phagocytosis and promoting inflammation via the release of cytokines [67]. Four SNPs (at codons 52, 54, and 57) in exon 1, the promoter, and 5′-untranslated regions (UTRs) of the *MBL2* gene are associated with low or nearly absent serum MBL levels and may contribute to pulmonary TB susceptibility [68], although this remains controversial. Therefore, more work is required to clarify the relationship between MBL variants and TB.

10.3.2.2 SP-A and -D

A lung surfactant is a complex structure of lipids (90–95%) and proteins (5–10%) that promotes lung expansion and reduces alveolar surface tension. Lung SPs, which are collagen-containing calcium-dependent lectins known as collectins, are structurally similar to MBL. Of the four known SPs (SP-A, -B, -C, and -D), SP-A and -D are predominantly expressed by alveolar type II epithelial cells and recognize mycobacteria via their lectin domains while activating immune cells through their collagen domain to promote the uptake of pathogens by phagocytes and modulate the oxidative burst and intracellular bacterial killing [69]. SP-A exists as two highly similar isoforms encoded by separate genes (*SP-A1* and *SP-A2*). Allelic variants of SP-A and SP-D have been shown to influence susceptibility to *Mtb* [70], and an association between intronic and exonic *SP-A1/A2* SNPs and pulmonary TB has also been reported [64]. These polymorphisms may affect splicing and/or mRNA maturation, although this remains to be confirmed.

10.3.2.3 DC-SIGN (CD209)

The *Mtb* receptor DC-SIGN (CD209) is a calcium-dependent carbohydrate-binding molecule that recognizes mannose-containing glycoconjugates, including those present in the mycobacterial cell wall. It is a type II transmembrane protein predominantly expressed by subsets of DCs and alveolar macrophages that directly mediates phagocytosis and interferes DC maturation. The cytoplasmic tail of DC-SIGN has three conserved motifs that are involved in ligand binding and receptor signaling, phagocytosis, and intracellular trafficking of ligand particles [53]. Two polymorphisms in the *DC-SIGN* promoter region (−871A/G and −336A/G) were found to be associated with TB susceptibility. In a separate study, SNPs within the 5′- and 3′-UTRs of *DCSIGN* and *DC-SIGNR*—a homolog expressed in endothelial cells—showed possible associations with TB, with higher genetic diversity observed among Africans as compared to non-Africans [71].

10.3.2.4 MRC1 (CD206)

MRC1, also known as CD206, is a member of the CTLR family and a type I transmembrane protein abundantly expressed by alveolar macrophages and DCs. The carbohydrate recognition domain of MRC1 binds to mycobacterial mannose-*N*-acetylglucosamine- and fucose-terminated glycoconjugates, lipoglycan, and mannose-capped lipoarabinomannan (ManLAM). The latter is a cellular component of *Mtb*, and this interaction leads to antigen presentation and elicits an immune response. MRC1 also promotes the phagocytosis of *Mtb* and serves as a molecular link between innate and adaptive immune responses [64]. Recent studies have shown that the MRC1-mediated uptake of live *Mtb* or ManLAM by macrophages leads to upregulation of the nuclear receptor peroxisome proliferator-activated receptor γ, which is linked to macrophage anti-inflammatory pathways. In a recent case-control study, six non-synonymous SNPs (1186G/A, 1195G/A, 1212T/C, 1221C/G, 1303C/T, and 1323C/T) in exon 7 of the *MRC1* gene were found to be associated with pulmonary TB in the Chinese population [72]. The frequency of the G allele and AA genotype of 1186G/A was significantly lower in pulmonary TB patients than in healthy controls, and a linkage disequilibrium analysis showed a significant correlation between GGTCCT or GGTCCC haplotypes and TB susceptibility [73]. While a genetic association between MRC1 and TB is plausible, the causative polymorphisms and underlying molecular mechanisms have yet to be elucidated.

10.3.3 Cytokines and Their Receptors

The outcome of *Mtb* infections depends on cytokine networks established and maintained by infected macrophages and T lymphocytes that coordinate the immune response. Polymorphisms in the promoter or coding regions of cytokine genes may modify transcription factor recognition sites, thereby altering transcriptional activation and cytokine production, which may in turn influence susceptibility to *Mtb*.

10.3.3.1 IFNγ

IFNγ is a critical regulatory cytokine in host resistance to *Mtb* infection. IFNγ levels were shown to influence susceptibility to and the outcome of TB. Thus, polymorphisms in the *IFNγ* gene may play a critical role in the anti-TB immune response. Several SNPs in the human *IFNγ* gene promoter (1616A/G, 874T/A, 3234C/T) were found to affect *Mtb* susceptibility in different ethnic groups [74]. In particular, the 874T/A mutation disrupted an NFκB binding site, resulting in low production of IFNγ and increased risk of developing active TB. However, these findings were not corroborated in Gambia or the Republic of Guinea, where two other *IFNγ* gene polymorphisms (−1616A/G and 3234C/T) were associated with TB [74]. A recent study of 77 TB patients in Japan revealed that the *IFNγ* gene 874 AA genotype was a strong independent predictor of the time to achieve negative conversion of sputum [75]. This indicates that the presence or absence of this SNP can provide useful information for public health decisions regarding the required duration of patient isolation and clinical course of treated TB patients.

10.3.3.2 TNFα and TNFR1

TNFα, one of 19 TNF family members, exerts its functions via two receptors—namely, TNFR1 and TNFR2—and mediates the protective immune response against *Mtb*. TNFα acts in synergy with IFNγ and stimulates the antimycobacterial activity macrophages to kill *Mtb*. Two SNPs in the promoter region of the *TNFα* gene (−238G/A and −308G/A) were associated with reduced *TNFα* transcription and increased risk of pulmonary TB in Colombia; however, no association was observed in studies from Turkey, India, or Cambodia [64]. There are several reports of a correlation between TB and TNFR1 or TNFR2 (the SNP rs3397 and 3′-UTR haplotype GTT) in African populations [76].

10.3.3.3 IL12 and IL12RB1

IL12 is mainly secreted by phagocytic cells (monocytes, macrophages, neutrophils, and DCs), and induces IFNγ production by T lymphocytes via signaling through IL12 receptors (IL12RB1 and IL12RB2) while promoting the differentiation of Th1 cells. IL12 regulates host defense against *Mtb* infection via the IL12/IFNγ axis. Polymorphisms in the *IL12B* gene encoding the IL12p40 subunit have been detected in the promoter, introns 2 and 4, exon 5, and 3′-UTR [64]. Polymorphisms located in the promoter and intron 2 were found to be strongly associated with pulmonary TB in Moroccan and Chinese populations, whereas the others did not confer protection against TB. Three missense non-synonymous polymorphisms (M365T, G378R, and Q214R) in the *IL12RB1* gene have been linked to lower IL12 response and increased susceptibility to *Mtb* in the Japanese population [77], but no such association was found in studies from Morocco or Korea. An *IL12B* 3′-UTR SNP (rs3212227) was identified as a risk factor for pulmonary TB, but no associations were observed in genotypic and allelic tests in a meta-analysis [78].

10.3.3.4 IL10

IL10 is a potent immunosuppressive cytokine produced by activated monocytes and/or macrophages, DCs, B cells, and regulatory T cell subsets that inhibits cell proliferation and the secretion of inflammatory cytokines against *Mtb*. IL10 also promotes *Mtb* persistence in humans by blocking phagosome maturation in macrophages. Two SNPs in the promoter region of *IL10* gene, i.e., −1082G/A and −592A/C, have been correlated with susceptibility to *Mtb*; the latter was shown to decrease risk of infection, but the significance of the −1082G/A polymorphism in TB is unclear [64].

10.3.3.5 MCP1 (CCL2)

MCP1 (CCL2) is a β-chemokine that is produced by and acts on monocytes and macrophages, resulting in the suppression of IL12p40 and stimulation of matrix metalloproteinase (MMP)1 production in these cells in response to mycobacterial antigens. Human MMP1 plays a key role in the granulomatous reaction and may promote the spread of *Mtb* and persistence of non-resolving inflammation. A polymorphism in the promoter region (−2518, genotype GG) of the *MCP1* gene was shown to be associated with increased susceptibility to TB in studies from Mexico and Korea; increased plasma MCP1 levels in response to *Mtb* infection were accompanied by TB progression in carriers of the susceptibility genotype. The two-locus genotype −2518 MCP1—MMP1 2G/2G in Peruvians increased the risk of progression from latent to active TB. MMP1 overexpression may activate MCP1 and *Mtb*-driven inflammatory responses via activation of protease-activated receptor 1, leading to severe pulmonary TB disease and delayed response to treatment [79].

10.3.4 VDR

Before the development of antibiotics, TB was treated by vitamin D supplementation either through the diet or by exposure to sunlight. VDR modulates the antimycobacterial response triggered by TLRs as well as cytokine responses via binding to its ligand, the active metabolite of vitamin D (1,25[OH]$_2$D$_3$). The activation of TLR1 and TLR2 on monocytes increased VDR expression and vitamin D1 hydroxylase genes, leading to the intracellular killing of *Mtb*. Several VDR polymorphisms

(*Fok*I, *Taq*I, *Bsm*I, and *Apa*I) have been linked to TB resistance [80]. A Gambian study demonstrated that the homozygous T/T *Taq*I genotype was correlated with higher circulating levels of 1,25$(OH)_2D_3$ and may confer protection against TB [81]. In contrast, studies in Cambodia and West and South Africa found no association between any VDR polymorphism with TB susceptibility [64]. The heterogeneity of the results could be due to several factors including different ethnic backgrounds, population admixture, different case and control definitions, or small sample sizes. A family-based study conducted in West Africa suggested that VDR haplotypes rather than individual alleles or genotypes are responsible for increased susceptibility to *Mtb* [82].

10.3.5 HLA Alleles

HLA—with its ever-increasing allelic diversity (12,482 and 4592, class I and II alleles, respectively; http://www.ebi.ac.uk/imgt/hla/stats.html [as of September 2017])—is the most polymorphic locus in the human genome. The HLA complex consists of class I (HLA-A, -B, and -C) and class II (HLA-DM, -DO, -DR, -DQ, and -DP) molecules that present pathogenic peptides to CD8+ and CD4+ T cells, respectively. Several HLA alleles—particularly of class II—have been implicated in *Mtb* susceptibility, although this is controversial. A recent meta-analysis showed that HLA-DRB1*04, *09, *10, *15, and *16 gene polymorphisms contribute to the risk of TB, especially in East Asians [83]. Two Cambodian studies demonstrated that the HLA-DQB1*0503 allele and other DQB1 alleles (*0301, *0303, *0401, *0402, *0503, *0601, *0602, and *0603) were linked to *Mtb* susceptibility [84, 85] and increased susceptibility to pulmonary TB, while the HLA-DQB1*0503 allele resulted in decreased production of IFNγ by CD4+ T cells and impaired immune response against *Mtb*. Case-control studies in India and Indonesia have reported a higher frequency of HLA-DR2 allele (DRB1*1501) in TB patients [86]; a positive correlation between TB and the DR2 allele was supported by a meta-analysis [87]. However, no association was found in Egypt, Cambodia, Hong Kong, or Brazil [64].

10.4 Conclusions

Mycobacterial disease is a multi-factorial disease resulting from a strong immune response to a persistent pathogen. Genetic aberrations in the innate immune pathway have been linked to partial or fatal defects in host defense against pulmonary mycobacterial infection. A better understanding of the role of genetic factors in mycobacterial disease will not only facilitate molecular diagnosis and the development of more effective drugs targeting *Mtb* but can also enable clinicians to recommend individualized prophylactic and treatment approaches and improved family screening.

References

1. Dye C. Global epidemiology of tuberculosis. Lancet. 2006;367(9514):938–40.
2. Namkoong H, et al. Epidemiology of pulmonary nontuberculous mycobacterial disease, Japan(1). Emerg Infect Dis. 2016;22(6):1116–7.
3. Vinnard C, et al. Deaths related to nontuberculous mycobacterial infections in the United States, 1999–2014. Ann Am Thorac Soc. 2016;13(11):1951–5.
4. Jouanguy E, et al. Interferon-gamma-receptor deficiency in an infant with fatal bacille Calmette-Guerin infection. N Engl J Med. 1996;335(26):1956–61.
5. Newport MJ, et al. A mutation in the interferon-gamma-receptor gene and susceptibility to mycobacterial infection. N Engl J Med. 1996;335(26):1941–9.
6. Dorman SE, et al. Clinical features of dominant and recessive interferon gamma receptor 1 deficiencies. Lancet. 2004;364(9451):2113–21.
7. Marazzi MG, et al. Disseminated Mycobacterium scrofulaceum infection in a child with interferon-gamma receptor 1 deficiency. Int J Infect Dis. 2010;14(2):e167–70.
8. Pierre-Audigier C, et al. Fatal disseminated Mycobacterium smegmatis infection in a child with inherited interferon gamma receptor deficiency. Clin Infect Dis. 1997;24(5):982–4.
9. Koscielniak E, et al. Disseminated Mycobacterium peregrinum infection in a child with complete interferon-gamma receptor-1 deficiency. Pediatr Infect Dis J. 2003;22(4):378–80.
10. de Vor IC, et al. Deletion of the entire interferon-gamma receptor 1 gene causing complete deficiency in three related patients. J Clin Immunol. 2016;36(3):195–203.
11. Bustamante J, et al. Mendelian susceptibility to mycobacterial disease: genetic, immunological, and clinical features of inborn errors of IFN-gamma immunity. Semin Immunol. 2014;26(6):454–70.
12. Dorman SE, et al. Viral infections in interferon-gamma receptor deficiency. J Pediatr. 1999;135(5):640–3.
13. Wu UI, Holland SM. Host susceptibility to non-tuberculous mycobacterial infections. Lancet Infect Dis. 2015;15(8):968–80.
14. Roesler J, et al. Listeria monocytogenes and recurrent mycobacterial infections in a child with complete interferon-gamma-receptor (IFNgammaR1) deficiency: mutational analysis and evaluation of therapeutic options. Exp Hematol. 1999;27(9):1368–74.
15. Jouanguy E, et al. In a novel form of IFN-gamma receptor 1 deficiency, cell surface receptors fail to bind IFN-gamma. J Clin Invest. 2000;105(10):1429–36.
16. Roesler J, et al. Hematopoietic stem cell transplantation for complete IFN-gamma receptor 1 deficiency: a multi-institutional survey. J Pediatr. 2004;145(6):806–12.
17. Chantrain CF, et al. Successful hematopoietic stem cell transplantation in a child with active disseminated Mycobacterium fortuitum infection and interferon-gamma receptor 1 deficiency. Bone Marrow Transplant. 2006;38(1):75–6.
18. Reuter U, et al. Correction of complete interferon-gamma receptor 1 deficiency by bone marrow transplantation. Blood. 2002;100(12):4234–5.
19. Martinez-Barricarte R, et al. Mycobacterium simiae infection in two unrelated patients with different forms of inherited IFN-gammaR2 deficiency. J Clin Immunol. 2014;34(8):904–9.
20. Sologuren I, et al. Partial recessive IFN-gammaR1 deficiency: genetic, immunological and clinical features of 14 patients from 11 kindreds. Hum Mol Genet. 2011;20(8):1509–23.
21. Vinh DC, et al. Refractory disseminated coccidioidomycosis and mycobacteriosis in interferon-gamma receptor 1 deficiency. Clin Infect Dis. 2009;49(6):e62–5.
22. Zerbe CS, Holland SM. Disseminated histoplasmosis in persons with interferon-gamma receptor 1 deficiency. Clin Infect Dis. 2005;41(4):e38–41.
23. Roesler J, et al. Meningoencephalitis caused by varicella-zoster virus reactivation in a child with dominant partial interferon-gamma receptor-1 deficiency. Pediatr Infect Dis J. 2011;30(3):265–6.
24. de Beaucoudrey L, et al. Revisiting human IL-12Rbeta1 deficiency: a survey of 141 patients from 30 countries. Medicine (Baltimore). 2010;89(6):381–402.

25. Tabarsi P, et al. Lethal tuberculosis in a previously healthy adult with IL-12 receptor deficiency. J Clin Immunol. 2011;31(4):537–9.
26. Ouederni M, et al. Clinical features of Candidiasis in patients with inherited interleukin 12 receptor beta1 deficiency. Clin Infect Dis. 2014;58(2):204–13.
27. Alangari AA, et al. Treatment of disseminated mycobacterial infection with high-dose IFN-gamma in a patient with IL-12Rbeta1 deficiency. Clin Dev Immunol. 2011;2011:691956.
28. Holland SM. Immunotherapy of mycobacterial infections. Semin Respir Infect. 2001;16(1):47–59.
29. Altare F, et al. Inherited interleukin 12 deficiency in a child with bacille Calmette-Guerin and Salmonella enteritidis disseminated infection. J Clin Invest. 1998;102(12):2035–40.
30. Prando C, et al. Inherited IL-12p40 deficiency: genetic, immunologic, and clinical features of 49 patients from 30 kindreds. Medicine (Baltimore). 2013;92(2):109–22.
31. MacLennan C, et al. Interleukin (IL)-12 and IL-23 are key cytokines for immunity against Salmonella in humans. J Infect Dis. 2004;190(10):1755–7.
32. Liu L, et al. Gain-of-function human STAT1 mutations impair IL-17 immunity and underlie chronic mucocutaneous candidiasis. J Exp Med. 2011;208(8):1635–48.
33. Kumar N, et al. Gain-of-function signal transducer and activator of transcription 1 (STAT1) mutation-related primary immunodeficiency is associated with disseminated mucormycosis. J Allergy Clin Immunol. 2014;134(1):236–9.
34. Dupuis S, et al. Impaired response to interferon-alpha/beta and lethal viral disease in human STAT1 deficiency. Nat Genet. 2003;33(3):388–91.
35. Chapgier A, et al. A partial form of recessive STAT1 deficiency in humans. J Clin Invest. 2009;119(6):1502–14.
36. Dupuis S, et al. Impairment of mycobacterial but not viral immunity by a germline human STAT1 mutation. Science. 2001;293(5528):300–3.
37. Uzel G, et al. Dominant gain-of-function STAT1 mutations in FOXP3 wild-type immune dysregulation-polyendocrinopathy-enteropathy-X-linked-like syndrome. J Allergy Clin Immunol. 2013;131(6):1611–23.
38. Salem S, Gros P. Genetic determinants of susceptibility to Mycobacterial infections: IRF8, a new kid on the block. Adv Exp Med Biol. 2013;783:45–80.
39. Hambleton S, et al. IRF8 mutations and human dendritic-cell immunodeficiency. N Engl J Med. 2011;365(2):127–38.
40. Fan JB, Zhang DE. ISG15 regulates IFN-gamma immunity in human mycobacterial disease. Cell Res. 2013;23(2):173–5.
41. Zhang X, et al. Human intracellular ISG15 prevents interferon-alpha/beta over-amplification and auto-inflammation. Nature. 2015;517(7532):89–93.
42. Salt BH, et al. IKBKG (nuclear factor-kappa B essential modulator) mutation can be associated with opportunistic infection without impairing Toll-like receptor function. J Allergy Clin Immunol. 2008;121(4):976–82.
43. Filipe-Santos O, et al. Inborn errors of IL-12/23- and IFN-gamma-mediated immunity: molecular, cellular, and clinical features. Semin Immunol. 2006;18(6):347–61.
44. Courtois G. The NF-kappaB signaling pathway in human genetic diseases. Cell Mol Life Sci. 2005;62(15):1682–91.
45. Doffinger R, et al. X-linked anhidrotic ectodermal dysplasia with immunodeficiency is caused by impaired NF-kappaB signaling. Nat Genet. 2001;27(3):277–85.
46. Bustamante J, et al. Germline CYBB mutations that selectively affect macrophages in kindreds with X-linked predisposition to tuberculous mycobacterial disease. Nat Immunol. 2011;12(3):213–21.
47. Haverkamp MH, van de Vosse E, van Dissel JT. Nontuberculous mycobacterial infections in children with inborn errors of the immune system. J Infect. 2014;68(Suppl 1):S134–50.
48. Hsu AP, et al. Mutations in GATA2 are associated with the autosomal dominant and sporadic monocytopenia and mycobacterial infection (MonoMAC) syndrome. Blood. 2011;118(10):2653–5.

49. Spinner MA, et al. GATA2 deficiency: a protean disorder of hematopoiesis, lymphatics, and immunity. Blood. 2013;123(6):809–21.
50. Cuellar-Rodriguez J, et al. Successful allogeneic hematopoietic stem cell transplantation for GATA2 deficiency. Blood. 2011;118(13):3715–20.
51. Kawai T, Akira S. The role of pattern-recognition receptors in innate immunity: update on Toll-like receptors. Nat Immunol. 2010;11(5):373–84.
52. Jo EK. Mycobacterial interaction with innate receptors: TLRs, C-type lectins, and NLRs. Curr Opin Infect Dis. 2008;21(3):279–86.
53. Azad AK, Sadee W, Schlesinger LS. Innate immune gene polymorphisms in tuberculosis. Infect Immun. 2012;80(10):3343–59.
54. Quesniaux VJ, et al. Toll-like receptor 2 (TLR2)-dependent-positive and TLR2-independent-negative regulation of proinflammatory cytokines by mycobacterial lipomannans. J Immunol. 2004;172(7):4425–34.
55. Ben-Ali M, et al. Toll-like receptor 2 Arg677Trp polymorphism is associated with susceptibility to tuberculosis in Tunisian patients. Clin Diagn Lab Immunol. 2004;11(3):625–6.
56. Dalgic N, et al. Arg753Gln polymorphism of the human Toll-like receptor 2 gene from infection to disease in pediatric tuberculosis. Hum Immunol. 2011;72(5):440–5.
57. Thuong NT, et al. A polymorphism in human TLR2 is associated with increased susceptibility to tuberculous meningitis. Genes Immun. 2007;8(5):422–8.
58. Ferwerda B, et al. The toll-like receptor 4 Asp299Gly variant and tuberculosis susceptibility in HIV-infected patients in Tanzania. AIDS. 2007;21(10):1375–7.
59. Pulido I, et al. The TLR4 ASP299GLY polymorphism is a risk factor for active tuberculosis in Caucasian HIV-infected patients. Curr HIV Res. 2010;8(3):253–8.
60. Velez DR, et al. Variants in toll-like receptors 2 and 9 influence susceptibility to pulmonary tuberculosis in Caucasians, African-Americans, and West Africans. Hum Genet. 2010;127(1):65–73.
61. Davila S, et al. Genetic association and expression studies indicate a role of toll-like receptor 8 in pulmonary tuberculosis. PLoS Genet. 2008;4(10):e1000218.
62. Sun Q, et al. Toll-like receptor polymorphisms and tuberculosis susceptibility: a comprehensive meta-analysis. J Huazhong Univ Sci Technolog Med Sci. 2015;35(2):157–68.
63. Hawn TR, et al. A polymorphism in Toll-interleukin 1 receptor domain containing adaptor protein is associated with susceptibility to meningeal tuberculosis. J Infect Dis. 2006;194(8):1127–34.
64. Fol M, et al. Immune response gene polymorphisms in tuberculosis. Acta Biochim Pol. 2015;62(4):633–40.
65. Lee HK, et al. Double-stranded RNA-mediated TLR3 activation is enhanced by CD14. Immunity. 2006;24(2):153–63.
66. Yuan Q, et al. The association between C-159T polymorphism in CD14 gene and susceptibility to tuberculosis: a meta-analysis. Mol Biol Rep. 2014;41(11):7623–9.
67. Takahashi K, Ezekowitz RA. The role of the mannose-binding lectin in innate immunity. Clin Infect Dis. 2005;41(Suppl 7):S440–4.
68. Yim JJ, Selvaraj P. Genetic susceptibility in tuberculosis. Respirology. 2010;15(2):241–56.
69. Haataja R, Hallman M. Surfactant proteins as genetic determinants of multifactorial pulmonary diseases. Ann Med. 2002;34(5):324–33.
70. Floros J, et al. Surfactant protein genetic marker alleles identify a subgroup of tuberculosis in a Mexican population. J Infect Dis. 2000;182(5):1473–8.
71. Boily-Larouche G, et al. DC-SIGN and DC-SIGNR genetic diversity among different ethnic populations: potential implications for pathogen recognition and disease susceptibility. Hum Immunol. 2007;68(6):523–30.
72. Zhang X, et al. The novel human MRC1 gene polymorphisms are associated with susceptibility to pulmonary tuberculosis in Chinese Uygur and Kazak populations. Mol Biol Rep. 2013;40(8):5073–83.

73. Alter A, et al. Genetic and functional analysis of common MRC1 exon 7 polymorphisms in leprosy susceptibility. Hum Genet. 2010;127(3):337–48.
74. Cooke GS, et al. Polymorphism within the interferon-gamma/receptor complex is associated with pulmonary tuberculosis. Am J Respir Crit Care Med. 2006;174(3):339–43.
75. Shibasaki M, et al. An influence of Interferon-gamma gene polymorphisms on treatment response to tuberculosis in Japanese population. J Infect. 2009;58(6):467–9.
76. Moller M, et al. A functional haplotype in the 3′untranslated region of TNFRSF1B is associated with tuberculosis in two African populations. Am J Respir Crit Care Med. 2010;181(4):388–93.
77. Akahoshi M, et al. Influence of interleukin-12 receptor beta1 polymorphisms on tuberculosis. Hum Genet. 2003;112(3):237–43.
78. Liu G, et al. Association between IL12B polymorphisms and tuberculosis risk: a meta-analysis. Infect Genet Evol. 2013;21:401–7.
79. Ganachari M, et al. Host gene-encoded severe lung TB: from genes to the potential pathways. Genes Immun. 2012;13(8):605–20.
80. Sun YP, Cai QS. Vitamin D receptor FokI gene polymorphism and tuberculosis susceptibility: a meta-analysis. Genet Mol Res. 2015;14(2):6156–63.
81. Bellamy R, et al. Tuberculosis and chronic hepatitis B virus infection in Africans and variation in the vitamin D receptor gene. J Infect Dis. 1999;179(3):721–4.
82. Bornman L, et al. Vitamin D receptor polymorphisms and susceptibility to tuberculosis in West Africa: a case-control and family study. J Infect Dis. 2004;190(9):1631–41.
83. Tong X, et al. Polymorphisms in HLA-DRB1 gene and the risk of tuberculosis: a meta-analysis of 31 studies. Lung. 2015;193(2):309–18.
84. Goldfeld AE, et al. Association of an HLA-DQ allele with clinical tuberculosis. JAMA. 1998;279(3):226–8.
85. Goldfeld AE. Genetic susceptibility to pulmonary tuberculosis in Cambodia. Tuberculosis (Edinb). 2004;84(1–2):76–81.
86. Bothamley GH, et al. Association of tuberculosis and M. tuberculosis-specific antibody levels with HLA. J Infect Dis. 1989;159(3):549–55.
87. Kettaneh A, et al. Human leukocyte antigens and susceptibility to tuberculosis: a meta-analysis of case-control studies. Int J Tuberc Lung Dis. 2006;10(7):717–25.

Chapter 11
Pulmonary Malignancies (1): Lung Cancer—What Are the Roles of Genetic Factors in Lung Cancer Pathogenesis?

Naozumi Hashimoto, Mitsuo Sato, and Yoshinori Hasegawa

Abstract Carcinogenesis, including that of lung cancer, has been shown to be caused by the accumulation of genetic alterations. Some of the genetic changes are germline mutations, inherited gene alterations, and single-nucleotide polymorphisms. Germline mutations and inherited gene alterations are related to the development of familial lung cancer, and certain single-nucleotide polymorphisms are associated with an increase in the risk of lung cancer. Other factors associated with an increase in the risk of lung cancer include environmental and genetic interactions. The inhalation of a number of environmental carcinogenic agents, such as tobacco smoke, asbestos, or air pollutants, may lead to the induction of gene mutations, misreading in gene replication, or damage of DNA repair mechanisms. Multiple mechanisms for the acquisition of genetic predisposition to lung cancer have been intensively investigated, and further scientific knowledge would be valuable in the development of new therapeutic targets for treating lung cancer.

Keywords Lung cancer · Familial lung cancer · Genetic factors
Environmental factors

11.1 Introduction

Epidemiological studies have shown that the incidence of lung cancer is age-dependent and that the age-specific incidence risk of lung cancer exceeds 1.0 for individuals (both males and females) aged >60 years; this risk has been estimated based on cancer incidence data for 2010 in Japan [1]. Pathological observations of

N. Hashimoto · M. Sato · Y. Hasegawa (✉)
Department of Respiratory Medicine, Nagoya University Graduate School of Medicine, Nagoya, Japan
e-mail: yhasega@med.nagoya-u.ac.jp

T. Kaneko (ed.), *Clinical Relevance of Genetic Factors in Pulmonary Diseases*, Respiratory Disease Series: Diagnostic Tools and Disease Managements,
https://doi.org/10.1007/978-981-10-8144-6_11

tumor tissues demonstrate a variety of abnormal tissue formations, such as dysplasia or atypical adenomatous hyperplasia in lung adenocarcinoma, from the precancerous state to invasive cancer. In addition, genomic analysis has revealed that lung cancer accumulates high amounts of genetic and epigenetic alterations [2], including gene mutations, rearrangements, loss of heterozygosity, and gene expression and copy number alterations. During research to discover tumor oncogenes and tumor suppressor genes, the notion that the increase in the number of gene alterations corresponds to tumor development, i.e., the "multistep tumor progression" model, has been established [3].

While discussing genetic factors associated with lung cancer pathogenesis, two factors that influence gene alterations should be considered. One involves cancer susceptibility genes that are acquired by inheritance, and the other is environmental factors, such as tobacco smoke, asbestos, and inhalation of environmental chemicals and dust, which promote genetic and epigenetic alterations. In particular, the causal relation between tobacco smoke and lung cancer has been well established. The risk of lung cancer is 4–5 times higher in smoking males and 2–3 times higher in smoking females compared with that in never-smokers [4]. International Agency for Research on Cancer (IARC) has classified six carcinogens in mainstream smoke as carcinogenic to humans (Group 1) [5]. In addition, there are a number of lung cancer patients among non-smokers. Some, not all, of them have lung cancer due to breathing in secondhand tobacco smoke. Occupational and environmental exposure and genetic susceptibility will be discussed.

11.2 Overview of Genes Associated with Lung Cancer

Lung cancer is a heterogeneous disease clinically, histologically, and molecularly. It is histologically classified into two major subtypes: non-small cell lung cancer (NSCLC) accounting for approximately 85% of the cases of lung cancer and small cell lung cancer (SCLC) accounting for approximately 15% of the cases. NSCLC is further classified into three subtypes: adenocarcinoma, squamous cell carcinoma, and large cell carcinoma. Lung cancer develops from normal epithelial cells, its presumed cellular origin, to overt cancer cells through a stepwise acquisition of growth-advantageous molecular alterations over some decades [6, 7]. The high heterogeneity of lung cancer is suggested to result from the diversity in the cell types based on their origins and in the types and numbers of molecular alterations it accumulates. The cellular origins of lung cancer are largely unknown, but at least three different types of cells belonging to distinct cellular lineages, namely, type II alveolar, basal, and neuroendocrine cells, are speculated to be the origins of three different histological subtypes, namely, adenocarcinoma, squamous cell carcinoma, and SCLC, respectively. Furthermore, as mentioned below, lung cancers classified as the same histological types can harbor subpopulations exhibiting extremely high diversity in terms of molecular alterations, which closely correlate with its biological aggressiveness.

Intensive molecular analysis of lung cancer began in the late 1980s and has revealed that lung cancer cells harbor numerous genetic and epigenetic alterations as well as copy number changes and rearrangements that result in the activation of oncogenes or inactivation of tumor suppressor genes. Furthermore, in the past decade, tremendous advances in high-throughput sequencing technologies have allowed comprehensive molecular profiling of lung cancer with high sensitivity and accuracy. For example, The Cancer Genome Atlas (TCGA), a project launched in 2005 to catalog genetic alterations responsible for human cancers, has completed characterization of more than 20 types of human cancers, including adenocarcinoma, squamous cell carcinoma, and SCLC [8–11]. Comprehensive analyses by TCGA and other groups have revealed that molecular alterations found in three histological subtypes of lung cancer differ significantly, with some common changes; this finding is consistent with that of previous studies [7–16] (Table 11.1). Furthermore, these groups have discovered several previously unacknowledged

Table 11.1 Major molecular alterations in lung cancer

	Adenocarcinoma	Squamous cell carcinoma	Small cell carcinoma
Genes in tumor suppressing pathways or TSGs			
The p53 pathway			
CDKN2A (p14)	Mutation or deletion (23%)	Mutation or deletion (44%)	Mutation (rare ~2%)
MDM2	Amplification (8%)	Amplification (2%)	
p53	Mutation or deletion (47%)	Mutation (94%)	Mutation (94%)
The p16/RB pathway			
CDKN2A (p16)	Mutation or deletion (23%)	Mutation or deletion (44%)	Mutation (rare ~2%)
RB1	Mutation or deletion (6%)	Mutation or deletion (7%)	Mutation (78%)
TSGs in chromosome 3p			
RASSF1A	Methylation (31%)	Methylation (43%)	Methylation (72–85%)
SEMA3B	Methylation (46%)	Methylation (47%)	
Genes in oncogenic pathways or oncogenes			
Receptor tyrosine kinase			
EGFR	Mutation (10%)	Mutation (1%)	Mutation (rare)
	Amplification (3%)	Amplification (5%)	Amplification (rare)
HER2	Mutation (1%)	Amplification (2%)	Mutation (rare)
	Amplification (3%)		Amplification (5–30%)
MET	Mutation (7%)	Mutation (1–2%)	Mutation (rare ~13%)
	Amplification (3–20%)	Amplification (1–21%)	Amplification (1–5%)
FGFR1/4	Mutation (rare)	Mutation (2%)	Mutation (1%)

(continued)

Table 11.1 (continued)

	Adenocarcinoma	Squamous cell carcinoma	Small cell carcinoma
	Amplification (1–4%), Fusion (1%)	Amplification (16–22%), fusion (4%)	Amplification (5–6%)
ALK	Fusion (3%)	Fusion (very rare)	
ROS1	Fusion (1–2%)	Fusion (very rare)	
RET	Fusion (1%)	Fusion (very rare)	
The RAS/RAF/MAP pathway			
KRAS	Mutation (10–35%)	Mutation (1%)	Mutation (very rare)
BRAF	Mutation (1–7%)	Mutation (2%)	Mutation (1%)
The PI3K/AKT/mTOR pathway			
PIK3CA	Mutation (2%)	Mutation (5%)	Mutation (1%)
	Amplification (2–6%)	Amplification (33–36%)	
AKT1	Mutation (1%), Amplification (1%)	Mutation (1%), Amplification (1%)	
AKT2	Amplification (1%)	Amplification (5%)	
PTEN	Mutation or deletion (3%)	Mutation or deletion (10%)	Mutation or deletion (6%)
LKB1 (STK11)	Mutation or deletion (14–60%)	Mutation (2–30%)	Mutation (rare)
MYC	Amplification (9%)	Amplification (5%)	Amplification (18–30%)
Lineage-specific oncogenes			
TITF1	Amplification (10–15%)	Amplification (3–15%)	Amplification (rare)
SOX2	Amplification (3%)	Amplification (23–42%)	Amplification (27%)

Frequencies are based on Refs. [7–16]
TSG tumor suppressor gene

recurrent alterations, including rearrangement of *TP73* and *TP73* delta ex2/3 exhibiting oncogenic functions that can potentially serve as therapeutic targets for lung cancer. Importantly, knowledge from epidemiological studies and experimental models recapitulating multistep carcinogenesis of lung cancer has suggested that only a handful (usually five to eight) of genes are "drivers," whereas others are only "passengers" (discussed later) [17–19]. This has important clinical implications because "drivers," but not "passengers," serve as therapeutic targets for lung cancer. The discovery of an activating mutation in epidermal growth factor receptor (*EGFR*) in adenocarcinoma that is strongly associated with response to *EGFR*-targeted tyrosine kinase inhibitors (TKIs) indicates the first success in applying molecular knowledge on lung cancer in the clinic, which was obtained in 2002 [20, 21]. In 2007, a gene rearrangement in lung cancer involving anaplastic lymphoma kinase (*ALK*) was also discovered, and ALK-targeted TKIs have shown remarkable clinical benefits [22]. These findings have afforded molecularly tailored medicine in lung cancer, thereby beginning a new era of lung cancer treatment.

Copy number analysis in lung cancer has identified some recurrent alterations shared by all histological subtypes or found in certain specific ones. Frequent loss of a copy of chromosome 3p in all histological subtypes of lung cancer as well as in premalignant lesions was identified in the late 1980s, suggesting that this region contains tumor suppressor genes, the loss of which greatly contributes to the initiation and progression of lung cancer. Thus, intensive research involving the identification and characterization of commonly deleted regions in chromosome 3p, as well as functional analysis with gene transferring methods, has been conducted, leading to the identification of multiple tumor suppressor genes, including *FHIT*, *RASSF1A*, *FUS1*, and *SEMA3B*. Unlike classical tumor suppressor genes, such as p53, these genes were inactivated very rarely by mutations but very frequently by promoter specific methylation [23, 24]. One of the *MYC* proto-oncogenes (*MYC*, *MYCN*, or *MYCL*) is amplified in both NSCLC and SCLC. *MYC* is amplified mostly in NSCLC, whereas all members of the *MYC* family are amplified in SCLC. The accuracy of tiling array comparative genomic hybridization has greatly improved, leading to the identification of some lineage-specific oncogenes, including *TTF1* (14q) amplified in adenocarcinoma and *SOX2* (3q) amplified in squamous cell carcinoma and SCLC [16, 25, 26].

The tumor suppressor gene p53 is the most frequently mutated gene in lung cancer; it is mutated in approximately 50% of adenocarcinoma, approximately 90% of squamous cell carcinoma, and approximately 100% of SCLC [8–10]. In response to cellular stresses, such as carcinogens and UV, that potentially cause DNA damage, p53 induces G1 cell cycle arrest to allow DNA repair or apoptosis, depending on the severity of DNA damage. In addition, either *CDKN2A* (p16) or *RB1*, both belonging to the same pathway that regulates G1–S transition in the cell cycle, is frequently inactivated in all three histological subtypes. Interestingly, using an alternate exon1, *CDKN2A* encodes another gene, p14 ARF, that functions as a tumor suppressor in the p53 pathway by suppressing MDM2, an E3 ubiquitin ligase that induces p53 degradation via the ubiquitin proteasome system. Notably, in nearly all SCLC tumors, both *p53* and *RB* are inactivated. These findings demonstrate that the inactivation of both the p53 and p16/RB pathways is a fundamental, universal genetic alteration in lung cancer of all histological subtypes, particularly SCLC. By contrast, most other alterations in lung cancer exhibit cell subtype specificity to varying extents. For example, alterations in genes encoding receptor tyrosine kinases (RTKs) occur almost exclusively in lung adenocarcinomas; these include activating mutations in *EGFR*, *HER2*, and *MET* as well as translocations involving *ALK*, *ROS*, *RET*, *NTRK1*, *NRG1*, and *ERBB4*. One exception is a gene rearrangement involving *FGFR* family genes that are exclusively found in squamous cell carcinoma. *RAS* family genes encoding proteins that are direct downstream effectors of these RTKs are mutated almost exclusively in adenocarcinoma. LKB1 (also known as STK11), a multifunctional serine/threonine kinase that functions as a TSG, in part, through suppressing mTOR, is mutated frequently in adenocarcinoma and less frequently in squamous cell carcinoma. As expected, genes associated with differentiation demonstrate histology-specific patterns of occurrence. For instance, mutations in the neuroendocrine differentiation genes *NOTCH1*, *NOTCH2*, and *NOTCH3* have been found in SCLC. Importantly, even in the same histological type, especially in adenocarcinoma, types of alterations as well as amount of mutational burden involving the entire genome significantly differ between tumors from smokers and from non-smokers. Studies have shown that NSCLC tumors from smokers exhibit tenfold higher mutation frequency than those from non-smokers. *p53* and Kirsten rat sarcoma viral oncogene (*KRAS*) mutations are more common in smokers than in non-smokers, whereas *EGFR* and *HER2* mutations and rearrangements involving *ALK* occur much more commonly in non-smokers than in smokers.

Multi-region deep sequencing of primary lung tumors has revealed remarkable heterogeneity along with common alterations, suggesting the existence of a tumor's evolutionary tree comprising the fundamental trunk (a stem clone) and branches (subclones) [27, 28]. Analysis has shown that driver mutations, such as those involving *p53*, *KRAS*, and *EGFR*, are usually observed in a stem clone, suggesting that single biopsy samples for searching for driver mutations are sufficient.

Smoking is the main cause of lung cancer, with accountability for approximately 80% of the cases. Nevertheless, the incidence of lung cancer in non-smokers is increasing worldwide, but its etiology is largely unknown. Recently, *APOBEC3B*, belonging to the APOBEC gene family, is emerging as a potential endogenous source of mutations [29]. Physiologically, APOBEC3B protects the genome from retroviral and retrotransposon propagation by deaminating cytosine, resulting in C to T transitions. Studies analyzing whole-genome sequencing data, including that of TCGA, have shown that *APOBEC3B*-associated mutations are prevalent throughout the genome, co-occurring with increased expression of *APOBEC3B* mRNA in several human cancers, including lung adenocarcinoma and squamous cell carcinoma, suggesting that *APOBEC3B* is a critical source of mutations in lung cancer. Moreover, multi-region deep sequencing of primary lung tumors has shown high intra-tumor heterogeneity in *APOBEC3B*-associated mutations, suggesting that *APOBEC3B* contributes to the generation of tumor heterogeneity in lung cancer.

Collectively, these detailed molecular findings in lung cancer have helped identify many genes as actionable therapeutic targets. Novel therapeutic agents targeting these genes are under development or are being tested in clinical trials.

11.3 Inherited Susceptibility of Lung Cancer

11.3.1 Familial Lung Cancer

Most cases of lung cancer are caused by the accumulation of somatic gene alterations found in tumor cells only and not by germline mutations or inherited gene alterations. In contrast, Li–Fraumeni syndrome is a representative hereditary cancer predisposition, which is linked to germline mutations of the p53 tumor suppressor gene [30, 31]. Li–Fraumeni syndrome is also termed SBLA, which stands for familial development of sarcoma (S); breast and brain tumor (B); leukemia, lung, and laryngeal cancer (L); and adrenal cortical carcinoma (A) [32]. Kleihues et al. reported that the incidence of lung cancer in patients with malignant transformation of Li–Fraumeni syndrome was not frequent and was 4–6% in 91 families [33].

On the other hand, Hwang et al. reported that lung cancer was the third most common tumor type in mutation carriers and that the standardized incidence ratio of lung cancer was 38.5 (95% CI, 16.6–76.0) [34]. In addition, the mean age when tumor develops in Li–Fraumeni syndrome is organ specific, and the cumulative risk of lung cancer increases in an age-dependent manner. Both reports indicated the mean age of lung cancer diagnosis is approximately 50 years.

As for another inherited susceptibility to lung cancer, a family in which members carry a germline EGFR T790M mutation has been reported [35]. Somatic mutation involving *EGFR* T790M is known as one of the activating mutations in lung cancer and also an acquired gatekeeper mutation that results in resistance to first-generation EGFR–TKI treatment [36]. This report has shown that some family members who carry a germline *EGFR* T790M mutation develop NSCLC with secondary activating *EGFR* mutations occurring in the same allele where the germline *EGFR* T790M mutation occurs. Although the mechanisms are not clear, a germline *EGFR* T790M mutation is one of the factors for inherited susceptibility to lung cancer.

11.3.2 Genome-Wide Association Study

The Genetic Epidemiology of Lung Cancer Consortium, funded by the National Cancer Institute in the United States, collected familial lung cancer cases and conducted a family-based linkage study. Over 1000 families with familial lung cancer have been enrolled [37], and extracted germline DNA of highly aggregated lung cancer families has been used for linkage studies and genotyping by the Center for Inherited Diseases Research using microsatellite markers. In 2004, Bailey-Wilson et al. reported a major susceptibility locus localized to chromosome 6q23-25 that influences the risk of lung cancer [38]. Thereafter, several genome-wide association studies (GWAS) have reported 5p15.33, 6p21.33, 6q23-25, and 15q24-25.1 to be associated with susceptibility gene loci for familial lung cancer.

In relation to cancer susceptibility, the gene locus 5p15.33 contains *TERT* and *CRR9/CLPTM1L* [39]. *TERT* is known as the gene that encodes the catalytic subunit of telomerase reverse transcriptase and plays an important role in genetic stability. *CRR9/CLPTM1L* is termed cisplatin resistance-related protein-9 (*CRR9*) or as cleft lip and palate transmembrane protein-1-like (*CLPTM1L*). It is overexpressed in NSCLC and is required for KRAS-induced lung tumorigenesis [40, 41]. The gene locus 6p21.33 encompasses HLA-B-associated transcript 3 (*Bat3*), which controls DNA damage-induced acetylation of p53 [42]. This gene locus contains *RGS17* that encodes a member of the regulator of G-protein signaling (RGS) family. *RGS17* knockdown inhibits tumor growth, and *RGS17* overexpression increases tumor growth [43]. The gene locus 15q24-25.1 encompasses the genes *IREB2*, *LOC123688*, *PSMA4*, *CHRNA5*, *CHRNA3*, and *CHRNB4* [44, 45]. *IREB2* encodes an iron regulatory protein 2 that regulates iron metabolism [46]. *LOC123688* is a putative gene, and its function is not known. *PSMA4* encodes proteasome alpha type subunit 4—a structural protein of the 20S proteasome core—and may regulate the proliferation of lung cancer cells [45, 47, 48]. *CHRNA5*, *CHRNA3*, and *CHRNB4* encode nicotinic acetylcholine receptor subunits (α5, α3, and β4, respectively) and have been shown to be associated with nicotine dependence and lung cancer risk [49, 50].

As mentioned above, intensive linkage analysis and single-nucleotide polymorphism analysis of these gene loci have been performed, and they have provided evidence of genetic influence on the risk of lung cancer. However, the mutation at individual gene loci seems to be a small effect on the cause of tumorigenesis. Cumulative effects of genetic predispositions to lung cancer may play an important role in inherited susceptibility to it.

11.4 Environment and Genetic Interactions

11.4.1 Tobacco Smoke and Genetic Susceptibility

The causal relationship between lung cancer and tobacco smoke has been well established, and smoking cessation in nationwide efforts can be beneficial to decrease the incidence of lung cancer [51]. Tobacco smoke contains 3000–4000 chemicals, more than 50 of which are identified as carcinogenic agents. In mainstream smoke, benzene, cadmium, 2-aminonaphthalene, nickel, chromium, and 4-aminobiphenyl are characterized as IARC Group 1 agents (carcinogenic to humans), and formaldehyde, 1,3-butadiene, and benzo[a]pyrene are listed as IARC Group 2A (probably carcinogenic to humans) [5]. Some of these agents have been shown to induce gene mutations, DNA damage, and chromosomal aberrations. Benzo[α]pyrene is known to directly attack a number of chemical sites and form DNA adducts [52]. Consequently, gene mutations, and misreading in gene replication, or genomic instability are induced. Carcinogenic agents also influence DNA repair mechanisms [53]. Individual susceptibility to these carcinogens may be dependent on the activity of detoxification enzymes, such as the genetically polymorphic cytochrome P450, or drug metabolism [54]. In addition, individual addictive smoking behavior may be partly influenced by genetic factors, such as dopamine receptor gene polymorphisms, but these relationships are weak as an association with smoking behavior [50].

11.4.2 Environmental Inhalation

In addition to tobacco smoke, several environmental carcinogenic agents interact with genes. One representative example is asbestos, in which six types of minerals belong to the serpentine class. Although the toxic effects of asbestos are dependent on the type of asbestos, size of fiber, and environment, exposure to it is well known to be a major risk factor for lung cancer and mesothelioma. Asbestos induces DNA damage by producing reactive oxygen species, resulting in mutations in proto-oncogenes, such as *KRAS* [55] and *p53* [56]. The latency periods for the development of lung cancer and mesothelioma after asbestos exposure are more than 20 and 30 years, respectively. In addition, smoking synergistically increases the risk of lung cancer. These findings also support the notion of "multistep tumor progression," i.e., the cumulative alterations of genes.

In addition to asbestos, air pollutants such as particular matter ($PM_{2.5}$ or PM_{10}) and diesel exhaust, radioactive materials such as indoor radon gas and X- and gamma rays, and chemicals such as arsenic, beryllium, silica, aluminum, and nickel have been reported as environmental risk factors for lung cancer development. In addition to genetic susceptibility to lung cancer, the interactions between genes and the environment may influence individual cancer susceptibility, including acquired, cumulative mutated genes and the detoxification enzymes which activities depend on genetic polymorphisms.

11.5 Driver and Passenger Mutations in Lung Cancer

Cancer genomes exhibit two types of somatic mutations arising from various processes: the "driver" mutation and the "passenger" mutation. A mutation of cancer genes that promotes cancer development and confers a selective growth advantage is defined as a "driver" mutation. Driver mutations tend to cause clonal expansions. Conversely, a "passenger" mutation is commonly accepted as a mutation that does not provide a growth advantage. The term "oncogenic addiction" describes a finding whereby cancer cells develop in line with the hallmarks of cancer, depending on genetic modifications, such as driver mutations and gene amplifications. This dependency provides clues to find new therapeutic strategies against cancer. Therefore, the strategy to distinguish oncogenic driver mutations from passenger mutations among cancer genomes is warranted. Indeed, the approach to reveal cancer genes displaying the nature of oncogene addiction has provided some notable successes. Protein kinases are frequently mutated in cancer, and inhibitors of this family have proven to be effective anticancer drugs. EGFR has a tyrosine protein kinase domain, and epithelial growth factor stimulation induces phosphorylation of this domain. Major mutations in this domain of EGFR are either in-frame deletions in exon 19 (exon 19 deletions) or an amino acid substitution at position 858 (exon 20 L858R), resulting in cluster formation around the adenosine triphosphate-binding pocket of the catalytic domain of tyrosine protein kinases. The common activating mutations of EGFR show an additive specific gain of function in lung cancer. The incidence of EGFR mutation might be associated with adenocarcinoma in never-smoking females among Asian populations, including the Japanese population [57]. Several inhibitors targeting EGFR mutations have been utilized to treat lung cancer. Small-molecule inhibitors of *ALK* rearrangement are also introduced in lung cancer with an *ALK* fusion gene. Although *KRAS* is the most commonly mutated gene, KRAS itself is not easily targetable.

A recent large-scale sequence analysis of cellular kinases in various types of cancers has identified more than 1000 mutations, indicating that numerous alterations in DNA sequence underlie the development of all tumors [58]. The incidence of passenger mutations is likely to be involved in somatic mutations detected in cancer [58, 59]. Combinations of some mutations that are less frequently detected in most lung adenocarcinomas may promote cancer phenotypes [59]. The analysis of known genes could not detect new high-frequency mutations in lung cancer in addition to gene mutations previously reported [58]. The existence of oncogenes, including *Src* or *KRAS*, is insufficient to develop cancer in animal models when tissue injury and subsequent tissue repair are not involved [60]. *KRAS* and *EGFR* mutations are frequently observed in adenocarcinoma. The incidence of *KRAS* mutations is approximately 30% in lung adenocarcinomas in Western population and approximately 10% in Asian population. The incidences of *KRAS* and *EGFR* mutations are also mutually exclusive. The frequency of EGFR mutations is more than 60% in female, non-smoking lung cancer patients among Asian populations [61].

Tumor suppressor genes, such as *p53* and phosphatase and tensin homologue deleted from chromosome 10 (*PTEN*), correct genomic instability, restraining aberrant growth and survival. Genetic alteration of tumor suppressor genes causes loss of function through inactivating mutations, deletion mutations, or epigenetic silencing, thereby accelerating cancer development accompanied by oncogene activation. Mutated tumor suppressor genes, including *p53* and *CDKN2A*, are frequently observed in lung adenocarcinoma and squamous cell carcinoma [8, 59]. A recent GWAS has demonstrated the impact of epigenetic factors on the development of lung adenocarcinoma with *EGFR* mutation [62, 63]. *TERT* at 5p15.33, *BTNL2* at 6p21.3, tumor protein p63 (*TP63*) at 3q28, bromodomain PHD finger transcription factor (*BPTF*) at 17q24.2, HLA class II at 6p21.32, and forkhead box P4 (*FOXP4*) at 6p21.1 are strongly associated with the development of lung adenocarcinoma with *EGFR* mutation in East Asian population [63]. Multiple genetic factors modulate the development of lung adenocarcinomas with *EGFR* mutations. Thus, cancer also develops in the tumor microenvironment where cancer cells and their stromal neighbors are orchestrated in oncogenic signaling networks.

11.6 Conclusion

Cancer is known as a genetic disease, which means that genetic alteration is a cause of carcinogenesis. The accumulation of genetic and epigenetic alterations, including gene mutations, rearrangements, loss of heterozygosity, and gene expression and copy number alterations, causes lung cancer. Some gene alterations involve cancer susceptibility genes acquired by inheritance, and others are affected by environmental factors. Although interactions between genes and the environment are complicated, multiple mechanisms for the acquisition of genetic predisposition to lung cancer have been revealed after intensive investigation, as mentioned in this chapter. These scientific findings would become powerful tools for discovering new therapeutic targets and preventing lung cancer.

References

1. Cancer statistics in Japan 2014. Foundation for Promotion of Cancer Research Source: estimated using the method by Wum LM et al., Estimating lifetime and age-conditional probabilities of developing cancer. Lifetime Data Anal. 1998;4:169–86.
2. Kandoth C, McLellan MD, Vandin F, Ye K, Niu B, Lu C, Xie M, Zhang Q, McMichael JF, Wyczalkowski MA, Leiserson MD, Miller CA, Welch JS, Walter MJ, Wendl MC, Ley TJ, Wilson RK, Raphael BJ, Ding L. Mutational landscape and significance across 12 major cancer types. Nature. 2013;502(7471):333–9.
3. Vogelstein B, Fearon ER, Kern SE, Hamilton SR, Preisinger AC, Nakamura Y, White R. Allelotype of colorectal carcinomas. Science. 1989;244(4901):207–11.
4. Wakai K, Inoue M, Mizoue T, Tanaka K, Tsuji I, Nagata C, Tsugane S, Research Group for the Development and Evaluation of Cancer Prevention Strategies in Japan. Tobacco smoking and lung cancer risk: an evaluation based on a systematic review of epidemiological evidence among the Japanese population. Jpn J Clin Oncol. 2006;36(5):309–24.
5. IARC Working Group on the Evaluation of Carcinogenic Risks to Humans. Tobacco smoke and involuntary smoking. IARC Monogr Eval Carcinog Risks Hum. 2004;83:78.
6. Sato M, Shames DS, Gazdar AF, Minna JD. A translational view of the molecular pathogenesis of lung cancer. J Thorac Oncol. 2007;2:327–43.
7. Larsen JE, Minna JD. Molecular biology of lung cancer: clinical implications. Clin Chest Med. 2011;32:703–40.
8. Cancer Genome Atlas Research Network. Comprehensive genomic characterization of squamous cell lung cancers. Nature. 2012;489:519–25.
9. Cancer Genome Atlas Research Network. Comprehensive molecular profiling of lung adenocarcinoma. Nature. 2014;511:543–50.
10. George J, Lim JS, Jang SJ, et al. Comprehensive genomic profiles of small cell lung cancer. Nature. 2015;524:47–53.
11. Vogelstein B, Papadopoulos N, Velculescu VE, Zhou S, Diaz LA Jr, Kinzler KW. Cancer genome landscapes. Science. 2013;339:1546–58.
12. Takeuchi K, Soda M, Togashi Y, et al. RET, ROS1 and ALK fusions in lung cancer. Nat Med. 2012;18:378–81.
13. Karachaliou N, Pilotto S, Lazzari C, Bria E, de Marinis F, Rosell R. Cellular and molecular biology of small cell lung cancer: an overview. Transl Lung Cancer Res. 2016;5:2–15.
14. Gao J, Aksoy BA, Dogrusoz U, et al. Integrative analysis of complex cancer genomics and clinical profiles using the cBioPortal. Sci Signal. 2013;6:pl1.
15. Cerami E, Gao J, Dogrusoz U, et al. The cBio cancer genomics portal: an open platform for exploring multidimensional cancer genomics data. Cancer Discov. 2012;2:401–4.
16. Rudin CM, Durinck S, Stawiski EW, et al. Comprehensive genomic analysis identifies SOX2 as a frequently amplified gene in small-cell lung cancer. Nat Genet. 2012;44:1111–6.
17. Armitage P, Doll R. The age distribution of cancer and a multi-stage theory of carcinogenesis. Br J Cancer. 1954;8:1–12.
18. Sato M, Vaughan MB, Girard L, et al. Multiple oncogenic changes (K-RAS(V12), p53 knockdown, mutant EGFRs, p16 bypass, telomerase) are not sufficient to confer a full malignant phenotype on human bronchial epithelial cells. Cancer Res. 2006;66:2116–28.
19. Sato M, Larsen JE, Lee W, et al. Human lung epithelial cells progressed to malignancy through specific oncogenic manipulations. Mol Cancer Res. 2013;11:638–50.
20. Lynch TJ, Bell DW, Sordella R, et al. Activating mutations in the epidermal growth factor receptor underlying responsiveness of non-small-cell lung cancer to gefitinib. N Engl J Med. 2004;350:2129–39.
21. Paez JG, Janne PA, Lee JC, et al. EGFR mutations in lung cancer: correlation with clinical response to gefitinib therapy. Science. 2004;304:1497–500.
22. Soda M, Choi YL, Enomoto M, et al. Identification of the transforming EML4-ALK fusion gene in non-small-cell lung cancer. Nature. 2007;448:561–6.

23. Dammann R, Li C, Yoon JH, Chin PL, Bates S, Pfeifer GP. Epigenetic inactivation of a RAS association domain family protein from the lung tumour suppressor locus 3p21.3. Nat Genet. 2000;25:315–9.
24. Zochbauer-Muller S, Fong KM, Virmani AK, Geradts J, Gazdar AF, Minna JD. Aberrant promoter methylation of multiple genes in non-small cell lung cancers. Cancer Res. 2001;61:249–55.
25. Bass AJ, Watanabe H, Mermel CH, et al. SOX2 is an amplified lineage-survival oncogene in lung and esophageal squamous cell carcinomas. Nat Genet. 2009;41:1238–42.
26. Weir BA, Woo MS, Getz G, et al. Characterizing the cancer genome in lung adenocarcinoma. Nature. 2007;450:893–8.
27. de Bruin EC, McGranahan N, Mitter R, et al. Spatial and temporal diversity in genomic instability processes defines lung cancer evolution. Science. 2014;346:251–6.
28. Zhang J, Fujimoto J, Zhang J, et al. Intratumor heterogeneity in localized lung adenocarcinomas delineated by multiregion sequencing. Science. 2014;346:256–9.
29. Burns MB, Temiz NA, Harris RS. Evidence for APOBEC3B mutagenesis in multiple human cancers. Nat Genet. 2013;45:977–83.
30. Li FP, Fraumeni JF. Soft-tissue sarcomas, breast cancer, and other neoplasms. A familial syndrome? Ann Intern Med. 1969;71:747–52.
31. Varley JM. Germline TP53 mutations and Li-Fraumeni syndrome. Hum Mutat. 2003;21:313–20.
32. Lynch HT, Guirgis HA. Childhood cancer and the SBLA syndrome. Med Hypotheses. 1979;5:15–22.
33. Kleihues P, Schäuble B, zur Hausen A, Estève J, Ohgaki H. Tumors associated with p53 germline mutations: a synopsis of 91 families. Am J Pathol. 1997;150(1):1–13.
34. Hwang SJ, Cheng LS, Lozano G, Amos CI, Gu X, Strong LC. Lung cancer risk in germline p53 mutation carriers: association between an inherited cancer predisposition, cigarette smoking, and cancer risk. Hum Genet. 2003;113(3):238–43.
35. Bell DW, Gore I, Okimoto RA, Godin-Heymann N, Sordella R, Mulloy R, Sharma SV, Brannigan BW, Mohapatra G, Settleman J, Haber DA. Inherited susceptibility to lung cancer may be associated with the T790M drug resistance mutation in EGFR. Nat Genet. 2005;37(12):1315–6.
36. Kobayashi S, Boggon TJ, Dayaram T, Jänne PA, Kocher O, Meyerson M, Johnson BE, Eck MJ, Tenen DG, Halmos B. EGFR mutation and resistance of non-small-cell lung cancer to gefitinib. N Engl J Med. 2005;352(8):786–92.
37. Genetic Epidemiology of Lung Cancer Consortium GWAS of Familial Lung Cancer. https://www.ncbi.nlm.nih.gov/projects/gap/cgi-bin/study.cgi?study_id=phs000629.v1.p1
38. Bailey-Wilson JE, Amos CI, Pinney SM, Petersen GM, de Andrade M, Wiest JS, Fain P, Schwartz AG, You M, Franklin W, Klein C, Gazdar A, Rothschild H, Mandal D, Coons T, Slusser J, Lee J, Gaba C, Kupert E, Perez A, Zhou X, Zeng D, Liu Q, Zhang Q, Seminara D, Minna J, Anderson MW. A major lung cancer susceptibility locus maps to chromosome 6q23-25. Am J Hum Genet. 2004;75(3):460–74.
39. Kachuri L, Amos CI, McKay JD, Johansson M, Vineis P, Bueno-de-Mesquita HB, Boutron-Ruault MC, Johansson M, Quirós JR, Sieri S, Travis RC, Weiderpass E, Le Marchand L, Henderson BE, Wilkens L, Goodman GE, Chen C, Doherty JA, Christiani DC, Wei Y, Su L, Tworoger S, Zhang X, Kraft P, Zaridze D, Field JK, Marcus MW, Davies MP, Hyde R, Caporaso NE, Landi MT, Severi G, Giles GG, Liu G, McLaughlin JR, Li Y, Xiao X, Fehringer G, Zong X, Denroche RE, Zuzarte PC, McPherson JD, Brennan P, Hung RJ. Fine mapping of chromosome 5p15.33 based on a targeted deep sequencing and high density genotyping identifies novel lung cancer susceptibility loci. Carcinogenesis. 2016;37(1):96–105.
40. Yamamoto K, et al. A novel gene, CRR9, which was up-regulated in CDDP-resistant ovarian tumor cell line, was associated with apoptosis. Biochem Biophys Res Commun. 2001;280:1148–54.
41. James MA, et al. CRR9/CLPTM1L regulates cell survival signaling and is required for Ras transformation and lung tumorigenesis. Cancer Res. 2014;74:1116–27.

42. Sasaki T, Gan EC, Wakeham A, Kornbluth S, Mak TW, Okada H. HLA-B-associated transcript 3 (Bat3)/Scythe is essential for p300-mediated acetylation of p53. Genes Dev. 2007;21(7):848–61.
43. You M, Wang D, Liu P, Vikis H, James M, Lu Y, Wang Y, Wang M, Chen Q, Jia D, Liu Y, Wen W, Yang P, Sun Z, Pinney SM, Zheng W, Shu XO, Long J, Gao YT, Xiang YB, Chow WH, Rothman N, Petersen GM, de Andrade M, Wu Y, Cunningham JM, Wiest JS, Fain PR, Schwartz AG, Girard L, Gazdar A, Gaba C, Rothschild H, Mandal D, Coons T, Lee J, Kupert E, Seminara D, Minna J, Bailey-Wilson JE, Amos CI, Anderson MW. Fine mapping of chromosome 6q23-25 region in familial lung cancer families reveals RGS17 as a likely candidate gene. Clin Cancer Res. 2009;15(8):2666–74.
44. Liu P, Vikis HG, Wang D, Lu Y, Wang Y, Schwartz AG, Pinney SM, Yang P, de Andrade M, Petersen GM, Wiest JS, Fain PR, Gazdar A, Gaba C, Rothschild H, Mandal D, Coons T, Lee J, Kupert E, Seminara D, Minna J, Bailey-Wilson JE, Wu X, Spitz MR, Eisen T, Houlston RS, Amos CI, Anderson MW, You M. Familial aggregation of common sequence variants on 15q24-25.1 in lung cancer. J Natl Cancer Inst. 2008;100(18):1326–30.
45. Liu Y, Liu P, Wen W, James MA, Wang Y, Bailey-Wilson JE, Amos CI, Pinney SM, Yang P, de Andrade M, Petersen GM, Wiest JS, Fain PR, Schwartz AG, Gazdar A, Gaba C, Rothschild H, Mandal D, Kupert E, Lee J, Seminara D, Minna J, Anderson MW, You M. Haplotype and cell proliferation analyses of candidate lung cancer susceptibility genes on chromosome 15q24-25.1. Cancer Res. 2009;69(19):7844–50.
46. LaVaute T, Smith S, Cooperman S, Iwai K, Land W, Meyron-Holtz E, Drake SK, Miller G, Abu-Asab M, Tsokos M, Switzer R III, Grinberg A, Love P, Tresser N, Rouault TA. Targeted deletion of the gene encoding iron regulatory protein-2 causes misregulation of iron metabolism and neurodegenerative disease in mice. Nat Genet. 2001;27(2):209–14.
47. Davoli R, Fontanesi L, Russo V, Cepica S, Musilová P, Stratil A, Rubes J. The porcine proteasome subunit A4 (PSMA4) gene: isolation of a partial cDNA, linkage and physical mapping. Anim Genet. 1998;29(5):385–8.
48. Nandi D, Woodward E, Ginsburg DB, Monaco JJ. Intermediates in the formation of mouse 20S proteasomes: implications for the assembly of precursor beta subunits. EMBO J. 1997;16(17):5363–75.
49. Hung RJ, McKay JD, Gaborieau V, Boffetta P, et al. A susceptibility locus for lung cancer maps to nicotinic acetylcholine receptor subunit genes on 15q25. Nature. 2008;452(7187):633–7.
50. Wang JC, Cruchaga C, Saccone NL, et al. Risk for nicotine dependence and lung cancer is conferred by mRNA expression levels and amino acid change in CHRNA5. Hum Mol Genet. 2009;18(16):3125–35.
51. Schottenfeld D. The etiology and epidemiology of lung cancer. In: Pass HI, et al., editors. Principles and practice of lung cancer. Philadelphia: Lippincott Williams & Wilkins; 2010. p. 3–22.
52. Weinberg RA. Cell genomes are under occasional attack from exogenous mutagens and their metabolites. The biology of cancer. 2nd ed. New York: Garland Science; 2014. p. 527–35.
53. Kazma R, Babron MC, Gaborieau V, Génin E, Brennan P, Hung RJ, McLaughlin JR, Krokan HE, Elvestad MB, Skorpen F, Anderssen E, Vooder T, Välk K, Metspalu A, Field JK, Lathrop M, Sarasin A, Benhamou S. ILCCO consortium. Lung cancer and DNA repair genes: multilevel association analysis from the International Lung Cancer Consortium. Carcinogenesis. 2012;33(5):1059–64.
54. Agundez JA. Cytochrome P450 gene polymorphism and cancer. Curr Drug Metab. 2004;5(3):211–24.
55. Nelson HH, Christiani DC, Wiencke JK, Mark EJ, Wain JC, Kelsey KT. K-ras mutation and occupational asbestos exposure in lung adenocarcinoma: asbestos-related cancer without asbestosis. Cancer Res. 1999;59(18):4570–3.
56. Panduri V, Surapureddi S, Soberanes S, Weitzman SA, Chandel N, Kamp DW. P53 mediates amosite asbestos-induced alveolar epithelial cell mitochondria-regulated apoptosis. Am J Respir Cell Mol Biol. 2006;34(4):443–52.

57. Mitsudomi T, Kosaka T, Endoh H, et al. Mutations of the epidermal growth factor receptor gene predict prolonged survival after gefitinib treatment in patients with non-small-cell lung cancer with postoperative recurrence. J Clin Oncol. 2005;23:2513–20.
58. Greenman C, Stephens P, Smith R, et al. Patterns of somatic mutation in human cancer genomes. Nature. 2007;446:153–8.
59. Ding L, Getz G, Wheeler DA, et al. Somatic mutations affect key pathways in lung adenocarcinoma. Nature. 2008;455:1069–75.
60. Grivennikov SI, Greten FR, Karin M. Immunity, inflammation, and cancer. Cell. 2010;140:883–99.
61. Dearden S, Stevens J, Wu YL, et al. Mutation incidence and coincidence in non small-cell lung cancer: meta-analyses by ethnicity and histology (mutMap). Ann Oncol. 2013;24:2371–6.
62. Shiraishi K, Kunitoh H, Daigo Y, et al. A genome-wide association study identifies two new susceptibility loci for lung adenocarcinoma in the Japanese population. Nat Genet. 2012;44:900–3.
63. Shiraishi K, Okada Y, Takahashi A, et al. Association of variations in HLA class II and other loci with susceptibility to EGFR-mutated lung adenocarcinoma. Nat Commun. 2016;7:12451.

Chapter 12
Pulmonary Malignancies (2): Mesothelioma—What Are the Roles of Genetic Factors in the Pathogenesis of Mesothelioma?

Takashi Nakano, Eisuke Shibata, Kozo Kuribayashi, Yoshie Yoshikawa, and Masaki Ohmuraya

Abstract Malignant pleural mesothelioma is a highly lethal and aggressive tumor, and its incidence is increasing because of widespread asbestos exposure in the last 50 years. Malignant mesothelioma is characterized by a long latency period of 40 years between initial exposure to asbestos and tumor development, indicating that multiple somatic genetic alterations contribute to its carcinogenesis. Molecular genetic studies have identified multiple chromosomal alterations in most mesothelioma tumor tissues and cell lines. In addition, these studies have identified several key genetic alterations. Mutation rates in *CDKN2A*, *NF2*, and *BAP1*, which are cancer suppressor genes, are high in mesothelioma cells. Moreover, diagnosis of a new familial cancer predisposition syndrome associated with germline *BAP1* mutation indicates the importance of genetic factors in mesothelioma susceptibility. In this chapter, we have summarized the clinicopathological aspects of mesothelioma and have discussed the roles of genetic factors in the development of malignant pleural mesothelioma.

Keywords Mesothelioma · Asbestos · *BAP1* · *NF2* · Genetic susceptibility · Cancer predisposition syndrome

T. Nakano (✉)
Center for Respiratory Medicine, Otemae Hospital, Osaka, Japan
e-mail: nakano@otemae.gr.jp

E. Shibata · K. Kuribayashi
Division of Respiratory Diseases, Department of Internal Medicine, Hyogo College of Medicine, Nishinomiya, Hyogo, Japan

Y. Yoshikawa · M. Ohmuraya
Department of Genetics, Hyogo College of Medicine, Nishinomiya, Hyogo, Japan

T. Kaneko (ed.), *Clinical Relevance of Genetic Factors in Pulmonary Diseases*, Respiratory Disease Series: Diagnostic Tools and Disease Managements,
https://doi.org/10.1007/978-981-10-8144-6_12

12.1 Introduction

Malignant mesothelioma primarily arises from mesothelial cells of serosal membranes consisting of the pleura, peritoneum, pericardium, and tunica vaginalis. In majority of cases, mesothelioma is of pleural origin (malignant pleural mesothelioma), followed by peritoneal origin (malignant peritoneal mesothelioma), which accounts for 7–13% of all mesothelioma cases. Development of mesothelioma is strongly associated with asbestos exposure. Malignant pleural mesothelioma is usually caused by occupational asbestos exposure but can also occur because of low-level asbestos exposure in the general environment. Approximately 10–15% patients with malignant mesothelioma have no apparent exposure to asbestos. A small fraction of cases of malignant peritoneal mesothelioma is associated with heavier and longer asbestos exposure than pleural mesothelioma. However, >60% patients with peritoneal mesothelioma have no history of asbestos exposure. Generally, mesothelioma develops as a sporadic malignant neoplasm in association with asbestos or other mineral particles exposure. Some studies have reported familial clustering of mesothelioma independent of asbestos exposure [1, 2]. Moreover, its clustering among blood relatives, in whom two or more individuals have malignant mesothelioma, suggests genetic susceptibility besides asbestos exposure.

BRCA1-associated protein 1 (*BAP1*) is a tumor suppressor gene located on chromosome 3p21.1 that encodes a deubiquitinating enzyme. BAP1 regulates cell cycle checkpoints, target gene transcription, and DNA damage repair. A recent study showed that germline *BAP1* mutations in two families were associated with a high incidence of malignant mesothelioma [3]. Moreover, germline *BAP1* mutations are associated with a novel hereditary cancer syndrome that occurs in family members with several cancer types, including malignant mesothelioma, uveal melanoma, cutaneous melanoma, renal cell carcinoma, and basal cell carcinoma. Germline *BAP1* mutations are rare in sporadic mesothelioma caused by asbestos exposure. However, a long latency period of 40 years suggests that multiple somatic mutations contribute to the carcinogenesis of mesothelioma.

12.2 Epidemiology of Malignant Mesothelioma

Malignant mesothelioma is a relatively uncommon disease. However, its incidence in Japan is increasing and is predicted to peak by 2030. At present, 1500 new mesothelioma cases are reported per year; this number has increased from 500 in 1995 (when ICD-10 was introduced) to 1550 in 2016. Incidence of mesothelioma is increasing globally because of large-scale asbestos consumption. In the USA and Sweden, which have tried to decrease asbestos exposure for nearly 50 years, the incidence of mesothelioma is declining after reaching a peak. However, the incidence of mesothelioma is yet to peak in Japan. In the USA, age-adjusted death rate of mesothelioma decreased from 13.96 per million in 1999 to 10.93 in 2015 [4]. Malignant mesothelioma develops after a very long latency period of approximately 40 years. Despite regulatory action against and prohibition of the use of asbestos, the number of mesothelioma patients is increasing substantially in many countries where asbestos has been widely used in the past. In Japan, current exposure to asbestos may occur during maintenance and rebuilding of old buildings containing asbestos.

12.3 Asbestos Consumption and Mesothelioma Incidence

Asbestos is regulated and/or is completely banned in developed countries but continues to be used in some developing countries. Asbestos consumption in China has increased sharply because of rapid industrialization, and similar trends have been observed in Thailand and Vietnam in Southeast Asia. In 2010, Asia accounted for 64% of the global asbestos consumption, which increased from 47% in 2000. Asbestos use in Vietnam and Thailand decreased by 27% and 8%, respectively, from 2012 to 2013. In contrast, asbestos consumption in China increased by 7% to 570,000 tons in 2013, thus making it the top consumer of asbestos.

In Japan, mesothelioma-associated mortality was low until the early 1990s, with less than 200 reported deaths in 1991. A retrospective reconfirmation study of mesothelioma-associated deaths reported in Japanese death certificate data (ICD-10) was performed between 2003 and 2008 [5]. This study investigated 2069 mesothelioma cases out of 6030 cases mentioned in death certificates to clarify the clinical and pathological diagnosis of mesothelioma [5]. Results of this study showed that 929 of 2069 cases were pathologically reconfirmed to be mesothelioma. Since 2006, all patients with pathologically proven mesothelioma have been legally compensated through Workers' Accident Insurance or Asbestos Health Damage Relief Law. Pathologically proven diagnosis is required to obtain a certificate for compensation. Therefore, ICD-10 data of mesothelioma obtained after 2006 may be more reliable than those obtained before 2005.

The annual number of mesothelioma-associated deaths closely corresponds to the trend of asbestos import after Korean War, with a latency period of approximately 40 years from the first exposure to mesothelioma development (Fig. 12.1). Asbestos consumption in Japan showed two peaks: 352,000 ton consumption in 1974 and 320,000 ton consumption in 1988. Therefore, mesothelioma incidence may peak twice 40 years after these consumption peaks. Analysis of the association between the incidence of mesothelioma and quantity of asbestos used showed that 70 tons of produced and consumed asbestos caused at least one death due to mesothelioma [6]. Therefore, mesothelioma-associated deaths are predicted to reach approximately 2000 per year from 2014 to 2028. Other studies indicate that mesothelioma-associated mortality in Japanese people aged 50–89 years may increase until 2027, totaling to 66,327 deaths from 2003 to 2050 [7].

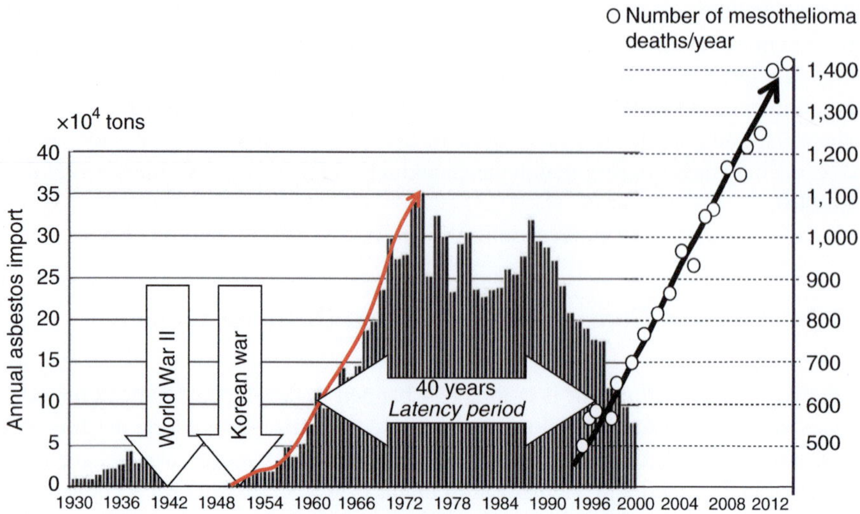

Fig. 12.1 Annual asbestos import and mesothelioma-associated deaths in Japan (death certificates from 1995 to 2013 were analyzed). Asbestos import ceased between 1942 and 1948 because of World War II. Recovery of Japanese industry has been accelerating since the Korean War (1950–1953), and asbestos import vastly increased in the late 1960s. Increased asbestos import after the Korean War closely corresponds to that of mesothelioma deaths since 1995, with a latency period of 40 years

12.4 Asbestos-Induced Carcinogenesis and Other Etiological Factors

Development of malignant mesothelioma is strongly associated with asbestos exposure. Asbestos is a generic term for a group of naturally occurring fibrous crystalline silicate minerals classified as group 1 carcinogens in humans by International Agency for Research on Cancer (IARC). Asbestos minerals are divided into two groups, namely, amphibole and serpentine, based on their crystalline structure. Amphibole forms crocidolite (blue asbestos) and amosite (brown asbestos) and serpentine form chrysotile (white asbestos) are widely used in insulation and fireproofing (Table 12.1). Crocidolite and amosite are considerably more persistent in the lung tissue than chrysotile. Inhaled chrysotile disappears rapidly from the lung tissue. However, cell culture studies have suggested that chrysotile is more toxic than some amphiboles. Chrysotile has a hollow central core, which acts as an ion reservoir, that may be responsible for its toxicity. Asbestos carcinogenicity depends on its fiber morphology, chemical composition, exposure concentration, exposure time, and biopersistence. Crocidolite induces mesothelioma at a high rate, and the relative mesothelioma risk for crocidolite, amosite, and chrysotile is a ratio of 500:100:1. Crocidolite is an iron-rich asbestos mineral that catalyzes the generation of reactive

Table 12.1 Chemical properties of fibrous minerals implicated to cause mesothelioma

Fiber type	Name	Chemical formula	Carcinogenic potential[a]
Amphibole			
	Crocidolite (blue asbestos)[a]	$Na_2(Fe^{3+})_2(Fe^{2+})_3Si_8O_{22}(OH)_2$	+++
	Amosite (brown asbestos)[a]	$(Mg < Fe^{2+})_7Si_8O_{22}(OH)_2$	++
	Tremolite	$Ca_2Mg_5Si_8O_{22}(OH)_2$	
	Anthophyllite	$Mg_7Si_8O_{22}(OH)_2$	
	Actinolite	$Ca_2(Mg, Fe^{2+})_5 Si_8O_{22}(OH)_2$	
Serpentine			
	Chrysotile (white asbestos)[a]	$Mg_6Si_4O_{10}(OH)_3$	+
Fibrous zeolite			
	Erionite	$(K_2Na_2Ca)MgAl_8Si_{28}O_{72}\cdot 28H_2O$	+++

[a]Commercial asbestos; specific ratio of relative risk for mesothelioma is 1 for chrysotile, 100 for amosite, and 500 for crocidolite

oxygen species in the presence of hydrogen peroxide and superoxide. Active oxygen and nitrogen species created by the surface charge on iron-rich fibers damage mesothelial cells. The shape of the fibers is also important. Fibers having a diameter of >0.25 μm and a length of ≥8 μm have the highest carcinogenic potency. These long thin asbestos fibers physically associate with the mitotic spindle apparatus in dividing cells to prevent proper segregation of chromosomes, resulting in chromosome damage [8]. Asbestos exposure may induce cytokine response to promote local and systemic immunosuppression. In addition, asbestos activates epidermal growth factor and mitogen-activated protein kinase signaling, thereby increasing the expression of transcription factors nuclear factor-kappa B (NF-κB) and activator protein 1 [9].

Fibrous minerals besides asbestos can also cause mesothelioma in humans. Erionite differs substantially from asbestos in terms of its structure and chemical composition. Moreover, its carcinogenic activity is higher than that of chrysotile and crocidolite. Erionite is classified as an IARC group 1 carcinogen in humans. Erionite has a very large surface area, most of which is internal. This internal area is connected with its fiber surface through tiny pores. These surface pores allow the passage of cations but are too small to allow the passage of large antioxidant molecules, which are produced to counteract the toxic effects of reactive oxygen species, to the most active regions of the fiber. Blockade of the surface pores with isopentane reduces the cytotoxicity of erionite by 50% [10]. Some villages in the Cappadocian region of Turkey show an extremely high incidence of malignant mesothelioma because erionite is present in volcanic tuffs used to cut blocks for building houses in these villages. Moreover, epidemiological and experimental studies have confirmed the high potential of erionite to induce malignant mesothelioma.

12.5 Molecular Pathogenesis of Malignant Mesothelioma

Genomic studies are limited for a small number of samples because mesothelioma is a rare tumor. Moreover, it is difficult to trace sequential accumulation of genetic/epigenetic alterations leading to mesothelioma development. Even though it has lagged behind other common malignancies, many researches to understand molecular pathogenesis have been done: cytogenetic testing, copy number analysis, genomic DNA sequencing, gene expression and epigenetic regulation analysis, transcript variant search, microRNA and noncoding RNA analysis, etc. Innovative molecular techniques, including next-generation sequencing (NGS), have provided new information on mutations associated with the development of malignant mesothelioma. However, results of these analyses do not provide information for developing effective molecular therapies to remarkably improve patient prognosis.

12.5.1 Chromosomal Changes

Cytogenetic testing can detect gain or loss of chromosomes or chromosome fragments. Cytogenetic analysis and classical comparative genomic hybridization (CGH) analysis (resolution: approximately 2–10 Mb) of malignant mesothelioma have detected complex and heterogeneous chromosomal changes and more loss of genetic material than gain in mesothelioma tissues. Loss of chromosomes 1p, 3p, 4q, 6q, 9p, 13, 14q, and 22 has been detected in majority of abnormal cases [11, 12]. The recurrent pattern of chromosomal loss suggests that these chromosomal regions correspond to locations of tumor suppressor genes whose loss or inactivation may play a pivotal role in mesothelioma tumorigenesis. Increased commercial availability of high-density oligonucleotide and single-nucleotide polymorphism (SNP) arrays has facilitated their use (average space between probes is approximately 3–8 kb for high-density oligonucleotide or SNP arrays). Development of array CGH confirmed that frequent homozygous deletion occurred in the genes *CDKN2A/2B* (cyclin-dependent kinase inhibitor 2A/2B) at 9p21.3, and the minimal common region of 22q loss carried *NF2* (neurofibromin 2) [13]. However, these two genes are the only driver genes known to be present in the genomic instability regions in malignant mesothelioma tissues to date. Significance of 3p21 deletion in malignant mesothelioma is under investigation. In 2011, a study found that *BAP1* is inactivated by somatic mutations [14]. The minimal common deletion region at 3p21.1 carry *BAP1* and *PBRM1* et al., but not *RASSF1A* and *TUSC2* that are lost in lung, breast, kidney and other cancers at 3p21.3 [15]. The genomic pattern of peritoneal mesothelioma is similar to that of pleural mesothelioma [16]. Recent studies targeting the 3p21 region by performing high-density array CGH (average probe interval: 254 bp) have detected multiple minute simultaneous biallelic deletions in this region, especially in *BAP1* (8/33, 24%), *SETD2* (7/33, 21%), *PBRM1* (3/33, 9%), and *SMARCC1*

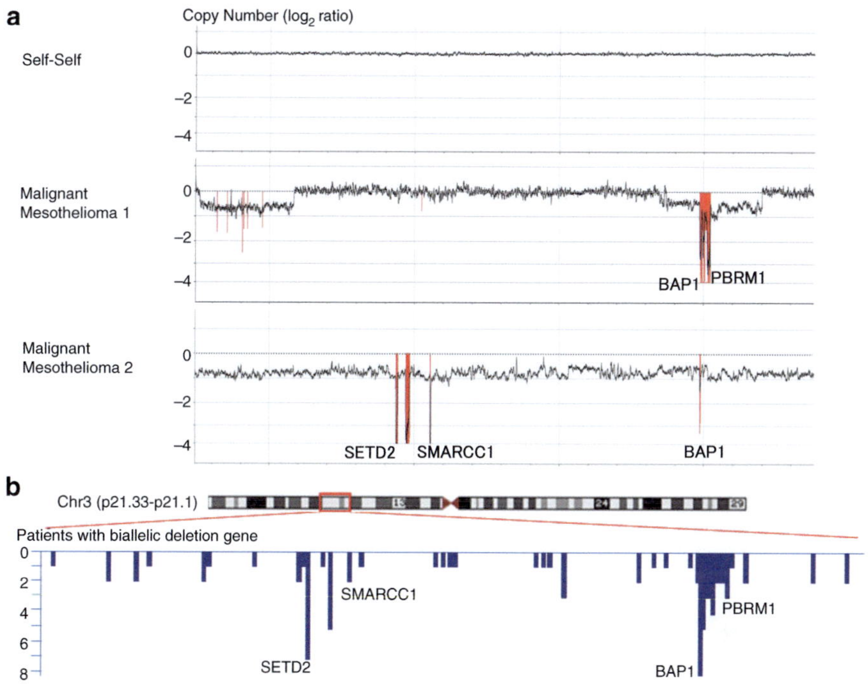

Fig. 12.2 Segmental copy number loss detected in the 3p21 region by performing high-density array CGH. (**a**) Self-self, which indicates the same genomic DNA, was used for labeling both Cy5 and Cy3 in the array CGH analysis and shows the performance of the array without any genetic signal. Representative copy number change in two mesothelioma specimens. Copy number is shown as a $\log_2$ ratio. Regions showing biallelic deletion are marked in red. (**b**) Frequency of biallelic deletion in 251 genes in the 3p21 region in 33 mesothelioma specimens. The genes have been aligned along the genome location on the vertical axis. The horizontal blue bars represent each of the 46 genes, and the length of the bar represents case frequency that showed biallelic deletions. Number of patients with a given biallelic deletion is shown on the *Y*-axis

(2/33, 6%) [17] (Fig. 12.2). In all, 46 genes in this region were found to contain biallelic deletions in at least one biopsy specimen out of 33 mesothelioma specimens examined; break points of these genomic deletions were different in different cases. Many of these deletions were not contiguous but alternated with segments showing oscillating copy number changes along the 3p21 region. This may be because of chromothripsis (derived from the Greek word "chromos" for chromosome and "thripsis" for shattering into pieces) [18], a phenomenon characterized by numerous genomic rearrangements caused by a single catastrophic event in multiple cancer samples.

The frequency of micronuclei formation is significantly higher in peripheral blood lymphocytes of patients with malignant mesothelioma than in peripheral blood lymphocytes of patients with lung cancer and benign respiratory diseases or healthy control subjects [19]. Micronucleus is the small nucleus that forms after failing to attach properly to the mitotic spindle and resulting not to be incorporated into one of the daughter nuclei during cell division. Micronuclei formation is thought to be an indicator of genotoxic events and chromosomal instability. A study has proposed that chromothripsis induces micronuclei formation [20].

12.5.2 Driver Genes Associated with Mesothelioma Development

Integrative OncoGenomics database (https://www.intogen.org/), a database of mutational cancer driver genes, shows that the top 5 mutated genes in 28 cancer types (6792 samples) are *TP53*, *PIK3CA*, *KRAS*, *BRAF*, and *PTEN*. Malignant mesothelioma rarely shows mutations in most of the well-known driver genes, including the abovementioned genes, but show abundant chromosomal abnormalities.

12.5.2.1 *CDKN2A* Deletion

Inactivation of *CDKN2A*, a tumor suppressor gene, is associated with the development of several cancer types. Homozygous deletion of 9p21.3 is the most frequently detected genetic alteration in malignant mesothelioma and occurs in >90% cell lines established from malignant mesothelioma. The deleted region contains *CDKN2A* and *CDKN2B* and often methylthioadenosine phosphorylase (*MTAP*) and *MIR31* present in adjacent regions. Transcription of *CDKN2A* produces three alternatively spliced variants that encode distinct proteins. Two encode structurally related isoforms, p16INK4A and p16gamma, and inhibit CDK4 kinase to prevent phosphorylation of the retinoblastoma protein (RB). The remaining transcript, which contains an alternate first exon located 20-kb upstream of the remainder of the gene, encodes an alternate reading frame (ARF) protein p14ARF. This protein stabilizes tumor suppressor protein p53 by interacting with E3 ubiquitin-protein ligase MDM2. Proteins encoded by this gene play an essential role in regulating cell cycle and senescence through two major tumor-suppressing pathways of RB and p53. In malignant mesothelioma, *CDKN2A* is inactivated mainly through deletion and less frequently through methylation [21] or heterozygous deletion/point mutation.

Mice lacking *CDKN2A* show expected Mendelian distribution and normal development, except for thymic hyperplasia [22]. Asbestos exposure induces iron overload. A rat model of iron-induced peritoneal mesothelioma was established by repeatedly injecting iron saccharate and nitrilotriacetate, an iron chelator, intraperitoneally; this mouse model showed homozygous deletion of *CDKN2A/2B* [23]. Results obtained using this mouse model suggest that oxidative stress induces the homozygous deletion of *CDKN2A/2B*, suggesting that it is a major target gene in mesothelioma development.

Several studies have assessed the homozygous deletion of *CDKN2A* for diagnosing mesothelioma. Fluorescence in situ hybridization (FISH) of *CDKN2A* is useful for differentiating between reactive and normal mesothelioma cells in pleural effusion smears.

Homozygous deletion of *CDKN2A* can be used for diagnosing malignant mesothelioma by using a combination of morphological markers specific to mesothelioma, including cell-in-cell engulfment with or without hump formation, multinucleate cell formation, and large berrylike cell aggregate formation [24]. Results of this study showed that 80/93 (86.0%) cases of sporadic mesothelioma showed homozygous deletion of *CDKN2A* and 15/93 (16.1%) cases of sporadic mesothelioma showed heterozygous deletion of *CDKN2A* by setting the cutoff value of homozygous/heterozygous deletion of this gene, namely, no deletion positive in reactive mesothelial cells, by FISH examination. In this condition, the overall survival of patients with mesothelioma who show homozygous *CDKN2A* deletion ($n = 24$) is significantly lower than that of patients with mesothelioma not showing *CDKN2A* deletion ($n = 5, p = 0.0002$). Also, low homozygous deletion/high heterozygous deletion cases ($n = 5$) had a significantly better prognosis than homozygous deletion ($\geq 30\%$) cases ($n = 17; p = 0.011$) [25].

12.5.2.2 Inactivation of *NF2* and Hippo Pathway

The *NF2* gene responsible for neurofibromatosis type 2 familial cancer syndrome, which is the most frequently mutated gene detected in mesothelioma, is located at chromosome 22q12. Homozygous or heterozygous deletion or point mutations inactivate this gene in 40–50% patients with malignant mesothelioma [26, 27]. *NF2*-encoded protein merlin, which contains a FERM domain, specifically binds to several target proteins localized both in the cytoplasm and nucleus. NF2 acts upstream of SAV1, LATS1/2, and yes-associated protein (YAP) in Hippo tumor suppressor pathway. This pathway plays vital roles in regulating organ size, cell contact inhibition, stem cell function, and regeneration. Disruption of the Hippo pathway inhibits the phosphorylation of YAP transcriptional cofactor, which then translocates to the nucleus. YAP interacts with a TEA domain-containing transcription factor to promote the transcription of cell proliferation-associated and anti-apoptotic genes.

NF2 homozygous mutant mice die early during embryonic development [28]. Hemizygous mice do not show clinical features of human NF2, a tumor spectrum that differs significantly from that observed in NF2 patients [29]. Intraperitoneal injection of crocidolite fibers in *NF2* heterozygous knockout mice induces mesothelioma development at a higher frequency than that in their wild-type counterparts [30]. Mesothelioma cell lines established from neoplastic ascites obtained from these heterozygous knockout mice do not express merlin because of the loss of the wild-type *NF2* allele. These results indicate an association between asbestos exposure and *NF2* inactivation in mesothelioma oncogenesis. SiRNA-induced knockdown of *NF2* and transfection of the gene encoding phosphorylation-resistant YAP (constitutively active) into immortalized human mesothelial cells promote their transformation to mesothelioma-like tumor cells after subcutaneous transplantation into nude mice [31]. This suggests that activated YAP plays a crucial role in oncogenic transformation.

Deletions and mutations in *SAV1* and *LATS2* are also observed in malignant mesothelioma cells [32]. Established 61 mesothelioma primary cultures showed the altered *LATS2* gene by point mutations and exon deletions in 11% of malignant mesothelioma [33]. In addition, coexisting mutation in *LATS2* and *NF2* was detected in the same mesothelioma specimens. The patient subgroup showing the similar gene expression pattern with ones having mutations in both genes presented a poor prognosis, but tumors of this subgroup showed higher sensitivity to dual PI3K/mTOR inhibitor (PF-04691502) [33]. Because *LATS2* and *NF2* are susceptible to exon-level deletion, the frequency of Hippo pathway disruption may be higher in malignant mesothelioma than that determined previously by performing sequence analysis of DNA obtained from tumor specimens. Studies with this pathway would hide the possibility of causing a new therapeutic strategy.

12.5.2.3 *BAP1* Mutation and Tumor Predisposition Syndrome

BAP1 encodes a nuclear ubiquitin carboxy-terminal hydrolase, which functions as a deubiquitinating enzyme. *BAP1* has gained attention because it frequently shows somatic mutations in malignant mesothelioma and melanoma cells and because germline mutations in this gene are associated with a new tumor predisposition syndrome. Frequent somatic mutations in *BAP1* have been observed in highly metastatic uveal melanomas; exome sequencing detected 26 of 31 (84%) metastasizing tumors and one of them was germline in origin [34]. Studies focused on the frequently deleted 3p21 region in malignant mesothelioma detected somatic *BAP1* mutations in 12 of 53 (23%) [14] and 14 of 23 (61%) tumor specimens [35]. The frequency of *BAP1* inactivation varies in malignant mesothelioma, with 20–30% inactivation frequency being determined by performing Sanger sequencing or NGS [14, 36] and higher frequency (>60%) being determined using integrated genomic approaches that combine sequencing with array CGH, multiple ligation-dependent probe amplification (MLPA), and immunohistochemistry [35, 37, 38]. Studies that assess cancer biopsy specimens by almost exclusively performing DNA sequencing, especially NGS, tend to overlook exon-level or whole-gene deletions. Somatic *BAP1* mutations occur predominantly in epithelioid or biphasic-type malignant mesothelioma [35, 39].

Germline *BAP1* mutations in two families with a high incidence of malignant mesothelioma and additional somatic alterations of this were identified in 2011, and the families were characterized as having mesothelioma and uveal melanoma [3]. Subsequent linkage analysis showed that *BAP1* is an inherited susceptibility locus on chromosome 3p21. Results of this study indicate that germline alterations affect the risk of mesothelioma, a cancer associated with environmental factors. Another study detected co-segregating germline mutations in *BAP1* in two unrelated families whose different members had melanocytic tumors, uveal melanoma, and cutaneous melanoma [40]. Moreover, meningioma, renal cell carcinoma, basal cell carcinoma, and other cancers are added to the tumor spectrum of this syndrome. New branches of families carrying *BAP1* mutations were identified by screening patients with a family history of multiple mesotheliomas and melanomas and/or multiple cancers caused by germline *BAP1* mutation; this screening identified four families that shared the same *BAP1* mutation [41]. These studies identified carriers of high-risk germline *BAP1* mutations that will benefit from genetic counseling and screening for early cancer detection. *BAP1* tumor predisposition syndrome is inherited in an autosomal dominant manner. Once a germline *BAP1* pathogenic variant has been identified in an affected family member, prenatal testing should be performed for determining the increased risk of this syndrome and preimplantation genetic diagnosis.

Earlier studies showed that BAP1 binds to the RING finger domain of BRCA1; however, recent studies have shown that BRCA1 is not the binding partner of BAP1 [42]. This contains binding domains for HCFC1, chromatin-associated transcriptional regulator regulating cell proliferation. Calypso, a *Drosophila* Polycomb group gene, also encodes the ubiquitin carboxy-terminal hydrolase BAP1. Biochemically purified calypso exists in a complex with Polycomb group protein ASX. In *Drosophila*, this complex (called Polycomb repressive deubiquitinase [PR-DUB]) binds to target genes belonging to the Polycomb group [43]. Reconstituted recombinant *Drosophila* and human PR-DUB complexes, containing human BAP1 and ASXL1, remove monoubiquitin from histone H2A but not from H2B in nucleosomes. *Drosophila* mutants lacking PR-DUB show increased levels of monoubiquitinated H2A. A mutation that disrupts the catalytic activity of calypso or absence of ASX abolishes H2A deubiquitination in vitro and represses the expression of HOX genes, which are master regulators of embryonic development, in vivo [43].

BAP1 deletion in mice induces embryogenic lethality. However, systemically or hematopoietically restricted *BAP1* deletion in adults recapitulates features of human myelodysplastic syndrome [44]. Unexposed mice showing *BAP1* heterozygous deletion do not develop spontaneous mesothelioma [45]. However, the frequency and rate of mesothelioma development are significantly higher in *BAP1*$^{+/-}$ mice exposed to asbestos than in their wild-type littermates.These findings suggest that high penetrance of malignant mesothelioma requires environmental exposure to asbestos or other carcinogenic fibers. Mesothelioma cells from *BAP1*$^{+/-}$ mice show biallelic inactivation of *BAP1*. It is interesting that mesothelioma from BAP1$^{+/-}$ mice did not require homozygous loss of *CDKN2A* unlike in wild-type mice.

12.5.2.4 Comprehensive Analysis of Genomic Alterations

Whole-exome studies (WES) have shown that each mesothelioma biopsy specimen has specific mutations and rarely has driver mutations. Two recent studies provided similar results. One study detected 490 mutated genes in 22 frozen biopsy specimens of mesothelioma; of these, 477 (97%) genes were mutated only in one biopsy specimen, with an average of 23 mutations per sample (range, 2–51) [46]. The other study was a WES (99 specimens) and identified an average of 24 ± 11 (mean ± s.d.) protein-coding alterations per sample; targeted NGS (460 genes in 103 cases of mesothelioma) performed in this study showed that majority of the detected mutations (85%; 2144/2529 protein-altering somatic mutations) were novel [47]. Mutations in human cancers range from as low as one base substitution per exome (<0.1/Mb) in some pediatric malignancies to several mutations per exome (~100/Mb) in adult malignancies such as lung cancer and melanoma [48]. Low level of mutations detected by NGS in malignant mesothelioma is unexpected and highly unusual. NGS often cannot detect medium- and large-sized DNA deletions (>30 bp), and conventional whole-genome array CGH cannot detect small- and medium-sized deletions (<3000 bp) in tumor biopsy specimens. Moreover, these analyses overlook genomic deletions of 30 and 3000 bp. Results of combined high-density array CGH (average probe interval: 254 bp in the 3p21 region) and targeted NGS showed that frequencies of biallelic deletions in *BAP1*, *SETD2*, *PBRM1*, and *SMARCC1* were equal to or higher than those of sequence-level mutations [17]. Genomic alterations in mesothelioma usually include genomic rearrangements that induce complex and multiple deletions. Digital MLPA, which analyzes the copy number of approximately 600 exons simultaneously by using NGS-based MLPA, might be a reliable method for high-throughput detection of multiple segmental deletions in small amounts of DNA in mesothelioma specimens.

A study in 2016 that performed comprehensive NGS, including transcriptome (n = 211), whole-exome (n = 99), and targeted exome analyses (n = 103), of 216 pleural malignant mesothelioma specimens provided new information about somatic mutations. For sequence-level alterations, significantly mutated genes (q-score, ≥0.8) were *BAP1* (23%, 46/202), *NF2* (19%, 38/202), *TP53* (8%, 17/202), *SETD2* (8%, 17/202), *DDX3X* (4%, 8/202), *RYR2* (4%, 4/99), *CFAP45* (3%, 3/99), *SETDB1* (3%, 7/202), *ULK2* (1%, 3/202), and *DDX51* (1%, 3/202) [47]. Moreover, this study identified mutations in *SF3B1* at a frequency of ~2% (4/216); these mutations were associated with specific alterations in mRNA splicing.

12.5.3 Aberrant Transcriptional Regulation

Studies have been performed to identify biomarkers for diagnosing and histologically classifying mesothelioma by using transcriptome analysis; however, a definitive diagnostic tool has not been established to date. Moreover, studies determining molecular targets for mesothelioma treatment are ongoing. Because mutations in genes encoding proteins associated with histone modification and chromatin remodeling, including *BAP1*, *SETD2*, and *PBRM1*, occur predominantly in mesothelioma, diverse gene expression changes induced by aberrant epigenetic regulation can be easily estimated.

12.5.3.1 Deregulated Gene Expression

Majority of deregulated genes in malignant mesothelioma belong to the following pathways: angiogenesis, cell adhesion, p53 signaling, integrin signaling, MAPK signaling, apoptosis, and cell cycle regulation. These genes play a crucial role in cancer development and progression but are deregulated in many cancers. Gene expression patterns of not only one or a few genes but of a special set of genes have been used for the differential diagnosis of mesothelioma. A set of 26 genes selected from 4 gene ratio-based tests showed high sensitivity and specificity to individually distinguish malignant pleural mesothelioma from (1) normal pleura, (2) sarcoma, (3) renal cell carcinoma, and (4) thymoma [49]. A recent study showed that two gene sets, one containing 22 genes and the other containing 40 genes, selected from 117 genes identified in previous studies could differentiate between malignant and benign pleural proliferations [50].

12.5.3.2 Fusion Transcripts and Altered Splicing

Recurrent gene fusions are usually associated with oncogenic activation. Gene fusions involving tumor suppressor genes have been recently reported in mesothelioma (13 fusions involving *NF2*, 7 involving *BAP1*, 8 involving *SETD2*, 7 involving *PBRM1*, 2 involving *PTEN*, and 6 involving other genes, as determined by performing transcriptome analysis; $n = 211$) [47]. The same study also identified aberrant splicing variants. Many of these fusions or aberrant splicing variants were derived from genes in chromosome regions 22q12, 3p21, 9p21.3, and 13q12, which are frequently deleted in malignant mesothelioma. These gene regions may be depredated by chromothripsis, leading to extensive rearrangement that produces fusion genes or aberrant splicing variants.

12.5.3.3 Altered Expression of MicroRNAs and New Biomarkers

MicroRNAs (miRNAs) are short noncoding RNAs containing approximately 18–22 nucleotides and function as posttranscriptional regulators of gene expression. Expression of miRNAs is dysregulated in human cancers through various mechanisms, including amplification or deletion of miRNA genes, abnormal transcriptional control of miRNAs, dysregulation of epigenetic changes, and defect in biogenesis components. Expression of miRNAs is globally suppressed in malignant mesothelioma similar to that in other cancer types. Expression of miR-31 is reduced in most patients with mesothelioma because of the deletion of its encoding gene along with that of *CDKN2A* in 9p21.3 region [51]. Expression of miR-34b and miR-34c, which share a common primary transcript, is silenced by methylation in majority (85%) of patients with malignant mesothelioma [52]. Members of miR-34 family mediate p53-induced tumor suppression. MiRNA mimics are small, double-stranded RNA molecules that mimic endogenous mature miRNAs when transfected into cells. Mimics of miR-31 and miR-34b/c reduce cell growth through cell cycle arrest and inhibit cell migration and invasion, respectively [51, 52]. Expression of miRNAs belonging to miR-15 family is significantly downregulated in malignant mesothelioma compared with that in normal pleura [53]. The miR-15 family includes related mir-15a and mir-15b as well as miR-16-1, miR-16-2, miR-195, and miR-497. Mimics of miR-15a, miR-15b, and miR-16 inhibit malignant mesothelioma cell proliferation and induce cell cycle arrest and apoptosis by regulating target genes, including *CCND1* and *BCL-2* [53]. Expression of miRNAs belonging to miR-193a-3p and miR-200 families is significantly downregulated in malignant mesothelioma specimens compared with that in normal pleura. Transfection of malignant mesothelioma cells with a miR-193a-3p mimic inhibits their growth and induces their apoptosis and necrosis by decreasing the expression of antiapoptotic protein MCL1 [54]. However, these finding should be validated independently to determine the true diagnostic value of changes in the expression of these miRNAs. Several studies have focused on identifying blood-based diagnostic markers. Decreased levels of miR-103 in the peripheral blood of patients with malignant mesothelioma might be a useful biomarker [55]. Levels of miR-126 are significantly lower in the serum samples of patients with malignant mesothelioma than in those of asbestos-exposed or healthy control subjects [56]. However, these findings should be validated in further studies.

12.6 Pathology of Malignant Pleural Mesothelioma

Malignant pleural mesothelioma can be divided into three distinct histological types, namely, epithelioid, biphasic, and sarcomatoid mesothelioma, with relative frequencies of 60%, 30%, and 10%, respectively. Pathological pattern is the most important prognostic factor of mesothelioma; patients with a pure epithelioid histology show the best prognosis, those with a pure sarcomatoid histology show the poorest prognosis, and those with a biphasic pattern show an intermediate prognosis. Pathologically, mesothelioma is diagnosed based on H&E staining and immunohistochemical analysis of positive and negative mesothelioma markers. Positive markers include calretinin, cytokeratin 5/6, WT-1, and D2-40, and negative markers include CEA, Ber-EP4, TTF-1, MOC-31, and Leu-M1.

12.7 Clinical Presentation: Staging and Clinical Features

The pleura forms a continuous layer over the thoracic structures and is divided into parietal and visceral pleura. The parietal pleura lines the thoracic wall, diaphragm, and mediastinum, and the visceral pleura covers the lungs. Both the pleurae meet at the hilum as the pulmonary ligament. Because clearance of asbestos fibers occurs in the pleural cavity, most mesothelioma researchers believe that malignant pleural mesothelioma initially arises from mesothelial cells in the parietal pleura. In the

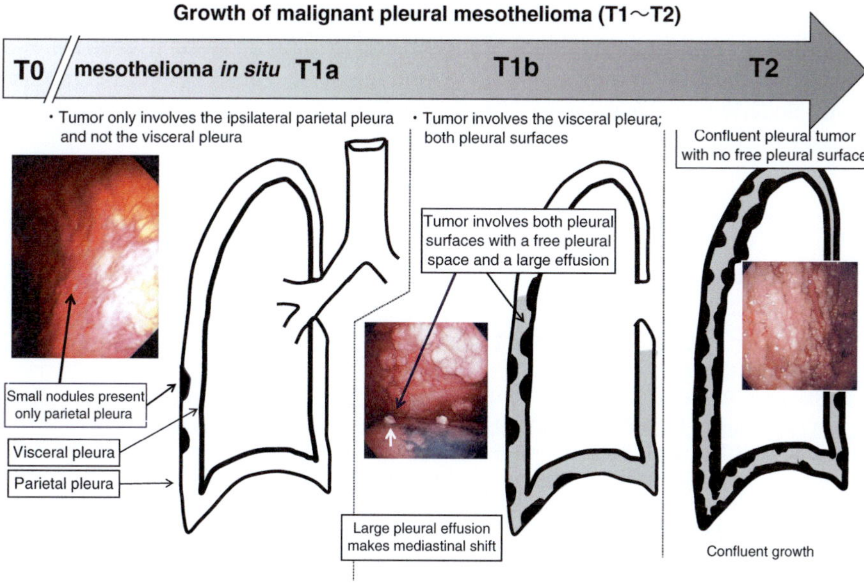

Fig. 12.3 Tumor growth of malignant pleural mesothelioma. T1a and T1b are International Mesothelioma Interest Group (IMIG) T-categories that are collapsed into a single T1 category in the eighth TNM classification proposed by IASLC (2016)

earliest clinical stage, tumors are localized in the parietal pleura of the hemithorax and not on the visceral pleura (T1a). Subsequently, tumors deposit on the visceral pleural surface (T1b). In advanced-stage mesothelioma, tumors grow diffusely in the visceral and parietal pleura, including the interlobar fissure (T2) (Fig. 12.3). In the eighth edition of TNM classification proposed by IASLC in 2016, T1a and T1b are collapsed into a single T1 category because no significant difference was observed in survival.

Most patients with early clinical stage of malignant pleural mesothelioma without symptom are discovered through the incidental observation of a pleural effusion or pleural thickening on chest X ray in high-risk group. Chest pain and shortness of breath are the most common clinical symptoms at the onset of mesothelioma. Mesothelioma cells form dissemination sites at a high rate along needle tracts and surgical wounds and then form palpable subcutaneous tumor nodules. Transdiaphragmatic extension to the liver and peritoneum is common. T3 indicates a locally advanced but potentially resectable tumor, and T4 indicates a very locally advanced and technically unresectable tumor.

12.8 Conclusion

Asbestos and non-asbestos fibrous minerals are strongly associated with the development of mesothelioma. Molecular mechanism underlying the development of mesothelioma has not been clearly understood despite intensive efforts. The finding that mesothelioma develops as a familial cancer syndrome with a *BAP1* germline mutation is surprising. Some mesothelioma susceptibility genes may contribute to the development of this rare neoplasm. A better understanding of molecular mechanisms underlying the pathogenesis of mesothelioma is important to develop curative treatment strategies for this devastating neoplasm.

References

1. Risberg B, Nickels J, Wågermark J. Familial clustering of malignant mesothelioma. Cancer. 1980;45:2422–7.
2. Hammar SP, Bockus D, Remington F, Freidman S, LaZerte G. Familial mesothelioma: a report of two families. Hum Pathol. 1989;20:107–12.
3. Testa JR, Cheung M, Pei J, Below JE, Tan Y, Sementino E, et al. Germline BAP1 mutations predispose to malignant mesothelioma. Nat Genet. 2011;43:1022–5.
4. Mazurek JM, Syamlal G, Wood JM, Hendricks SA, Weston A. Malignant mesothelioma mortality - United States, 1999–2015. MMWR Morb Mortal Wkly Rep. 2017;66:214–8.
5. Gemba K, Fujimoto N, Kato K, Aoe K, Takeshima Y, Inai K, et al. National survey of malignant mesothelioma and asbestos exposure in Japan. Cancer Sci. 2012;103:483–90.
6. Tossavainen A. Global use of asbestos and the incidence of mesothelioma. Int J Occup Environ Health. 2004;10:22–5.
7. Myojin T, Azuma K, Okumura J, Uchiyama I. Future trends of mesothelioma mortality in Japan based on risk function. Ind Health. 2012;50:197–204.
8. Ault JG, Cole RW, Jensen CG, Jensen LC, Bachert LA, Rieder CL. Behavior of crocidolite asbestos during mitosis in living vertebrate lung epithelial cells. Cancer Res. 1995; 55:792–8.
9. Altomare DA, Testa JR. Cytogenetic and molecular genetic changes in malignant mesothelioma. In: O'Byne K, Rusch V, editors. Malignant pleural mesothelioma. Oxford: Oxford University Press; 2006. p. 239–50.
10. King JE, Hasleton PS. The epidemiology and etiology of malignant mesothelioma. In: O'Byne K, Rusch V, editors. Malignant pleural mesothelioma. Oxford: Oxford University Press; 2006. p. 1–18.
11. Taguchi T, Jhanwar SC, Siegfried JM, Keller SM, Testa JR. Recurrent deletions of specific chromosomal sites in 1p, 3p, 6q, and 9p in human malignant mesothelioma. Cancer Res. 1993;53:4349–55.
12. Bjorkqvist AM, Tammilehto L, Anttila S, Mattson K, Knuutila S. Recurrent DNA copy number changes in 1q, 4q, 6q, 9p, 13q, 14q and 22q detected by comparative genomic hybridization in malignant mesothelioma. Br J Cancer. 1997;75:523–7.
13. Lindholm PM, Salmenkivi K, Vauhkonen H, Nicholson AG, Anttila S, Kinnula VL, et al. Gene copy number analysis in malignant pleural mesothelioma using oligonucleotide array CGH. Cytogenet Genome Res. 2007;119(1–2):46–52.
14. Bott M, Brevet M, Taylor BS, Shimizu S, Ito T, Wang L, et al. The nuclear deubiquitinase BAP1 is commonly inactivated by somatic mutations and 3p21.1 losses in malignant pleural mesothelioma. Nat Genet. 2011;43:668–72.
15. Yoshikawa Y, Sato A, Tsujimura T, Morinaga T, Fukuoka K, Yamada S, et al. Frequent deletion of 3p21.1 region carrying semaphorin 3G and aberrant expression of the genes participating in semaphorin signaling in the epithelioid type of malignant mesothelioma cells. Int J Oncol. 2011;39:1365–74.
16. Chirac P, Maillet D, Lepretre F, Isaac S, Glehen O, Figeac M, et al. Genomic copy number alterations in 33 malignant peritoneal mesothelioma analyzed by comparative genomic hybridization array. Hum Pathol. 2016;55:72–82.

17. Yoshikawa Y, Emi M, Hashimoto-Tamaoki T, Ohmuraya M, Sato A, Tsujimura T, et al. High-density array-CGH with targeted NGS unmask multiple noncontiguous minute deletions on chromosome 3p21 in mesothelioma. Proc Natl Acad Sci U S A. 2016;113:13432–7.
18. Stephens PJ, Greenman CD, Fu B, Yang F, Bignell GR, Mudie LJ, et al. Massive genomic rearrangement acquired in a single catastrophic event during cancer development. Cell. 2011;144:27–40.
19. Bolognesi C, Filiberti R, Neri M, Perrone E, Landini E, Canessa PA, et al. High frequency of micronuclei in peripheral blood lymphocytes as index of susceptibility to pleural malignant mesothelioma. Cancer Res. 2002;62:5418–9.
20. Zhang CZ, Spektor A, Cornils H, Francis JM, Jackson EK, Liu S, et al. Chromothripsis from DNA damage in micronuclei. Nature. 2015;522(7555):179–84.
21. Kobayashi N, Toyooka S, Yanai H, Soh J, Fujimoto N, Yamamoto H, et al. Frequent p16 inactivation by homozygous deletion or methylation is associated with a poor prognosis in Japanese patients with pleural mesothelioma. Lung Cancer. 2008;62:120–5.
22. Sharpless NE, Bardeesy N, Lee KH, Carrasco D, Castrillon DH, Aguirre AJ, et al. Loss of p16Ink4a with retention of p19Arf predisposes mice to tumorigenesis. Nature. 2001;413(6851):86–91.
23. Hu Q, Akatsuka S, Yamashita Y, Ohara H, Nagai H, Okazaki Y, et al. Homozygous deletion of CDKN2A/2B is a hallmark of iron-induced high-grade rat mesothelioma. Lab Investig. 2010;90(3):360–73.
24. Nabeshima K, Matsumoto S, Hamasaki M, Hida T, Kamei T, Hiroshima K, et al. Use of p16 FISH for differential diagnosis of mesothelioma in smear preparations. Diagn Cytopathol. 2016;44:774–80.
25. Hamasaki M, Matsumoto S, Abe S, Hamatake D, Kamei T, Hiroshima K, et al. Low homozygous/high heterozygous deletion status by p16 FISH correlates with a better prognostic group than high homozygous deletion status in malignant pleural mesothelioma. Lung Cancer. 2016;99:155–61.
26. Bianchi AB, Mitsunaga SI, Cheng JQ, Klein WM, Jhanwar SC, Seizinger B, et al. High frequency of inactivating mutations in the neurofibromatosis type 2 gene (NF2) in primary malignant mesotheliomas. Proc Natl Acad Sci U S A. 1995;92:10854–8.
27. Sekido Y, Pass HI, Bader S, Mew DJ, Christman MF, Gazdar AF, et al. Neurofibromatosis type 2 (NF2) gene is somatically mutated in mesothelioma but not in lung cancer. Cancer Res. 1995;55:1227–31.
28. McClatchey AI, Saotome I, Ramesh V, Gusella JF, Jacks T. The Nf2 tumor suppressor gene product is essential for extraembryonic development immediately prior to gastrulation. Genes Dev. 1997;11:1253–65.
29. McClatchey AI, Saotome I, Mercer K, Crowley D, Gusella JF, Bronson RT, et al. Mice heterozygous for a mutation at the Nf2 tumor suppressor locus develop a range of highly metastatic tumors. Genes Dev. 1998;12(8):1121–33.
30. Fleury-Feith J, Lecomte C, Renier A, Matrat M, Kheuang L, Abramowski V, et al. Hemizygosity of Nf2 is associated with increased susceptibility to asbestos-induced peritoneal tumours. Oncogene. 2003;22(24):3799–805.
31. Kakiuchi T, Takahara T, Kasugai Y, Arita K, Yoshida N, Karube K, et al. Modeling mesothelioma utilizing human mesothelial cells reveals involvement of phospholipase-C beta 4 in YAP-active mesothelioma cell proliferation. Carcinogenesis. 2016. pii: bgw084.
32. Murakami H, Mizuno T, Taniguchi T, Fujii M, Ishiguro F, Fukui T, et al. LATS2 is a tumor suppressor gene of malignant mesothelioma. Cancer Res. 2011;71:873–83.
33. Tranchant R, Quetel L, Tallet A, Meiller C, Renier A, de Koning L, et al. Co-occurring mutations of tumor suppressor genes, LATS2 and NF2, in malignant pleural mesothelioma. Clin Cancer Res. 2016. https://doi.org/10.1158/1078-0432.CCR-16-1971.
34. Harbour JW, Onken MD, Roberson ED, Duan S, Cao L, Worley LA, et al. Frequent mutation of BAP1 in metastasizing uveal melanomas. Science. 2010;330(6009):1410–3.
35. Yoshikawa Y, Sato A, Tsujimura T, Emi M, Morinaga T, Fukuoka K, et al. Frequent inactivation of the BAP1 gene in epithelioid-type malignant mesothelioma. Cancer Sci. 2012;103:868–74.

36. Zauderer MG, Bott M, McMillan R, Sima CS, Rusch V, Krug LM, et al. Clinical characteristics of patients with malignant pleural mesothelioma harboring somatic BAP1 mutations. J Thorac Oncol. 2013;8:1430–3.
37. Nasu M, Emi M, Pastorino S, Tanji M, Powers A, Luk H, et al. High incidence of somatic BAP1 alterations in sporadic malignant mesothelioma. J Thorac Oncol. 2015;10:565–76.
38. Emi M, Yoshikawa Y, Sato C, Sato A, Sato H, Kato T, et al. Frequent genomic rearrangements of BRCA1 associated protein-1 (BAP1) gene in Japanese malignant mesothelioma-characterization of deletions at exon level. J Hum Genet. 2015;60:647–9.
39. Cigognetti M, Lonardi S, Fisogni S, Balzarini P, Pellegrini V, Tironi A, et al. BAP1 (BRCA1-associated protein 1) is a highly specific marker for differentiating mesothelioma from reactive mesothelial proliferations. Mod Pathol. 2015;28:1043–57.
40. Wiesner T, Obenauf AC, Murali R, Fried I, Griewank KG, Ulz P, et al. Germline mutations in BAP1 predispose to melanocytic tumors. Nat Genet. 2011;43:1018–21.
41. Carbone M, Flores EG, Emi M, Johnson TA, Tsunoda T, Behner D, et al. Combined genetic and genealogic studies uncover a large BAP1 cancer syndrome kindred tracing back nine generations to a common ancestor from the 1700s. PLoS Genet. 2015;11(12):e1005633. https://doi.org/10.1371/journal.pgen.1005633. eCollection 2015
42. Nishikawa H, Wu W, Koike A, Kojima R, Gomi H, Fukuda M, et al. BRCA1-associated protein 1 interferes with BRCA1/BARD1 RING heterodimer activity. Cancer Res. 2009;69:111–9.
43. Scheuermann JC, de Ayala Alonso AG, Oktaba K, Ly-Hartig N, McGinty RK, Fraterman S, et al. Histone H2A deubiquitinase activity of the Polycomb repressive complex PR-DUB. Nature. 2010;465(7295):243–7.
44. Dey A, Seshasayee D, Noubade R, French DM, Liu J, Chaurushiya MS, et al. Loss of the tumor suppressor BAP1 causes myeloid transformation. Science. 2012;337(6101):1541–6.
45. Xu J, Kadariya Y, Cheung M, Pei J, Talarchek J, Sementino E, et al. Germline mutation of Bap1 accelerates development of asbestos-induced malignant mesothelioma. Cancer Res. 2014;74:4388–97.
46. Guo G, Chmielecki J, Goparaju C, Heguy A, Dolgalev I, Carbone M, et al. Whole-exome sequencing reveals frequent genetic alterations in BAP1, NF2, CDKN2A, and CUL1 in malignant pleural mesothelioma. Cancer Res. 2015;75:264–9.
47. Bueno R, Stawiski EW, Goldstein LD, Durinck S, De Rienzo A, Modrusan Z, et al. Comprehensive genomic analysis of malignant pleural mesothelioma identifies recurrent mutations, gene fusions and splicing alterations. Nat Genet. 2016;48:407–16.
48. Garraway LA, Lander ES. Lessons from the cancer genome. Cell. 2013;153:17–37.
49. De Rienzo A, Richards WG, Yeap BY, Coleman MH, Sugarbaker PE, Chirieac LR, et al. Sequential binary gene ratio tests define a novel molecular diagnostic strategy for malignant pleural mesothelioma. Clin Cancer Res. 2013;19:2493–502.
50. Bruno R, Ali G, Giannini R, Proietti A, Lucchi M, Chella A, et al. Malignant pleural mesothelioma and mesothelial hyperplasia: a new molecular tool for the differential diagnosis. Oncotarget. 2017;8:2758–70.
51. Ivanov SV, Goparaju CM, Lopez P, Zavadil J, Toren-Haritan G, Rosenwald S, et al. Pro-tumorigenic effects of miR-31 loss in mesothelioma. J Biol Chem. 2010;285:22809–17.
52. Kubo T, Toyooka S, Tsukuda K, Sakaguchi M, Fukazawa T, Soh J, et al. Epigenetic silencing of microRNA-34b/c plays an important role in the pathogenesis of malignant pleural mesothelioma. Clin Cancer Res. 2011;17:4965–74.
53. Reid G, Pel ME, Kirschner MB, Cheng YY, Mugridge N, Weiss J, et al. Restoring expression of miR-16: a novel approach to therapy for malignant pleural mesothelioma. Ann Oncol. 2013;24:3128–35.
54. Williams M, Kirschner MB, Cheng YY, Hanh J, Weiss J, Mugridge N, et al. miR-193a-3p is a potential tumor suppressor in malignant pleural mesothelioma. Oncotarget. 2015;6:23480–95.
55. Weber DG, Johnen G, Bryk O, Jockel KH, Bruning T. Identification of miRNA-103 in the cellular fraction of human peripheral blood as a potential biomarker for malignant mesothelioma—a pilot study. PLoS One. 2012;7(1):e30221.
56. Tomasetti M, Staffolani S, Nocchi L, Neuzil J, Strafella E, Manzella N, et al. Clinical significance of circulating miR-126 quantification in malignant mesothelioma patients. Clin Biochem. 2012;45(7–8):575–81.

Chapter 13
Genetic Factors in Sleep Disorders: What Are the Roles of Genetic Factors in the Pathogenesis of Sleep Disorders?

Kiminobu Tanizawa and Kazuo Chin

Abstract Most normal sleep traits and sleep disorders have a familial aggregation, suggesting significant effects of genetic factors. Obstructive sleep apnea (OSA) is a common and complex sleep disorder and has heritability. A recent genome-wide association study (GWAS) identified some genetic risks for OSA with genome-wide levels of significance for the first time. Congenital central hypoventilation syndrome has causative mutations in the paired-like homeobox 2B (*PHOX2B*) gene, and its phenotypes are associated with *PHOX2B* genotypes. GWASs have revealed several genetic variances for restless legs syndrome (RLS), whereas these variances have left most of the heritability in RLS unexplained. Narcolepsy is strongly associated with HLA DQ-B1*06:02, and the results of GWASs indicate an autoimmune pathogenesis of narcolepsy. Insomnia has significant heritability, and findings of GWASs have suggested common genetic predispositions with psychiatric disorders and sleep reactivity. Familial fatal insomnia is an autosomal-dominant genetic disorder caused by a mutation in the prion protein (*PRNP*) gene. Although advances in genetics have resulted in identification of genetic causes of some sleep disorders, further studies are required to elucidate the cellular and molecular mechanisms from genetic risks to clinical manifestations.

Keywords SNP · GWAS · Sleep apnea · Narcolepsy · Restless legs syndrome

13.1 Introduction

Sleep is a physiological necessity, and inadequate sleep quantity and quality have been associated with a wide range of adverse physical, mental, and behavioral outcomes [1]. Abnormal sleep duration and quality were reported to increase risks for obesity, hypertension, metabolic syndrome, type 2 diabetes, cardiovascular disease,

K. Tanizawa (✉) · K. Chin
Department of Respiratory Care and Sleep Control Medicine, Graduate School of Medicine, Kyoto University, Kyoto, Japan
e-mail: tanizawa@kuhp.kyoto-u.ac.jp

T. Kaneko (ed.), *Clinical Relevance of Genetic Factors in Pulmonary Diseases*, Respiratory Disease Series: Diagnostic Tools and Disease Managements,
https://doi.org/10.1007/978-981-10-8144-6_13

stroke, and even cancer [2]. Sleep disturbances have been associated with psychiatric disorders, suicides, accidents, injuries, reduced quality of life, and increased mortality [2].

A variety of sleep disorders have been reported, because sleep is a complex phenomenon with several traits such as recurrent behaviors, characteristic electroencephalogram (EEG) patterns, timing of the initiation and completion of sleep during 24 h, and responses to deprivation [3]. The recent international classification, *International Classification of Sleep Disorders* – Third Edition (ICSD-3), includes more than 60 sleep disorders [4]. ICSD-3 classifies sleep disorders into seven major categories: insomnias, sleep-related breathing disorders, central disorders of hypersomnolence, circadian rhythm sleep-wake disorders, sleep-related movement disorders, parasomnias, and other sleep disorders.

Normal sleep traits and sleep disorders have been considered to be affected by genetic factors as well as comorbidities and environmental factors, although there is no single gene for sleep [3, 5]. The investigations of genetic effects on sleep began with comparative studies of EEG patterns between monozygotic twins, dizygotic twins, and unrelated controls [6–8]. These studies showed that the spectral characteristics of EEGs were more similar in monozygotic twins, suggesting the heritability of EEG patterns during normal sleep. Several studies that followed revealed that many sleep parameters and sleep disorders are heritable, including sleep duration, chronotype, obstructive sleep apnea, restless legs syndrome, insomnia, parasomnia, and neurobehavioral response to sleep deprivation [5]. Based on the inheritability established in twin and family studies, the genetic risks for individual sleep disorders have been explored through linkage analysis, candidate gene analysis, and hypothesis-free genome-wide association studies (GWASs) [3, 5]. In some sleep disorders, identification of candidate genes has provided insights into the pathogenesis of diseases, although most of the cellular and molecular mechanisms remain uncovered.

This chapter will provide clinicians and researchers with a current overview of genetics in sleep disorders. Sleep disorders are often accompanied by congenital, neurological and psychiatric disorders, such as sleep disordered breathing in Prader-Willi syndrome and insomnia in depression [9–11]. Those sleep disorders assumed to be secondary to other underlying diseases or conditions are beyond the scope of this chapter, although the causative relationships between underlying diseases and sleep disorders have been unrevealed in most cases.

13.2 Obstructive Sleep Apnea

Obstructive sleep apnea (OSA) is one of the most common sleep disorders with a prevalence of around 15% in men and 5% in women [12–14]. OSA is characterized by repeated episodes of pharyngeal collapse leading to partial or complete obstruction of the upper airways during sleep. This disorder is associated with an increased risk for many adverse health outcomes, including cardiovascular events, hypertension, diabetes, metabolic syndrome, obesity, atrial fibrillation, stroke, cognitive impairment, motor vehicle accidents, and even mortality [15–24]. Repeated episodes of nocturnal apnea or hypopnea cause intermittent hypoxia, sympathetic activation, and sleep fragmentation, which are supposed to result in various outcomes [25, 26]. As OSA is a complex disorder with multiple predisposing factors such as obesity, age, male sex, and craniofacial abnormalities, it is unlikely that a single genetic predisposition can account for all of these traits [3]. On the other hand, some of the predisposing factors, including anatomic abnormalities and obesity, would be determined genetically [27].

Genetic studies of OSA began with studying familial forms of OSA. The prevalence of OSA in first-degree relatives of patients with OSA was reported to range between 21% and 84%, and the estimated odds ratio ranged from 2 to 46 [28–30]. Symptoms and anatomical risk factors were also shown to be inheritable [5]. As a whole, inherited factors were likely to account for about 40% of the risk [28]. On the other hand, obesity, a significant risk factor for OSA, also has a high familial aggregation. Twin and family studies revealed that the estimated heritability of body mass index (BMI) was 50–90% and 20–80%, respectively [31, 32]. The Cleveland Family Study (CFS) addressed this issue for the first time and demonstrated that the first-degree relatives of patients with OSA and obesity had an independent risk for pediatric and adolescent OSA as did African-American ethnicity [33]. Another family study including participants with BMI <30 (without obesity) showed that maxillofacial anatomy was a significant trait that contributed to familial aggregation of OSA [34]. In whites and African-Americans in the CFS, the heritability of AHI was 36.3% and 32.3%, respectively, and decreased to 32.3% and 23.7% after adjustment for BMI [35, 36]. The corresponding estimates for BMI were 52.8% for whites and 53.7% for African-Americans, and those for upper airway dimensions were 34% for whites and 39% for African-Americans [37]. A recent population-based study in Brazil reported that the heritability of the apnea-hypopnea index (AHI), the index for the severity of OSA, was 23–25% in a rural population with low levels of obesity [38].

Despite of high heritability, thus far no linkage analysis or candidate gene analysis has identified risk loci with a genome-wide level of statistical significance ($P < 5 \times 10^{-8}$) [5, 39]. Several candidate loci or genetic variants were reported in individual studies. Reported candidate genetic variances for OSA include those in *APOE* (apolipoprotein E), *CRP* (C-reactive protein), *GDNF* (glial cell-line derived neurotrophic factor), *HTRA2A* (serotonin receptor 2a), *LPAR1* (lysophosphatidic acid receptor 1), *PLEK* (pleckstrin), *PTGER2* (prostaglandin E2 receptor), *PPARGC1B* (peroxisome proliferator-activated receptor gamma coactivator 1-beta), *NRG1* (neuregulin 1), *FTO* (fat mass and obesity-associated protein), *TRABD2B* (TraB domain containing 2B), *SLC6A4* (solute carrier family 6 member 4), *LEPR* (leptin receptor), and *TNF* (tumor necrosis factor) [3, 5, 39–41]. However, most studies were underpowered with small sample sizes, and the results were not replicated across races and studies. To overcome the small sample size, some meta-analyses were conducted (Table 13.1) [42–46]. These meta-analyses identified some candidate genes, but the statistical significance did not reach a genome-wide level.

Table 13.1 Results of meta-analysis for the associations between genetic variances and obstructive sleep apnea

Authors [reference]: participants	Gene	Variance	Cases/ controls	Odds ratio (95% CI)	Heterogeneity P_Q/I^2	*P* value
Varvarigou et al. [42]: all	*TNFA*	rs1800629	309/370	1.82 (1.26–2.61)	0.25/28%	0.001
Xu et al. [43]	5-HTR	1438G/A	466/551	2.33 (1.48–3.66)	22.96/83%	<0.01
5-HTR and *5-HTT*	*5-HTT*	LPR L/S	593/479	1.24 (1.04–1.49)	0.02/0%	0.02
		STin2 VNTR 10/12	593/479	2.87 (1.38–5.97)	10.18/80%	<0.01
Qin et al. [44]	*5-HT2A*	1438G/A	728/566	2.33 (1.49–3.66)	0/82.0%	NR
5-HT2A, *5-HTT*, and *LEPR*	*5-HTT*	LPR S/L	521/755	0.80 (0.67–0.95)	0.995/0%	NR
		STin2 VNTR 10/12	521/755	2.08 (1.58–2.73)	0.346/9.4%	NR
	LEPR	GG/AA	292/167	0.39 (0.17–0.88)	0.818/0.0%	NR
Sun et al. [45]	*TNFA*	308G/A	864/430	2.15 (1.39–3.31)	0.18/36.9%	NR
Chinese population	*5-HTT*	LPR S/L	596/756	1.32 (1.12–1.55)	0.80/0%	NR
		STin2 VNTR 10/12	572/708	1.86 (1.12–3.08)	0.03/66.5%	NR
	APOE	NR	436/562	1.79 (1.10–2.92)	0.86/0%	NR
Lv et al. [46]	*LEPR*	Gln 223 Arg	102/77	0.35 (0.14–0.85)	NR	0.02
Leptin and *LEPR*		(Only in European)				

Abbreviations: P_Q *p*-value for chai-squared-based *Q* statistical test, I^2 *I*-squared index, *CI* confidence interval, *TNFA* tumor necrosis factor-α, *5-HTR* 5-hydroxytryptamine receptor, *5-HTT* 5-Hydroxytryptamine transporter, *LPR S/L* linked promoter region short or long, *STin2 VNTR* serotonin transporter intron 2 variable number tandem repeat, *LEPR* leptin receptor, *APOE* apolipoprotein E, *NR* not reported

There have been two GWASs on OSA so far (Table 13.2) [41, 47]. The first GWAS was conducted using the cohorts of the National Heart, Lung, and Blood Institute (NHLBI) sponsored Candidate Gene Association Resource (CARe) project [47]. It identified different genetic variances associated with OSA and AHI for African-Americans and individuals of European ancestry, although no variance met a genome-wide level of statistical significance. The second GWAS, published in 2016, reported the first genome-level significant findings for OSA-related physiologic traits in any population [41]. This study is the largest genetic analysis of OSA to date in any population and utilized genome-wide data from as many as 12,558 individuals focusing exclusively on Hispanic/Latino Americans. Of note, several

Table 13.2 Results of genome-wide analysis study for obstructive sleep apnea

Patel et al. [47]							
Ethnicity	*Traits*	*SNP*		*Gene*	*N*	*β (SE)*	*P value*
						BMI adjusted	BMI adjusted
						BMI unadjusted	BMI unadjusted
African-American	AHI	rs7030789		*LPAR1*	1657	0.109 (0.023) 0.129 (0.028)	1.50×10^{-6} 4.58×10^{-6}
African-American	AHI	rs7972342		*ITPR2*	1657	−0.113 (0.024) −0.134 (0.030)	2.33×10^{-6} (6.97×10^{-6})
Ethnicity	*Traits*	*SNP*		*Gene*	*N*	*OR (95% CI)*	*P value*
						BMI adjusted	BMI adjusted
						BMI unadjusted	BMI unadjusted
African-American	OSA	rs11126184		*PLEK*	1657	0.43 (0.31, 0.60) 0.45 (0.33, 0.62)	1.54×10^{-6} 1.41×10^{-6}
European Ancestry	OSA	rs11126184		*PTGER3*	4699	2.14 (1.58, 2.90) 1.77 (1.30, 2.41)	1.01×10^{-6} 2.21×10^{-4}
Cade et al. [41]							
Ethnicity	*Traits*	*SNP*	*SNPs*	*Genes in*	*N*	*β (SE)*	*P value*
		In region		Region		BMI adjusted	BMI adjusted
						BMI unadjusted	BMI unadjusted
Hispanic/Latino	AHI	rs116791765 T	28	*GPR83, MRE11A, LINC01171*	11,774	−0.329 (0.057) −0.345 (0.061)	1.90×10^{-8} 1.84×10^{-8}
	AHI	rs999944 A	1		12,557	−0.095 (0.019) −0.104 (0.020)	4.53×10^{-7} 2.48×10^{-7}
	Sleep SpO_2	rs75108997 A	4		11.809	−0.291 (0.055) −0.296 (0.058)	1.40×10^{-7} 3.52×10^{-7}

(continued)

Table 13.2 (continued)

Patel et al. [47]							
	Sleep SpO_2	rs116133558 T	1	*ATP2B4*	11.351	0.291 (0.056) 0.231 (0.059)	2.18×10^{-7} 9.09×10^{-5}
	Average event duration	rs35424364 A	3	*C6ORF183, CCDC162P*	10,240	0.030 (0.006) 0.032 (0.006)	4.88×10^{-8} 1.82×10^{-8}
	Average event duration	rs74472562 T	1	*RP11-45A12.2, TSPAN18*	10,240	−0.034 (0.006) −0.035 (0.006)	1.05×10^{-7} 6.47×10^{-8}
	Average event duration	rs2743173 T	1	*PLCB1*	10,240	0.019 (0.004) 0.019 (0.004)	3.85×10^{-7} 2.23×10^{-7}
	Average event duration	rs72699765 A	4	*AC124997.1*	10,240	0.029 (0.006) 0.029 (0.006)	3.93×10^{-7} 5.20×10^{-8}
	Average event duration	rs2033354 T	5		10,240	0.019 (0.004) 0.019 (0.004)	4.77×10^{-7} 3.65×10^{-7}

Abbreviations: *SNP*, single nucleotide polymorphism; *SE*, standard error; *BMI*, body mass index; *AHI*, apnea-hypopnea index; *OSA*, obstructive sleep apnea; *LPAR1*, lysophosphatidic acid receptor 1; *ITPR2*, inositol 1,4,5-trisphosphate receptor type 2; *OSA*, obstructive sleep apnea; *OR*, odds ratio; *CI*, confidence interval; *PLEK*, pleckstrin; *PTGER3*, prostaglandin E receptor 3; *GPR83*, G protein-coupled receptor 83; *MRE11A*, MRE11 homolog, double strand break repair nuclease; *LINC01171*, chromosome 11 open reading frame 97; *ATP2B4*, ATPase plasma membrane Ca^{2+} transporting 4; *C6ORF183*, chromosome 6 open reading frame 183; *CCDC162P*, coiled-coil domain containing 162, pseudogene; *TSPAN18*, tetraspanin 18; *PLCB1*, phospholipase C beta

genes in the identified regions have reported biological plausibility such as inflammatory, hypoxia signaling, and sleep pathways.

Another unrevealed issue is the effects of genetic factors on the consequences of OSA. Some studies suggest different relationships between OSA and cardiovascular consequences across races [39]. An analysis of National Health and Nutrition Examination Survey data showed a stronger association of self-reported OSA with hypertension in overweight African-Americans (OR, 4.74; 95% CI, 1.86–12.03) than in overweight Hispanic/Latinos (OR, 2.01; 95% CI, 1.16–3.49) or overweight whites (OR, 1.65; 95% CI, 1.06–2.57) [48]. In addition, among patients with stroke, Hispanics had a higher risk for questionnaire-based OSA than whites and African-Americans [49]. These racial differences suggest the genetic effects on cardiovascular outcomes of OSA, although there has been no prospective study assessing the relationship between polysomnographically diagnosed OSA and cardiovascular comorbidities across different races or ethnicities [39]. Of candidate genes for OSA, *ACE* (angiotensin-converting enzyme) polymorphisms have been also studied as candidate risk factors for hypertension with inconsistent results [50]. Similarly, the risk allele for hypertension in OSA in the Wisconsin Sleep Cohort turned out to be protective in Cleveland Family Study [51, 52], showing mixed results.

OSA is a common and complex disorder and includes different phenotypes [53]. Given the wide range of components and outcomes of OSA, further advances in the genetics are critical for a comprehensive understanding of its pathogenesis and pathophysiology. Identification of genetic traits would be helpful for risk stratification and for novel therapeutic innovations for more personalized medicine.

13.3 Congenital Central Hypoventilation Syndrome

Congenital central hypoventilation syndrome (CCHS) is a genetically inherited disorder with decreased tidal volumes and monotonous respiratory rates awake and asleep [54]. Alveolar hypoventilation is the most profound in non-rapid eye movement (NREM) sleep, although it is also observed during REM sleep and wakefulness usually to a milder degree [55]. Patients with CCHS have hypercapnia and hypoxemia caused by hypoventilation, but they do not respond to these abnormalities in terms of ventilation and arousal from sleep [55, 56]. Patients also cannot perceive asphyxia during wakefulness with and without exercise.

CCHS is a lifelong and life-threatening disorder [55]. It is typically diagnosed during the newborn period, although it can be diagnosed in childhood and even adulthood, described as "later-onset CCHS (LO-CCHS)." Regardless of age at presentation, the diagnosis of CCHS requires the absence of primary lung, cardiac, or neuromuscular disease or an identifiable brain stem lesion that may account for the entire phenotype [55]. CCHS is often associated with complications of the autonomic nervous system (ANS), including various autonomic nervous system dysfunctions (ANSDs), Hirschsprung disease (HSCR) in 20% of cases, and neural crest tumors (neuroblastoma, ganglioneuroblastoma, and ganglioneuroma) in 5–10% of cases [54].

Since the paired-like homeobox 2B (*PHOX2B*) gene was identified as the disease-defining gene for CCHS in 2003 [57, 58], CCHS has been recognized as a model for genetically defined sleep disorders [54–56]. The American Thoracic Society (ATS) statement in 2010 declared that a *PHOX2B* mutation is requisite to confirmation of a diagnosis of CCHS [54]. This statement mentioned that (1) about 90% of individuals with the CCHS phenotype are heterozygous for a polyalanine expansion repeat mutation in the *PHOX2B* gene; (2) the remaining 10% are heterozygous for a missense, nonsense, or frameshift mutation in the *PHOX2B* gene; and (3) a non-CCHS diagnosis should be sought if a *PHOX2B* mutation is negative.

The *PHOX2B* gene on chromosome 4p12 has a 20-alanine repeat in exon 3. CCHS is caused by (1) polyalanine repeat mutations (PARMs) in the 20-alanine repeat resulting in 25–35 alanine tracts or (2) non-polyalanine repeat mutations

(NPARMs) causing nucleotide deletions at the end of exon 2 or in exon 3 [54, 56]. NPARMs include predominantly frameshift mutations but also nonsense and missense with stop codon alterations [58]. In individuals with CCHS, PARMs manifest as heterogeneous genotypes of *PHOX2B*$^{20/25-25}$. Interestingly, 1–1.5% of the general population has the *PHOX2B*$^{20/15}$ genotype with loss of alanines [58], but this mutation is not diagnostic even when hypoventilation is observed [54, 56].

The inherence of CCHS is basically considered to have an autosomal-dominant pattern with incomplete penetrance [54, 58, 59]. Most parents of children with CCHS do not have a mutation at all, suggesting that most mutations occur de novo in affected individuals [54, 60, 61]. However, 5–10% of affected children inherit the mutation from a typically unaffected mosaic parent [58, 61]. Asymptomatic parental mosaicism is restricted to PARMs of genotypes 20/26 to 20/33 and severe NPARMs [54]. In addition, PARMs of genotypes 20/24 and 20/25 and some NPARMs are found in asymptomatic parents, indicating incomplete penetrance [54, 60–62]. Variable penetrance has been postulated to be due to other modifier mutations such as *HASH1*, *RET*, *GFRA1*, and *PHOX2A* [63]. In fact, family members of CHHS patients have a higher incidence of ANSD, HSCR, neuroblastoma, and sudden infant death syndrome, which can be associated with the candidate genes for modifiers [60, 64, 65]. Based on the presence of mosaicism and a nonpenetrant carrier state, a screening test for *PHOX2B* mutations is recommended for both asymptomatic parents of affected children [54].

The *PHOX2B* gene codes for a transcription factor that plays a central role in the specification of the fate of cells during development [55]. PHOX2B protein is necessary for the development of several neurons in the central and peripheral nervous systems. Functionally, *PHOX2B* is expressed by a chain of neurons involved in the integration of peripheral and central chemoreception [66–68]. This chain includes the carotid bodies, chemoreceptor afferents, chemoresponsive projections of the nucleus tractus solitarius (NTS) to the ventrolateral medulla, and central chemoreceptors in the retrotrapezoid nucleus (RTN). The RTN is a group of chemosensitive glutamatergic neurons that is located near the parafacial respiratory group and critical to central chemoreception, although the RTN in humans has not been definitely identified.

The molecular mechanisms through which *PHOX2B* mutations cause alveolar hypoventilation have not been entirely revealed. PARMs can reduce transcriptional activities of PHOX2B proteins to the PHOX2A promotor and dopamine β-hydroxylase (*DβH*) promotor [69]. This can be done through the localization of mutated proteins in cytoplasm and the aggregate formation in the nucleus. On the other hand, a *PHOX2B* frameshift mutation, one of the NPARMs that activates the PHOX2A promotor and DβH promotor, and the mutated proteins are exclusively localized to the nuclei as well as intact proteins [56]. These findings suggest that PARMs and NPARMs may lead to alveolar hypoventilation through distinct pathways, which may cause the different phenotypes associated with each of PARMs and NPARMs [70], as mentioned below.

CCHS patients have a wide spectrum of severity in terms of hypoventilation and other ANSDs. Of note, the CCHS phenotypes are significantly associated with *PHOX2B* genotypes. In general, longer polyalanine expansions in PARMs and

NPARMs are associated with more severe disease [54–56]. Continuous ventilator support is needed in 35% of patients with PARMs and 67% of those with NPARMs. $PHOX2B^{20/28–20/33}$ patients usually require continuous ventilator support, and $PHOX2B^{20/26}$ patients need variable support while awake. Late-onset cases with $PHOX2B^{20/25}$ have the mildest hypoventilation, which manifests primarily after exposure to respiratory depressants or severe respiratory infection, and can be managed with nocturnal support only. HSCR is seen in 19% of PARM cases and 80% of NPARM cases, and neural crest tumors are also more common in NPARM cases: 1% of PARM and 41% of NPARM patients. Cardiac systoles (sinus pauses of 3 s or longer) are seen in 19% and 83% of patients with $PHOX2B^{20/26}$ and $PHOX2B^{20/27}$, respectively, whereas they are observed in none with $PHOX2B^{20/25}$. In addition, in cases with PARMs, the number of polyalanine repeats is positively correlated with the number of ANSD symptoms and the degree of facial dysmorphology. Based on these findings, the ATS statement recommends different schedules of testing for CCHS cases with different genotypes (Table 13.3) [54].

Table 13.3 Testing schedules for congenital central hypoventilation syndrome stratified by *PHOX2B* genotype [54]

PHOX2B genotype	Annual in-hospital comprehensive physiologic testing (awake and asleep), exogenous and endogenous gas challenges and autonomic testing[a]	Assessment for Hirschsprung disease	Annual neurocognitive assessment[a]	Annual 72-h Holter recording and echocardiogram[a]	Annual imaging to assess for tumors of neural crest origin
PARM					
20/24 and 20/25	×		×	×	
20/26	×	×	×	×	
20/27	×	×	×	×	
20/28–20/33	×	×	×	×	×[b]
NPARM	×	×	×	×	×[c]

Cite: Weese-Mayer DE, Berry-Kravis EM, Ceccherini I, Keens TG, Loghmanee DA, Trang H, et al. (2010) An official ATS clinical policy statement: Congenital central hypoventilation syndrome: genetic basis, diagnosis, and management. *American Journal of Respiratory and Critical Care Medicine* 181: 626–44

The *American Journal of Respiratory and Critical Care Medicine* is an official journal of the American Thoracic Society

Abbreviations: *PARM* polyalanine repeat expansion mutation, *NPARM* nonpolyalanine repeat expansion mutation (missense, nonsense, frameshift)

[a]Infants under the age of 3 years should undergo comprehensive evaluations every 6 months

[b]Annual chest and abdominal imaging to identify ganglioneuromas and ganglioneuroblastomas

[c]Abdominal imaging and urine cathecholamines every 3 months in the first 2 years, then every 6 months until 7 years of age to identify neuroblastomas

Despite being a rare sleep disorder, clinical and genetic investigations of CCHS have shed light on the cellular and genetic basis of central respiratory control. The proposed pathogenesis of CCHS is a selective defect of central chemosensory integration rather than respiratory central pattern generator (rCPG) dysfunction because ventilation can adequately respond to volitional stimulus or exercise during wakeful status [55, 56]. Worsened symptoms during sleep suggest the existence of neurons that selectively mediate the chemical drive to breathing and play a critical role during sleep. Following the identification of *PHOX2B* as the disease-defining gene for CCHS, it was also demonstrated that *PHOX2B* was expressed on the neuronal chain involved in chemosensory integration but not on the serotonergic system including the rCPG [71, 72]. This expression pattern well fits with the pathogenesis speculated from clinical manifestations, a selective defect of the central chemosensory system.

Mouse models of CCHS were obtained by a knock-in approach to add a 7 alanine expansion to the 20-residue polyalanine tract (the $Phox2b^{27Ala}$ allele). Constitutive $Phox2b^{27Ala/+}$ mice reproduced two characteristics of human neonates with CCHS: blunted or unstable breathing with apneas and absence of a ventilator response to hypercapnia [73]. These $Phox2b^{27Ala/+}$ mice showed loss of RTN neurons and precursor populations by embryonic day 15.5, suggesting the link between RTN disruption and absent chemosensitivity to hypercapnia. Furthermore, conditional $Phox2b^{27Ala/+}$ mice, which had a massive loss of RTN neurons with intact downstream components of the RTN neural network, also had markedly defective chemosensitivity, demonstrating a stronger association between chemosensation and *PHOX2B* mutations at functional and neuroanatomical levels [74]. On the other hand, the conditional $Phox2b^{27Ala/+}$ mice recovered their ventilatory response to hypercapnia incompletely (to 40% of the normal value) and could survive to adulthood. These findings suggest a greater potential for respiratory plasticity and also call into question the necessity of the CO_2 drive to sustain life.

13.4 Restless Legs Syndrome/Willis-Ekbom Disease

Restless legs syndrome/Willis-Ekbom disease (RLS/WED) is a neurological and sleep-related disorder [75]. It often profoundly disturbs sleep and quality of life with various sensory and motor manifestations. The International Restless Legs Syndrome Study Group (IRLSSG) defined five essential diagnostic criteria for RLS/WED: (1) an urge to move the legs, usually accompanied by uncomfortable and unpleasant sensations in the legs, (2) symptoms that begin or worsen during periods of rest or inactivity, (3) relief of symptoms by movement, (4) occurrence or worsening in the evening or night, and (5) symptoms that are not solely accounted for as primary to another medical or behavioral condition [76]. The IRLSSG consensus criteria also classify the clinical course of RLS/WED into chronic-persistent (occurring on average at least twice weekly for the past year) and intermittent (occurring on average <2/week for the past year, with at least five lifetime events). The prevalence of RLS/WED is estimated to be about 7% in the European and

American population, and two thirds of these patients have mild and often intermittent RLS/WED [75]. A large-scale epidemiological study in Western Europe showed that the prevalence of chronic-persistent RLS/WED was 4.4%, that of medically significant RLS/WED was 2.7%, and that of RLS/WED having a high impact on health was 0.8% [77]. Although most cases of RLS/WED are mild, more severe cases can cause a 20–50% reduction in work capacity and thus an increase in social cost [78]. In addition, some studies suggested that RLS/WED could significantly increase the risk for cardiovascular disease [75].

A strong family clustering of RLS/WED has been identified. Of patients with RLS/WED, 40–65% have a family history of RLS/WED, and a positive family history may be associated with the onset of symptoms at an earlier age than those without a family history. A Canadian twin study revealed that the concordant rate of RLS was 54% and 19% in monozygotic and heterozygotic twins, respectively, and disease heritability was 69.4% [79]. Segregation analyses in families suggested an autosomal-dominant mode of inherence with a single major gene and fairly high penetrance, which was in line with twin studies [80, 81].

Based on these observations from twin and family studies, genome-wide linkage studies using cohorts of RLS families were conducted and have identified several linkage regions [82–84]. Linkage regions include RLS-1 on chromosome 12q22-23.3, RLS-2 on chromosome 14q13-22, RLS-3 on chromosome 9p24-22, RLS-4 on chromosome 2q33, and RLS-5 on chromosome 20p13. Although the linkage studies showed that RLS has Mendelian forms, mostly an autosomal-dominant mode, the genetic model is not simple because the model consists of additional genes with smaller effect and modifier genes as well as major loci. In addition, the identified linkage regions were so large and included such a large number of genes that only a small number of genes in the regions were sequenced to identify the candidate genes for RLS.

When GWASs became feasible, RLS/WED was one of the first disorders that benefited from this new method. Four GWASs between 2007 and 2011 identified some risk variants in six genes: *MEIS1* (myeloid ecotropic viral integration site 1 homolog) on chromosome 2, *BTBD9* (BTB/POZ domain-containing protein) on chromosome 6p, mitogen-activated protein kinase 5 (MAP2K5) and the adjacent *SKOR1* (SKI family transcriptional corepressor 1) on chromosome 15q, *PTPRD* (protein tyrosine phosphatase receptor type D) on chromosome 9p, and *TOX3* (TOX high mobility group box family member 3) on chromosome 16q [85]. *MEIS1* is involved with limb axis formation and neuronal differentiation [86–88] and *MAP2K5* with muscle cellular differentiation [89]. *SKOR1* plays a critical role in the development of sensory pathways in the dorsal horn of the spinal cord that relay pain and touch [90]. *PTPRD* is also involved with neuronal development [85, 91]. Thus, the associations between these genes and RLS/WED in GWASs suggest that RLS/WED may be caused by defects in the early development of the neuromuscular system.

Among these genes, variants in *MEIS1* conferred the highest risks with odds ratios around 2.7 [85, 92–94]. The risk allele in *MEIS1* was associated with a decrease of its expression at the levels of mRNA and protein [27]. *MEIS1* was also reported to regulate the expression of ferritins [27], and changes in iron metabolism have been proposed as a possible mechanism in the pathogenesis of RLS/WED [95]. In addition, rs3923809 in *BTBD9* was associated with RLS/WED in the first GWAS, and this association was replicated in the second GWAS exclusively in cases with restless leg movements (RLMs), not in those with only sensory symptoms [94]. The risk allele in rs3923809 caused a 13% decrease in serum ferritin, although *BTBD9* was not associated with iron metabolism and iron-related gene expression [96, 97]. In contrast, variants in *MAP2K5/SKOR1* and *TOX3* were associated with only RLS but not RLMs without sensory symptoms [40]. These findings collectively suggest that different genes may play different roles between motor and sensory aspects of RLS: *BTBD9* for motor and *MAP2K5/SKOR1* and *TOX3* for sensory.

Recently, two population-based cohort studies examined the associations between RLS-associated single nucleotide polymorphisms (SNPs) identified in GWASs and RLMs [98, 99]. The first study replicated significant results within *BTBD9*, *MEIS1*, *MAP2K5/SKOR1*, *PRPRD*, and *TOX3* and the second within *BTBD9*, *MEIS1*, and *MAP2K5/SKOR1*. Overall, GWASs and population-based studies showed repeatedly that variants in BTBD9 and MEIS1 are associated with RLS and RLMs. For other risk loci, the evidence is conflicting, partially because of different study populations, phenotyping and genotyped SNPs.

Despite the successful results in GWASs, it should be noted that SNPs identified in GWASs can account for less than 10% of the total heritability across different study populations [93]. GWAS is based on the "common disease-common variant" hypothesis, which means that many common genetic variations, each with a small to moderate effect, determine the genetic risks for common but complex diseases including RLS [100]. Thus, this "missing heritability" of RLS may be caused by rare variants that have not been addressed in GWASs but can account for the majority of genetic variations and have larger effects than common variances. In fact, a case-control sequencing study showed an excess of rare variants in *MEIS1* in cases [101]. Exome sequencing for a family with RLS identified a variant of the protocadherin alpha cluster, complex locus (*PCDHA3*) as a candidate, although its role in the pathogenesis remained unclear [102].

In conclusion, strong effects of genetic predisposition have been established in RLS/WED based on observations of family clustering and high heritability. However, the majority of heritability in RLS/WED remains unexplained, although recent GWASs provide some insight into it. The next-generation sequencing technology may be capable of detecting genetic risk variances and thus fill out the "missing heritability" links. In-depth analysis and epigenetic research also can be helpful in uncovering the pathogenesis of this disease.

13.5 Narcolepsy

Narcolepsy is a sleep disorder characterized by chronic sleepiness (hypersomnolence), sudden episodes of partial or complete paralysis of voluntary muscles (cataplexy), hypnagogic hallucinations, and sleep paralysis [103]. This disorder usually begins with the sudden onset of persistent hypersomnolence in the teen years. The severe sleepiness easily recurs even after adequate nighttime sleep and often causes serious problems such as poor performance at school and work and motor vehicle accidents. It affects 1 in 2000–4000 individuals in the general population [104, 105]. Although it is one of the most common causes of hypersomnolence, it is often diagnosed only after severe sleepiness has caused serious problems. Another characteristic of narcolepsy is dysregulated rapid eye movement (REM) sleep. While REM sleep occurs only during the sleep period in healthy people, it can occur at any time and often interrupts wakefulness in patients with narcolepsy. This disordered REM sleep causes cataplexy when it is triggered by strong emotions during wakefulness and hypnagogic hallucinations and sleep paralysis at the borders between wakefulness and sleep.

Orexin-A and orexin-B, neuropeptides also referred as hypocretin-1 and hypocretin-2, have been considered as key molecules for narcolepsy [3]. A narcolepsy-like phenotype was mimicked in mice and dogs with dysfunction of orexin pathway [106, 107], and orexin-producing neurons were markedly decreased in the brains of patients with narcolepsy [108]. Currently, it is recognized that narcolepsy has two phenotypes [103]. Type 1 narcolepsy is characterized by cataplexy and a very low level of orexin-A in cerebrospinal fluid. This type is caused by severe but highly selective loss of orexin-producing neurons. On the other hand, type 2 narcolepsy is characterized by less severe sleepiness, lack of cataplexy, and normal levels of orexin-A in cerebrospinal fluid. Although this type may be caused by less extensive injury to orexin-producing neurons, its pathophysiology has been unclear. Thus, the two types of narcolepsy may have different mechanisms although their phenotypes are partially similar.

Familial clustering has been reported in narcolepsy, although most cases are sporadic. First-degree relatives have 10- to 40-fold higher risks of narcolepsy than the general population, and its prevalence is 0.9–2.3% [109]. On the other hand, the concordance in monozygotic twins is as low as 32% [105], suggesting other mechanisms than genetic predispositions.

Genetically, narcolepsy is strongly associated with specific human leukocyte antigens (HLAs). More than 98% of patients with type 1 narcolepsy have a class II HLA antigen, HLA-DQB1*06:02, regardless of ethnic group [110, 111]. A recent study of a European cohort showed that the odds ratio of DQB1*06:02 for narcolepsy was as high as 251 [111]. This association is the strongest between an HLA and a disease that has ever been known, although this allele is not specific to narcolepsy. Additionally, 35–56% of patients with type 2 narcolepsy also have DQB1*06:02, while 12–38% of the general population have it [3, 103]. Two alleles (homozygotes) confer a two- to fourfold greater risk for narcolepsy than one allele (heterozygotes) and are also associated with more severe symptoms [112, 113].

Several other alleles in the HLA system may also contribute to genetic susceptibility to narcolepsy. DQA1*01:02 is almost always linked with DQB1*06:02, and a heterodimer produced by these linked genes presents antigens to T-cell receptors (TCRs) on CD4 T cells [114]. When the effects of other HLA class II alleles were examined in heterozygotes carrying a single allele of DQB1*06:02, six alleles predisposed to narcolepsy: DQA1*06, DQB1*03:01, DRB1*04, DRB1*08, DRB1*11, and DRB1*12 [115]. Three alleles were protective: DQA1*01 (except for DQA1*01:02), DQB1*05:01, and DQB1*06:01. In a European cohort, four alleles (DQB1*02, DQB1*05:01, DQB1*06:03, and DQB1*06:09) remained protective even after adjustment for DQB1*06:02 [111]. Another study showed the predisposing effect of HLA-DPB1*05:01 and the protective effects of HLA-DPA1*01:03-DPB1*04:01 and HLA-DPA1*01:03-DPB1*04:02 in Asians after matching of HLA-DR and HLA-DQ and the predisposing effects of HLA-A*11:01, HLA-B*35:03, and HLA-B*51:01 that were independent of HLA class II and ethnic group [114].

Recently, GWASs have explored the associations of SNPs in some genes with narcolepsy. Three SNPs (rs1154155, rs12587781, and rs1263646) in T-cell receptor alpha (*TRA*) locus were identified as conferring a genetic predisposition to narcolepsy in Caucasians with replication in Asians, although they were not significant in African-Americans [116]. The *TRA* locus encodes the α-chain of TCRαβ heterodimer expressed on T lymphocytes. TCR is a unique protein that interacts with both HLA class I (CD8 in cytotoxic T cells) and HLA class II (CD4 in helper T cells); the HLA class II protein includes the DQαβ heterodimer encoded by DQB1*06:02 and the closely linked DQA1*01:02. Of these SNPs, only the predisposing effect of rs1154155 within the *TRA* locus was replicated in another European GWAS [117].

Another SNP replicated in this European GWAS was a protective one near HLA-DQA2 (rs285884). This SNP was originally identified in the European population heterozygous for DRB1*15:01-DQB1*06:02. It was strongly linked to two HLA types of DRB1*03-DQB1*02 and DRB1*13:01-DQB1*06:03, and a trans DRB1*13:01-DQB1*06:03 haplotype was also protective against narcolepsy.

Other SNPs reported to be associated with narcolepsy include rs2305795 in the purinergic receptor subtype (*P2RY11*) gene, rs5770917 between *CPT1B* (carnitine palmitoyltransferase 1B) and *CHKB* (choline kinase β) genes, rs34593439 in the cathepsin H (*CTSH*) gene, and rs75537111 in the tumor necrosis factor superfamily member 4 (*TNFSF4*, also called *OX40L*) gene [114, 118–121]. The risk allele of rs2305795 in *P2RY11* for narcolepsy was associated with reduced expression of *P2RY11* in CD8 T cells and natural killer (NK) cells; CD8 T cells and NK cells with reduced expression of *P2RY11* were more susceptible to ATP-induced cell death because *P2RY11* proteins mediate the resistance to cell death [120]. A Japanese GWAS found that rs5770917 between *CPT1B* and *CHKB* provided a predisposition to narcolepsy in both Japanese and other ancestry groups [121]. The risk allele was associated with decreased expression of *CPT1B* and *CHKB*.

Of note, all of these factors for genetic predispositions to narcolepsy, including HLA haplotypes, are related to the immune system. These findings, in addition to epidemiological data, support an autoimmune pathogenesis of narcolepsy, although the mechanism of the destruction of orexin-producing neurons remains undetermined [103]. Epidemiologically, the onset of narcoleptic symptoms occurs most commonly in the late spring, suggesting the pathogenesis is triggered by winter infections [122]. Higher titers of antibodies against antistreptolysin O are commonly observed during the initial phase of narcolepsy [123]. In European children and teenagers, an increased occurrence of narcolepsy was reported after vaccination against the pandemic H1N1 influenza in the winter of 2009–2010 but only when they had the DQB1*06:02 allele [124, 125]. The pandemic of H1N1 influenza in the same season also resulted in a threefold increase in newly developed narcolepsy in China in the following year [122]. In addition, antibodies against a protein in orexin-producing neurons, Tribbles homolog 2 (Trib2), were identified in patients with newly diagnosed narcolepsy, although there has been no evidence that these antibodies can directly damage orexin-producing neurons [3, 126, 127]. Thus, it is possible that some immune stimuli such as infection or vaccination trigger autoimmune responses in young persons with genetic susceptibilities and lead to the destruction of orexin-producing neurons, probably because of some molecular mimicry [128]. On the other hand, it should be noted that no inflammatory sign has been detected in patients with narcolepsy, and immunomodulatory agents had little effect on narcoleptic symptoms in clinical trials [103].

The discovery of orexin as a key molecule and the identification of genetic predispositions have made great advances in understanding narcolepsy and developing effective therapies. However, the pathologic process that destroys orexin-producing neurons and the subsequent pathways leading to narcoleptic symptoms remain unrevealed. Further exploration of neurobiologic mechanisms in narcolepsy may lead to new preventive and therapeutic opportunities.

13.6 Insomnia

Insomnia is clinically defined as difficulty falling asleep, difficulty initiating or maintaining sleep, or non-restorative sleep at least three times a week for a minimum of 90 days and causing clinically significant distress according to the Diagnostic and Statistical Manual of Mental Disorders (DSM-5) [129]. About one third of the adult population experiences at least one of its symptoms, and the estimated prevalence of insomnia is between 6% and 10% [130–133]. Insomnia also can be defined as a quantitative trait of one or more sleep parameters based on questionnaires or sleep diaries, such as sleep latency or time of being awake during the night [5].

Several twin and family studies have shown that insomnia is moderately heritable, although the definitions of insomnia vary across studies. Actually, most studies used symptomatic definitions rather than the more strict ones based on disorder phenotypes. The estimated heritability of insomnia ranges between 22% and 59% in adults, and the range in studies of children is as wide as 14–71% [134–136]. Some recent longitudinal twin studies have integrated multiple waves of data into models to explore genetic contributions to insomnia in a more detailed way. One study showed that heritability estimates were 22–25% at single time points in adults [137]. When two time points were incorporated, the estimates increased to 38% for males and 59% for females, suggesting for the first time a significantly larger genetic effect in females. Another longitudinal twin study with four waves of data across childhood and adolescence found that genetic effects could account for 24–38% of the variance across waves, and the heritability estimate was 14% [138]. Genetic contributions to insomnia were stable throughout early childhood, while new genetic contributors were added at the average age of 10 and remained significant after then. These twin and family studies have strongly supported the presence of genetic predispositions to insomnia, although they cannot identify any specific gene.

Various genes have been studied as candidate genes for insomnia based on findings of neurobiological pathways. Of circadian genes (*CLOCK*, *Timeless*), the *Per 2* genotype was associated with the risk of insomnia, and the genetic effect was increased by high stress work [139]. *Per 3* genotype was also associated with insomnia in patients with alcohol dependence [140]. Insomnia has a bidirectional relationship with psychiatric disorders, and the serotonin transporter polymorphic region (*5-HTTLPR*) is one of the most common genetic factors studied in psychiatric disorders. Thus, the effects of the *5-HTTLPR* polymorphism on insomnia also have been examined. Recent studies found that each short allele (S allele) conferred an 80% or more increase in risk for insomnia [141, 142]. Additionally, individuals with the SS genotype had a higher risk under high job-related stress, suggesting the role of *5-HTTLPR* in stress reactivity mechanisms [143]. Other candidate genes studied include catecholamine-*O*-methyltransferase (*COMT*), dopamine receptor D4 (*DRD4*), dopamine transporter 1 (*DAT1*), apolipoprotein E (*APOE*, *ε4* allele), proliferator-activated receptor-γ coactivator-1α (*PCG-1α*), and aryl hydrocarbon receptor (*AHR*) [131]. A *COMT* polymorphism was not associated with any sleep and circadian parameters [144], while the variable number of tandem repeats in *DRD4* and a polymorphism had a significant association with daytime sleepiness [144]. *APOE ε4* and *PCG-1α* polymorphisms increase the risk for insomnia, and *PCG-1α* had a significant genetic contribution to insomnia even after adjustment for the *APOE ε4* genotype [145]. *CLOCK* and *AHR* polymorphisms and their combinations had protective effects on insomnia [146].

There have been five GWASs of insomnia so far [147–151]. The first GWAS was conducted in a large Korean cohort using self-report questionnaires to diagnose insomnia and found no genome-wide significant associations, although top SNPs of interest included rs11208305 in *PCLB1* (prior associations with schizophrenia) and rs718712 in *ROR1* (prior associations with bipolar disorder) [147]. The second GWAS in an Australian twin cohort also found no genetic variance that reached genome-wide significance [148]. The most significant result in the second study was an association of rs7316184 in *CACNA1C* with sleep quality and latency; this SNP was also associated with bipolar disorder and schizophrenia in previous studies. A British GWAS replicated the association between another SNP (rs16929277) in *CACNA1C* and sleep quality [149]. Spada et al. used objective sleep phenotypes measured with actigraphy for a GWAS of insomnia for the first time [150]. Their study showed a genome-wide significant association of rs75842709 in *UFL1* with sleep efficiency on weekdays that of chr9:864,201:D in *DMRT1* with sleep latency and rs2919869 in *SMYD1* with sleep offset, although these associations were not corrected for analysis of multiple phenotypes. A recent GWAS of self-reported sleep latency meta-analyzed the combination of seven European cohorts and identified three correlated SNPs (rs9900428, rs9907432, and rs7211029) in *RBFOX3* that passed the genome-wide significance threshold and could be also replicated [151]. Functional analyses showed the involvement of the *RBFOX3* gene in GABA and monoamine release, suggesting a role in sleep onset [151].

Although these GWASs have identified several novel candidate genes for insomnia, the same genes are not always significant across studies. This can be due to, in part, the inconsistent phenotyping of insomnia. Additionally, results of GWASs have left much of the heritability in insomnia unexplained, probably because GWASs cannot detect the effects of rare variants. Multiple testing and size power also remain significant problems in GWASs. Further GWASs with larger cohorts and meta-analyses with combined data across research groups can produce more significant results.

Advances in our understanding of the genetics of insomnia suggest two directions for future research. Epidemiologically insomnia is strongly related to other psychiatric orders, traits, and symptoms. Several genes identified through GWASs of insomnia also appear to be associated with other psychiatric disorders, and genes from other diseases may contribute to genetic risks for insomnia [152, 153]. Many of these genes are related to intrinsic neuronal excitability [131, 154, 155]. These findings suggest that changes in neural excitability in wake-promoting or sleep-inhibiting neurons may cause hyperarousal and difficulty sleeping and thus insomnia [131]. This hyperexcitability could also underlie a greater sleep reactivity, which means easier sleep disruption after a challenge, often a stressful event [156]. There is evidence that sleep reactivity is a greater risk factor for insomnia than a family history of insomnia [157], and it also has a moderate degree of heritability [156, 157]. Additionally, the genetic effects in sleep reactivity significantly overlap with those in insomnia [156]. These findings collectively suggest that sleep reactivity may be a potential mechanism of insomnia with common genetic predispositions. Furthermore, the examination of overlaps between insomnia and other psychiatric traits or even nonpsychiatric traits can also expand the unpredicted potential candidate genes and account for unexplained heritability of insomnia. Another genetic approach beyond GWASs is gene expression studies including pathway, epigenetics, and omics analyses. This approach can be applied not only to identify insomnia-related genes but also to explore molecular mechanisms of different responses to environments and treatments among individuals.

13.7 Fatal Familial Insomnia

Fatal familial insomnia (FFI) is an autosomal-dominant genetic neurodegenerative disease initially reported in 1986 [158]. It is caused by the mutation of the prion protein gene (*PRNP*) at position 178 (D178N) together with the presence of a methionine at the codon 129 polymorphic site on the mutated allele (cis-129M) [159, 160]. In individuals having the same mutation but valine at position 129 of the mutated allele, familial Creutzfeldt-Jakob disease (fCJD) is usually manifested [161].

Clinical manifestations in FFI are heterogenous [158, 162, 163]. FFI is characterized by insomnia, sleep fragmentation, altered arousal, daytime dreamlike automatism, and dysautonomia. These symptoms are followed by cognitive impairment and motor disorders, leading to terminal dementia. The age at clinical onset ranges between 36 and 62 years (average 51 years) [158]. The first symptoms are often nonspecific and insomnia cannot be noticed at first. Patients are unable to sleep even when they feel tired or slept badly the previous night. While dreamlike stupor, hallucinations, and behavioral abnormalities are common, social behavior is generally preserved [162–164]. Cognitive and attention impairments may fluctuate at their onset. As the disease progresses, patients suffer from memory impairment and loss of language and skills, accompanied by pyramidal and extrapyramidal signs including worsening ataxia and dystonia, and eventually become completely dependent [165, 166]. Survival from clinical onset is 12 months on average, ranging between 8 and 11 months for codon 129 homozygotes and between 17 and 72 months for heterozygotes [167, 168].

Major regions in FFI are the mediodorsal and anterior ventral nuclei of the thalamus and the pulvinar and the ventral anterior, ventral medial, and inferior olives [158, 169, 170]. These lesions show marked neuronal loss and astrocytic gliosis microscopically. Affected regions also include the inner part of the temporal cortex, CA1 region of the hippocampus, cingulate cortex, and other cortical areas, where spongiform changes, as well as neuron loss, astrocytic gliosis, and microglial activation, are observed. Immunohistochemistry shows very scanty or absent protein K-resistant prion protein (PrPres) in the thalamus and inferior olives, while small granular deposits and synaptic-like PrPres deposition are seen in affected cortical areas [158]. Gel electrophoresis and Western blotting of total brain homogenates reveal a weak band of non-glycosylated PrPres of 19KDa (PrP type 2) and strong mono-glycosylated and di-glycosylated PrPres bands, suggesting that PrPres in FFI is highly glycosylated [169, 171–173].

The diagnosis of genetic CJD, including FFI, is based on the presence of a definite relative with CJD in combination with neuropsychiatric disorder and disease-specific PrP gene mutation in the proband [158]. FFI is diagnosed when an individual with familial antecedents of FFI or CJD has neurological alterations consistent with FFI and a D178N mutation. A recent diagnostic algorithm had the sensitivity of 81% and can help to identify candidates for genetic screening (Table 13.4) [174]. As biomarkers in cerebrospinal fluids are not diagnostic for FFI, a genetic analysis has been mandatory for the diagnosis of FFI so far [163].

The mechanism by which PrP D178N causes a spontaneous misfolding of protein is still unclear. The D178N mutation is supposed to (1) cause conformational alterations affecting the intermolecular contacts between different PrP molecules; (2) interfere with salt bridges and S-S bridges, resulting in protein structural instability; and (3) increase aggregation [175–177]. Gene expression profiling in FFI showed deregulated genes mostly in the thalamus followed by the parietal cortex [178]. Altered functions in FFI include mitochondrial-associated processes (oxidative phosphorylation and mitochondrial electron transport), protein synthesis, regulation of transcription, RNA splicing, and signal transduction. Another study

Table 13.4 Diagnostic algorithm for fatal familial insomnia [174]

A	Organic sleep disturbances. If not clinically apparent, a polysomnography has to be performed
B	At least two of the following "CJD-like symptoms/signs"
	1. Psychiatric: visual hallucinations, personality change, depression, anxiety, aggressiveness, disinhibition, and listlessness
	2. Ataxia
	3. Visual
	4. Myoclonus
	5. Cognitive/mnestic deficits
C	At least one of the following "relatively disease-specific symptoms/signs"
	1. Loss of weight with a cutoff point of >10 kg during the last 6 months
	2. Vegetative: hyperhidrosis, newly diagnosed arterial hypertonia, tachycardia, obstipation, and hyperthermia
	3. Husky voice

Adapted by permission from BMJ Publishing Group Limited. [A Krasnianski, P Sanchez Juan, Claudia Ponto, M Bartl, U Heinemann, et al. (2014) A proposal of new diagnostic pathway for fatal familial insomnia. *Journal of Neurology, Neurosurgery & Psychiatry* 85:654–9]
When A, B, and C are fulfilled, the next diagnostic step is a genetic analysis of *PRNP*
Abbreviations: *CJD* Creutzfeldt-Jakob disease, *PRNP* prion protein

revealed severe downregulation of the genes and proteins that are associated with the mitochondrial respiratory chain and protein synthesis machinery [179]. This was in parallel with massive neuronal loss, gliosis, and increased oxidative stress. These findings indicate that mitochondrial damage and altered protein synthesis machinery are the major pathological events at the terminal stage of FFI, although it remains to be clarified whether these changes are a cause or consequence of FFI.

13.8 Circadian Rhythm Sleep Disorders/Familial Advanced Sleep Phase Syndrome

Circadian rhythm refers to 24-h oscillations that occur in the absence of external timing information [180]. In mammals, the core of circadian oscillations is a cell-autonomous transcriptional-translational feedback loop (TTFL) present in most cells. The circadian rhythm is controlled by light input transmitted from the retina to the suprachiasmatic nucleus in the hypothalamus, and cells within the suprachiasmatic nucleus have a TTFL with a cycle of about 24 h. Genes involved in the TTFL include *Clock*; *BMAIL1*; *CRY1* and *2* (cryptochrome 1 and 2); *PER1*, *2*, and *3* (Period 1, 2 and 3); *REV-ERB-α* and *β*; *ROR1*, *2*, and *3*; and *CK1ε*. Regulated transcriptional and posttranscriptional events generate endogenous 24-h rhythms in the mRNA and protein levels of most of these transcriptional regulators.

As an increasing number of genes involved in the molecular generation of circadian rhythms have been identified, circadian rhythm sleep disorders (CRSDs) have been addressed as the potential results of mutations of these genes. Among CRSDs, familial advanced sleep phase syndrome (fASPS) is an autosomal-dominant genetic disorder characterized by a regular sleep cycle that occurs 4 h earlier (advanced) than that of unaffected family members [3]. The first familial study showed a serine to glycine mutation in the casein kinase epsilon-binding regions of the *PER2* gene on chromosome 2q as the causative mutation for fASPS [181], although this result was not replicated in the second study [182]. The other familial study of fASPS showed a missense mutation in the casein kinase 1δ (*CK1δ*) gene, but this mutation led to opposing phenotypes between transgenic *Drosophila* and mouse models [183].

Chronotype is an individual circadian trait and can be associated with CRSDs [5]. It includes morningness (advanced rhythms) and eveningness ("night owls"). Twin and family studies showed a moderate degree of heritability of the chronotype, ranging between 14% and 54%, and genetic factors can account for about 50% of the variability of chronotypes [6, 184, 185]. Some polymorphisms in the circadian rhythm-related genes were reported to be associated with the chronotype: those in *PER1* and *PER2* with morningness [186, 187], 3111C allele in the *CLOCK* gene; those in the *PER3* with eveningness [188, 189]; and those in *PER3* and *ARNTL2* with chronotype [190]. As results were mixed across the studies, probably because of the small sample sizes, further larger studies would be required to determine the genetic predispositions to chronotype.

13.9 Conclusion

The goal of research on the genetic basis of sleep disorders is to identify genetic risks for these diseases and to reveal how the genetic variants affect the pathogenesis and pathophysiology of the diseases [3]. In terms of understanding cellular and molecular mechanisms in relation to genetic factors and disease manifestations, genetic studies of sleep disorders have just started.

Much work to identify the genetic variants that confer disease risks has been done, whereas most results of this work are inconclusive because of inadequate study design such as small sample size and liberal phenotyping and lack of replication across studies [5]. The genetic research has been most advanced in CCHS, narcolepsy, and RLS/WED. It is partly due to clearer phenotyping and relatively large sample sizes. OSA is a common but complex sleep disorder with multiple phenotypic components such as obesity, neuronal control of respiration, and craniofacial features. These multiple pathways have complicated identification of the genetic determinants of OSA. In insomnia, variable definitions and comorbidities, particularly psychiatric disorders, are supposed to be the major concerns. To detect common genetic factors across various phenotypes of insomnia, the identification of clinical features shared by several phenotypes of insomnia may be the first process.

Most sleep disorders have been shown to have significant heritability. However, genetic variances identified so far can account for only a little heritability. It partially reflects the limitations of GAWS approach because GAWSs typically focus on common genetic variances with small effects and neglect rare variances with potentially larger effects. Thus, candidate genes for sleep disorders should be explored beyond several GWASs. Rare variant analysis using whole-exome or whole-genome sequencing methods may resolve the problem of "missing heritability" in sleep disorders.

Moreover, functional studies are always necessary to elucidate the pathways from genetic predispositions to disease manifestations. Functional analysis using cellular and animal models can clarify the underlying mechanisms of sleep disorders as well as those of sleep, breathing, and other vital functions in healthy individuals. Translational research using omics and system biology methods also can help to understand what happens in patients with sleep disorders. Posttranscriptional modifications of gene expression can be potential players in sleep disorders. These functional analyses may be useful for identification of biomarkers and therapeutic targets.

In conclusion, although observational studies, candidate gene analysis, and GWASs have shed some light on the genetic aspects of sleep disorders, most risks and subsequent pathways remain unrevealed. Further genetic research and functional analysis using clinically well-defined study participants are critical for developing novel preventive and therapeutic interventions in sleep disorders.

References

1. Luyster FS, Strollo PJ Jr, Zee PC, Walsh JK, Boards of Directors of the American Academy of Sleep Medicine and the Sleep Research Society. Sleep: a health imperative. Sleep. 2012;35:727–34.
2. Alexander M, Ray MA, Hebert JR, Youngstedt SD, Zhang H, Steck SE, et al. The National Veteran Sleep Disorder Study: descriptive epidemiology and secular trends, 2000–2010. Sleep. 2016;39:1399–410.
3. Parish JM. Genetic and immunologic aspects of sleep and sleep disorders. Chest. 2013;143:1489–99.
4. Sateia MJ. International classification of sleep disorders-third edition: highlights and modifications. Chest. 2014;146:1387–94.
5. Gehrman PR, Keenan BT, Byrne EM, Pack AI. Genetics of sleep disorders. Psychiatr Clin North Am. 2015;38:667–81.
6. Andretic R, Franken P, Tafti M. Genetics of sleep. Annu Rev Genet. 2008;42:361–88.
7. Partinen M, Kaprio J, Koskenvuo M, Putkonen P, Langinvainio H. Genetic and environmental determination of human sleep. Sleep. 1983;6:179–85.
8. De Gennaro L, Marzano C, Fratello F, Moroni F, Pellicciari MC, Ferlazzo F, et al. The electroencephalographic fingerprint of sleep is genetically determined: a twin study. Ann Neurol. 2008;64:455–60.
9. Nixon GM, Brouillette RT. Sleep and breathing in Prader-Willi syndrome. Pediatr Pulmonol. 2002;34:209–17.
10. Tsuno N, Besset A, Ritchie K. Sleep and depression. J Clin Psychiatry. 2005;66:1254–69.
11. Alcantara C, Biggs ML, Davidson KW, Delaney JA, Jackson CL, Zee PC, et al. Sleep disturbances and depression in the multi-ethnic study of atherosclerosis. Sleep. 2016;39:915–25.

12. Young T, Palta M, Dempsey J, Peppard PE, Nieto FJ, Hla KM. Burden of sleep apnea: rationale, design, and major findings of the Wisconsin Sleep Cohort study. WMJ. 2009;108:246–9.
13. Peppard PE, Young T, Barnet JH, Palta M, Hagen EW, Hla KM. Increased prevalence of sleep-disordered breathing in adults. Am J Epidemiol. 2013;177:1006–14.
14. Nakayama-Ashida Y, Takegami M, Chin K, Sumi K, Nakamura T, Takahashi K, et al. Sleep-disordered breathing in the usual lifestyle setting as detected with home monitoring in a population of working men in Japan. Sleep. 2008;31:419–25.
15. Chin K, Oga T, Takahashi K, Takegami M, Nakayama-Ashida Y, Wakamura T, et al. Associations between obstructive sleep apnea, metabolic syndrome, and sleep duration, as measured with an actigraph, in an urban male working population in Japan. Sleep. 2010;33:89–95.
16. Young T, Blustein J, Finn L, Palta M. Sleep-disordered breathing and motor vehicle accidents in a population-based sample of employed adults. Sleep. 1997;20:608–13.
17. Teran-Santos J, Jimenez-Gomez A, Cordero-Guevara J. The association between sleep apnea and the risk of traffic accidents. Cooperative Group Burgos-Santander. N Engl J Med. 1999;340:847–51.
18. Young T, Peppard PE, Gottlieb DJ. Epidemiology of obstructive sleep apnea: a population health perspective. Am J Respir Crit Care Med. 2002;165:1217–39.
19. Quan SF, Wright R, Baldwin CM, Kaemingk KL, Goodwin JL, Kuo TF, et al. Obstructive sleep apnea-hypopnea and neurocognitive functioning in the Sleep Heart Health Study. Sleep Med. 2006;7:498–507.
20. Marin JM, Carrizo SJ, Vicente E, Agusti AG. Long-term cardiovascular outcomes in men with obstructive sleep apnoea-hypopnoea with or without treatment with continuous positive airway pressure: an observational study. Lancet. 2005;365:1046–53.
21. Yeboah J, Redline S, Johnson C, Tracy R, Ouyang P, Blumenthal RS, et al. Association between sleep apnea, snoring, incident cardiovascular events and all-cause mortality in an adult population: MESA. Atherosclerosis. 2011;219:963–8.
22. Shahar E, Whitney CW, Redline S, Lee ET, Newman AB, Nieto FJ, et al. Sleep-disordered breathing and cardiovascular disease: cross-sectional results of the Sleep Heart Health Study. Am J Respir Crit Care Med. 2001;163:19–25.
23. Gami AS, Pressman G, Caples SM, Kanagala R, Gard JJ, Davison DE, et al. Association of atrial fibrillation and obstructive sleep apnea. Circulation. 2004;110:364–7.
24. Yaggi HK, Concato J, Kernan WN, Lichtman JH, Brass LM, Mohsenin V. Obstructive sleep apnea as a risk factor for stroke and death. N Engl J Med. 2005;353:2034–41.
25. Arnardottir ES, Mackiewicz M, Gislason T, Teff KL, Pack AI. Molecular signatures of obstructive sleep apnea in adults: a review and perspective. Sleep. 2009;32:447–70.
26. Shamsuzzaman AS, Gersh BJ, Somers VK. Obstructive sleep apnea: implications for cardiac and vascular disease. JAMA. 2003;290(14):1906.
27. Xiong L, Catoire H, Dion P, Gaspar C, Lafreniere RG, Girard SL, et al. MEIS1 intronic risk haplotype associated with restless legs syndrome affects its mRNA and protein expression levels. Hum Mol Genet. 2009;18:1065–74.
28. Redline S, Tishler PV. The genetics of sleep apnea. Sleep Med Rev. 2000;4:583–602.
29. Redline S, Tosteson T, Tishler PV, Carskadon MA, Millman RP. Studies in the genetics of obstructive sleep apnea. Familial aggregation of symptoms associated with sleep-related breathing disturbances. Am Rev Respir Dis. 1992;145:440–4.
30. Redline S, Tishler PV, Tosteson TD, Williamson J, Kump K, Browner I, et al. The familial aggregation of obstructive sleep apnea. Am J Respir Crit Care Med. 1995;151:682–7.
31. Maes HH, Neale MC, Eaves LJ. Genetic and environmental factors in relative body weight and human adiposity. Behav Genet. 1997;27:325–51.
32. Silventoinen K, Kaprio J. Genetics of tracking of body mass index from birth to late middle age: evidence from twin and family studies. Obes Facts. 2009;2:196–202.
33. Redline S, Tishler PV, Schluchter M, Aylor J, Clark K, Graham G. Risk factors for sleep-disordered breathing in children. Associations with obesity, race, and respiratory problems. Am J Respir Crit Care Med. 1999;159:1527–32.

34. Mathur R, Douglas NJ. Family studies in patients with the sleep apnea-hypopnea syndrome. Ann Intern Med. 1995;122:174–8.
35. Palmer LJ, Buxbaum SG, Larkin EK, Patel SR, Elston RC, Tishler PV, et al. Whole genome scan for obstructive sleep apnea and obesity in African-American families. Am J Respir Crit Care Med. 2004;169:1314–21.
36. Palmer LJ, Buxbaum SG, Larkin E, Patel SR, Elston RC, Tishler PV, et al. A whole-genome scan for obstructive sleep apnea and obesity. Am J Hum Genet. 2003;72:340–50.
37. Patel SR, Frame JM, Larkin EK, Redline S. Heritability of upper airway dimensions derived using acoustic pharyngometry. Eur Respir J. 2008;32:1304–8.
38. de Paula LK, Alvim RO, Pedrosa RP, Horimoto AR, Krieger JE, Oliveira CM, et al. Heritability of OSA in a rural population. Chest. 2016;149:92–7.
39. Dudley KA, Patel SR. Disparities and genetic risk factors in obstructive sleep apnea. Sleep Med. 2016;18:96–102.
40. Winkelmann J, Schormair B, Xiong L, Dion PA, Rye DB, Rouleau GA. Genetics of restless legs syndrome. Sleep Med. 2017;31:18–22.
41. Cade BE, Chen H, Stilp AM, Gleason KJ, Sofer T, Ancoli-Israel S, et al. Genetic associations with obstructive sleep apnea traits in Hispanic/Latino Americans. Am J Respir Crit Care Med. 2016;194:886–97.
42. Varvarigou V, Dahabreh IJ, Malhotra A, Kales SN. A review of genetic association studies of obstructive sleep apnea: field synopsis and meta-analysis. Sleep. 2011;34:1461–8.
43. Xu H, Guan J, Yi H, Yin S. A systematic review and meta-analysis of the association between serotonergic gene polymorphisms and obstructive sleep apnea syndrome. PLoS One. 2014;9:e86460.
44. Qin B, Sun Z, Liang Y, Yang Z, Zhong R. The association of 5-HT2A, 5-HTT, and LEPR polymorphisms with obstructive sleep apnea syndrome: a systematic review and meta-analysis. PLoS One. 2014;9:e95856.
45. Sun J, Hu J, Tu C, Zhong A, Xu H. Obstructive sleep apnea susceptibility genes in Chinese population: a field synopsis and meta-analysis of genetic association studies. PLoS One. 2015;10:e0135942.
46. Lv D, Tan L, Wu Y, Cao C, Deng Z. Leptin and leptin receptor gene polymorphisms in obstructive sleep apnea: a HuGE review and meta-analysis. Sleep Breath. 2015;19:1073–8.
47. Patel SR, Goodloe R, De G, Kowgier M, Weng J, Buxbaum SG, et al. Association of genetic loci with sleep apnea in European Americans and African-Americans: the Candidate Gene Association Resource (CARe). PLoS One. 2012;7:e48836.
48. Sands-Lincoln M, Grandner M, Whinnery J, Keenan BT, Jackson N, Gurubhagavatula I. The association between obstructive sleep apnea and hypertension by race/ethnicity in a nationally representative sample. J Clin Hypertens (Greenwich). 2013;15:593–9.
49. Ramos AR, Guilliam D, Dib SI, Koch S. Race/ethnic differences in obstructive sleep apnea risk in patients with acute ischemic strokes in south Florida. Sleep Breath. 2014;18:165–8.
50. Padmanabhan S, Caulfield M, Dominiczak AF. Genetic and molecular aspects of hypertension. Circ Res. 2015;116:937–59.
51. Lin L, Finn L, Zhang J, Young T, Mignot E. Angiotensin-converting enzyme, sleep-disordered breathing, and hypertension. Am J Respir Crit Care Med. 2004;170:1349–53.
52. Patel SR, Larkin EK, Mignot E, Lin L, Redline S. The association of angiotensin converting enzyme (ACE) polymorphisms with sleep apnea and hypertension. Sleep. 2007;30:531–3.
53. Edwards BA, Eckert DJ, McSharry DG, Sands SA, Desai A, Kehlmann G, et al. Clinical predictors of the respiratory arousal threshold in patients with obstructive sleep apnea. Am J Respir Crit Care Med. 2014;190:1293–300.
54. Weese-Mayer DE, Berry-Kravis EM, Ceccherini I, Keens TG, Loghmanee DA, Trang H, et al. An official ATS clinical policy statement: congenital central hypoventilation syndrome: genetic basis, diagnosis, and management. Am J Respir Crit Care Med. 2010;181:626–44.
55. Ramanantsoa N, Gallego J. Congenital central hypoventilation syndrome. Respir Physiol Neurobiol. 2013;189:272–9.

56. Moreira TS, Takakura AC, Czeisler C, Otero JJ. Respiratory and autonomic dysfunction in congenital central hypoventilation syndrome. J Neurophysiol. 2016;116:742–52.
57. Amiel J, Laudier B, Attie-Bitach T, Trang H, de Pontual L, Gener B, et al. Polyalanine expansion and frameshift mutations of the paired-like homeobox gene PHOX2B in congenital central hypoventilation syndrome. Nat Genet. 2003;33:459–61.
58. Weese-Mayer DE, Berry-Kravis EM, Zhou L, Maher BS, Silvestri JM, Curran ME, et al. Idiopathic congenital central hypoventilation syndrome: analysis of genes pertinent to early autonomic nervous system embryologic development and identification of mutations in PHOX2b. Am J Med Genet A. 2003;123A:267–78.
59. Trochet D, O'Brien LM, Gozal D, Trang H, Nordenskjold A, Laudier B, et al. PHOX2B genotype allows for prediction of tumor risk in congenital central hypoventilation syndrome. Am J Hum Genet. 2005;76:421–6.
60. Berry-Kravis EM, Zhou L, Rand CM, Weese-Mayer DE. Congenital central hypoventilation syndrome: PHOX2B mutations and phenotype. Am J Respir Crit Care Med. 2006;174:1139–44.
61. Trochet D, Hong SJ, Lim JK, Brunet JF, Munnich A, Kim KS, et al. Molecular consequences of PHOX2B missense, frameshift and alanine expansion mutations leading to autonomic dysfunction. Hum Mol Genet. 2005;14:3697–708.
62. Matera I, Bachetti T, Puppo F, Di Duca M, Morandi F, Casiraghi GM, et al. PHOX2B mutations and polyalanine expansions correlate with the severity of the respiratory phenotype and associated symptoms in both congenital and late onset Central Hypoventilation syndrome. J Med Genet. 2004;41:373–80.
63. Sasaki A, Kanai M, Kijima K, Akaba K, Hashimoto M, Hasegawa H, et al. Molecular analysis of congenital central hypoventilation syndrome. Hum Genet. 2003;114:22–6.
64. Devriendt K, Fryns JP, Naulaers G, Devlieger H, Alliet P. Neuroblastoma in a mother and congenital central hypoventilation in her daughter: variable expression of the same genetic disorder? Am J Med Genet. 2000;90:430–1.
65. Weese-Mayer DE, Silvestri JM, Marazita ML, Hoo JJ. Congenital central hypoventilation syndrome: inheritance and relation to sudden infant death syndrome. Am J Med Genet. 1993;47:360–7.
66. Goridis C, Brunet JF. Central chemoreception: lessons from mouse and human genetics. Respir Physiol Neurobiol. 2010;173:312–21.
67. Guyenet PG, Mulkey DK. Retrotrapezoid nucleus and parafacial respiratory group. Respir Physiol Neurobiol. 2010;173:244–55.
68. Guyenet PG, Stornetta RL, Abbott SB, Depuy SD, Fortuna MG, Kanbar R. Central CO2 chemoreception and integrated neural mechanisms of cardiovascular and respiratory control. J Appl Physiol (1985). 2010;108:995–1002.
69. Bachetti T, Matera I, Borghini S, Di Duca M, Ravazzolo R, Ceccherini I. Distinct pathogenetic mechanisms for PHOX2B associated polyalanine expansions and frameshift mutations in congenital central hypoventilation syndrome. Hum Mol Genet. 2005;14:1815–24.
70. Wu HT, Su YN, Hung CC, Hsieh WS, Wu KJ. Interaction between PHOX2B and CREBBP mediates synergistic activation: mechanistic implications of PHOX2B mutants. Hum Mutat. 2009;30:655–60.
71. Ikeda K, Takahashi M, Sato S, Igarashi H, Ishizuka T, Yawo H, et al. A Phox2b BAC transgenic rat line useful for understanding respiratory rhythm generator neural circuitry. PLoS One. 2015;10:e0132475.
72. Ruffault PL, D'Autreaux F, Hayes JA, Nomaksteinsky M, Autran S, Fujiyama T, et al. The retrotrapezoid nucleus neurons expressing Atoh1 and Phox2b are essential for the respiratory response to CO(2). elife. 2015;4. https://doi.org/10.7554/eLife.07051.
73. Dubreuil V, Ramanantsoa N, Trochet D, Vaubourg V, Amiel J, Gallego J, et al. A human mutation in Phox2b causes lack of CO2 chemosensitivity, fatal central apnea, and specific loss of parafacial neurons. Proc Natl Acad Sci U S A. 2008;105:1067–72.

74. Ramanantsoa N, Hirsch MR, Thoby-Brisson M, Dubreuil V, Bouvier J, Ruffault PL, et al. Breathing without CO(2) chemosensitivity in conditional Phox2b mutants. J Neurosci. 2011;31:12880–8.
75. Garcia Borreguero D, Winkelmann J, Allen RP. Introduction: towards a better understanding of the science of RLS/WED. Sleep Med. 2017;31:1–2.
76. Allen RP, Picchietti DL, Garcia-Borreguero D, Ondo WG, Walters AS, Winkelman JW, et al. Restless legs syndrome/Willis-Ekbom disease diagnostic criteria: updated International Restless Legs Syndrome Study Group (IRLSSG) consensus criteria—history, rationale, description, and significance. Sleep Med. 2014;15:860–73.
77. Allen RP, Stillman P, Myers AJ. Physician-diagnosed restless legs syndrome in a large sample of primary medical care patients in western Europe: Prevalence and characteristics. Sleep Med. 2010;11:31–7.
78. Allen RP, Bharmal M, Calloway M. Prevalence and disease burden of primary restless legs syndrome: results of a general population survey in the United States. Mov Disord. 2011;26:114–20.
79. Xiong L, Jang K, Montplaisir J, Levchenko A, Thibodeau P, Gaspar C, et al. Canadian restless legs syndrome twin study. Neurology. 2007;68:1631–3.
80. Lazzarini A, Walters AS, Hickey K, Coccagna G, Lugaresi E, Ehrenberg BL, et al. Studies of penetrance and anticipation in five autosomal-dominant restless legs syndrome pedigrees. Mov Disord. 1999;14:111–6.
81. Winkelmann J, Muller-Myhsok B, Wittchen HU, Hock B, Prager M, Pfister H, et al. Complex segregation analysis of restless legs syndrome provides evidence for an autosomal dominant mode of inheritance in early age at onset families. Ann Neurol. 2002;52:297–302.
82. Desautels A, Turecki G, Montplaisir J, Sequeira A, Verner A, Rouleau GA. Identification of a major susceptibility locus for restless legs syndrome on chromosome 12q. Am J Hum Genet. 2001;69:1266–70.
83. Bonati MT, Ferini-Strambi L, Aridon P, Oldani A, Zucconi M, Casari G. Autosomal dominant restless legs syndrome maps on chromosome 14q. Brain. 2003;126:1485–92.
84. Winkelmann J, Lichtner P, Schormair B, Uhr M, Hauk S, Stiasny-Kolster K, et al. Variants in the neuronal nitric oxide synthase (nNOS, NOS1) gene are associated with restless legs syndrome. Mov Disord. 2008;23:350–8.
85. Schormair B, Kemlink D, Roeske D, Eckstein G, Xiong L, Lichtner P, et al. PTPRD (protein tyrosine phosphatase receptor type delta) is associated with restless legs syndrome. Nat Genet. 2008;40(8):946.
86. Mercader N, Leonardo E, Azpiazu N, Serrano A, Morata G, Martinez C, et al. Conserved regulation of proximodistal limb axis development by Meis1/Hth. Nature. 1999;402:425–9.
87. Dasen JS, Tice BC, Brenner-Morton S, Jessell TM. A Hox regulatory network establishes motor neuron pool identity and target-muscle connectivity. Cell. 2005;123:477–91.
88. Maeda R, Mood K, Jones TL, Aruga J, Buchberg AM, Daar IO. Xmeis1, a protooncogene involved in specifying neural crest cell fate in Xenopus embryos. Oncogene. 2001;20:1329–42.
89. Dinev D, Jordan BW, Neufeld B, Lee JD, Lindemann D, Rapp UR, et al. Extracellular signal regulated kinase 5 (ERK5) is required for the differentiation of muscle cells. EMBO Rep. 2001;2:829–34.
90. Gross MK, Dottori M, Goulding M. Lbx1 specifies somatosensory association interneurons in the dorsal spinal cord. Neuron. 2002;34:535–49.
91. Uetani N, Chagnon MJ, Kennedy TE, Iwakura Y, Tremblay ML. Mammalian motoneuron axon targeting requires receptor protein tyrosine phosphatases sigma and delta. J Neurosci. 2006;26:5872–80.
92. Winkelmann J, Schormair B, Lichtner P, Ripke S, Xiong L, Jalilzadeh S, et al. Genome-wide association study of restless legs syndrome identifies common variants in three genomic regions. Nat Genet. 2007;39:1000–6.

93. Winkelmann J, Czamara D, Schormair B, Knauf F, Schulte EC, Trenkwalder C, et al. Genome-wide association study identifies novel restless legs syndrome susceptibility loci on 2p14 and 16q12.1. PLoS Genet. 2011;7:e1002171.
94. Stefansson H, Rye DB, Hicks A, Petursson H, Ingason A, Thorgeirsson TE, et al. A genetic risk factor for periodic limb movements in sleep. N Engl J Med. 2007;357:639–47.
95. Earley CJ, Connor J, Garcia-Borreguero D, Jenner P, Winkelman J, Zee PC, et al. Altered brain iron homeostasis and dopaminergic function in Restless Legs Syndrome (Willis-Ekbom Disease). Sleep Med. 2014;15:1288–301.
96. Oexle K, Ried JS, Hicks AA, Tanaka T, Hayward C, Bruegel M, et al. Novel association to the proprotein convertase PCSK7 gene locus revealed by analysing soluble transferrin receptor (sTfR) levels. Hum Mol Genet. 2011;20:1042–7.
97. Oexle K, Schormair B, Ried JS, Czamara D, Heim K, Frauscher B, et al. Dilution of candidates: the case of iron-related genes in restless legs syndrome. Eur J Hum Genet. 2013;21(4):410.
98. Moore H IV, Winkelmann J, Lin L, Finn L, Peppard P, Mignot E. Periodic leg movements during sleep are associated with polymorphisms in BTBD9, TOX3/BC034767, MEIS1, MAP2K5/SKOR1, and PTPRD. Sleep. 2014;37:1535–42.
99. Winkelman JW, Blackwell T, Stone K, Ancoli-Israel S, Tranah GJ, Redline S, et al. Genetic associations of periodic limb movements of sleep in the elderly for the MrOS sleep study. Sleep Med. 2015;16:1360–5.
100. Risch N, Merikangas K. The future of genetic studies of complex human diseases. Science. 1996;273:1516–7.
101. Schulte EC, Kousi M, Tan PL, Tilch E, Knauf F, Lichtner P, et al. Targeted resequencing and systematic in vivo functional testing identifies rare variants in MEIS1 as significant contributors to restless legs syndrome. Am J Hum Genet. 2014;95:85–95.
102. Weissbach A, Siegesmund K, Bruggemann N, Schmidt A, Kasten M, Pichler I, et al. Exome sequencing in a family with restless legs syndrome. Mov Disord. 2012;27:1686–9.
103. Scammell TE. Narcolepsy. N Engl J Med. 2015;373:2654–62.
104. Longstreth WT Jr, Koepsell TD, Ton TG, Hendrickson AF, van Belle G. The epidemiology of narcolepsy. Sleep. 2007;30:13–26.
105. Mignot E. Genetic and familial aspects of narcolepsy. Neurology. 1998;50:S16–22.
106. Mignot E. Sleep, sleep disorders and hypocretin (orexin). Sleep Med. 2004;5(Suppl 1):S2–8.
107. Chemelli RM, Willie JT, Sinton CM, Elmquist JK, Scammell T, Lee C, et al. Narcolepsy in orexin knockout mice: molecular genetics of sleep regulation. Cell. 1999;98:437–51.
108. Thannickal TC, Moore RY, Nienhuis R, Ramanathan L, Gulyani S, Aldrich M, et al. Reduced number of hypocretin neurons in human narcolepsy. Neuron. 2000;27:469–74.
109. Chabas D, Taheri S, Renier C, Mignot E. The genetics of narcolepsy. Annu Rev Genomics Hum Genet. 2003;4:459–83.
110. Rogers AE, Meehan J, Guilleminault C, Grumet FC, Mignot E. HLA DR15 (DR2) and DQB1*0602 typing studies in 188 narcoleptic patients with cataplexy. Neurology. 1997;48(6):1550.
111. Tafti M, Hor H, Dauvilliers Y, Lammers GJ, Overeem S, Mayer G, et al. DQB1 locus alone explains most of the risk and protection in narcolepsy with cataplexy in Europe. Sleep. 2014;37:19–25.
112. Pelin Z, Guilleminault C, Risch N, Grumet FC, Mignot E. HLA-DQB1*0602 homozygosity increases relative risk for narcolepsy but not disease severity in two ethnic groups. US Modafinil in Narcolepsy Multicenter Study Group. Tissue Antigens. 1998;51:96–100.
113. Hong SC, Lin L, Lo B, Jeong JH, Shin YK, Kim SY, et al. DQB1*0301 and DQB1*0601 modulate narcolepsy susceptibility in Koreans. Hum Immunol. 2007;68:59–68.
114. Ollila HM, Ravel JM, Han F, Faraco J, Lin L, Zheng X, et al. HLA-DPB1 and HLA class I confer risk of and protection from narcolepsy. Am J Hum Genet. 2015;96:136–46.
115. Mignot E, Lin L, Rogers W, Honda Y, Qiu X, Lin X, et al. Complex HLA-DR and -DQ interactions confer risk of narcolepsy-cataplexy in three ethnic groups. Am J Hum Genet. 2001;68:686–99.

116. Hallmayer J, Faraco J, Lin L, Hesselson S, Winkelmann J, Kawashima M, et al. Narcolepsy is strongly associated with the T-cell receptor alpha locus. Nat Genet. 2009;41:708–11.
117. Hor H, Kutalik Z, Dauvilliers Y, Valsesia A, Lammers GJ, Donjacour CE, et al. Genome-wide association study identifies new HLA class II haplotypes strongly protective against narcolepsy. Nat Genet. 2010;42(9):786.
118. Han F, Faraco J, Dong XS, Ollila HM, Lin L, Li J, et al. Genome wide analysis of narcolepsy in China implicates novel immune loci and reveals changes in association prior to versus after the 2009 H1N1 influenza pandemic. PLoS Genet. 2013;9:e1003880.
119. Faraco J, Lin L, Kornum BR, Kenny EE, Trynka G, Einen M, et al. ImmunoChip study implicates antigen presentation to T cells in narcolepsy. PLoS Genet. 2013;9:e1003270.
120. Kornum BR, Kawashima M, Faraco J, Lin L, Rico TJ, Hesselson S, et al. Common variants in P2RY11 are associated with narcolepsy. Nat Genet. 2011;43:66–71.
121. Miyagawa T, Kawashima M, Nishida N, Ohashi J, Kimura R, Fujimoto A, et al. Variant between CPT1B and CHKB associated with susceptibility to narcolepsy. Nat Genet. 2008;40:1324–8.
122. Han F, Lin L, Warby SC, Faraco J, Li J, Dong SX, et al. Narcolepsy onset is seasonal and increased following the 2009 H1N1 pandemic in China. Ann Neurol. 2011;70:410–7.
123. Aran A, Lin L, Nevsimalova S, Plazzi G, Hong SC, Weiner K, et al. Elevated anti-streptococcal antibodies in patients with recent narcolepsy onset. Sleep. 2009;32:979–83.
124. Nohynek H, Jokinen J, Partinen M, Vaarala O, Kirjavainen T, Sundman J, et al. AS03 adjuvanted AH1N1 vaccine associated with an abrupt increase in the incidence of childhood narcolepsy in Finland. PLoS One. 2012;7:e33536.
125. Partinen M, Saarenpaa-Heikkila O, Ilveskoski I, Hublin C, Linna M, Olsen P, et al. Increased incidence and clinical picture of childhood narcolepsy following the 2009 H1N1 pandemic vaccination campaign in Finland. PLoS One. 2012;7:e33723.
126. Donadio V, Liguori R, Vandi S, Pizza F, Dauvilliers Y, Leta V, et al. Lower wake resting sympathetic and cardiovascular activities in narcolepsy with cataplexy. Neurology. 2014;83:1080–6.
127. Mignot EJ. A practical guide to the therapy of narcolepsy and hypersomnia syndromes. Neurotherapeutics. 2012;9:739–52.
128. Mahlios J, De la Herran-Arita AK, Mignot E. The autoimmune basis of narcolepsy. Curr Opin Neurobiol. 2013;23:767–73.
129. American Psychiatric Association. Diagnostic and statistical manual of mental disorders. 5th ed. Arlington, VA: American Psychiatric Association; 2013.
130. Morin CM. Epidemiology of insomnia. Sleep Med Clin. 2013;8:281–97.
131. Lind MJ, Gehrman PR. Genetic pathwaysto insomnia. Brain Sci. 2016;6. https://doi.org/10.3390/brainsci6040064.
132. Ohayon MM. Epidemiology of insomnia: what we know and what we still need to learn. Sleep Med Rev. 2002;6:97–111.
133. Roth T. Insomnia: definition, prevalence, etiology, and consequences. J Clin Sleep Med. 2007;3:S7–10.
134. Heath AC, Kendler KS, Eaves LJ, Martin NG. Evidence for genetic influences on sleep disturbance and sleep pattern in twins. Sleep. 1990;13:318–35.
135. Beaulieu-Bonneau S, LeBlanc M, Merette C, Dauvilliers Y, Morin CM. Family history of insomnia in a population-based sample. Sleep. 2007;30:1739–45.
136. McCarren M, Goldberg J, Ramakrishnan V, Fabsitz R. Insomnia in Vietnam era veteran twins: influence of genes and combat experience. Sleep. 1994;17:456–61.
137. Lind MJ, Aggen SH, Kirkpatrick RM, Kendler KS, Amstadter AB. A longitudinal twin study of insomnia symptoms in adults. Sleep. 2015;38:1423–30.
138. Barclay NL, Gehrman PR, Gregory AM, Eaves LJ, Silberg JL. The heritability of insomnia progression during childhood/adolescence: results from a longitudinal twin study. Sleep. 2015;38:109–18.
139. Li J, Huang C, Lan Y, Wang Y. A cross-sectional study on the relationships among the polymorphism of period2 gene, work stress, and insomnia. Sleep Breath. 2015;19:1399–406.

140. Brower KJ, Wojnar M, Sliwerska E, Armitage R, Burmeister M. PER3 polymorphism and insomnia severity in alcohol dependence. Sleep. 2012;35:571–7.
141. Brummett BH, Krystal AD, Ashley-Koch A, Kuhn CM, Zuchner S, Siegler IC, et al. Sleep quality varies as a function of 5-HTTLPR genotype and stress. Psychosom Med. 2007;69:621–4.
142. Bouvette-Turcot AA, Pluess M, Bernier A, Pennestri MH, Levitan R, Sokolowski MB, et al. Effects of genotype and sleep on temperament. Pediatrics. 2015;136:e914–21.
143. Harvey CJ, Gehrman P, Espie CA. Who is predisposed to insomnia: a review of familial aggregation, stress-reactivity, personality and coping style. Sleep Med Rev. 2014;18:237–47.
144. Jawinski P, Tegelkamp S, Sander C, Hantzsch M, Huang J, Mauche N, et al. Time to wake up: no impact of COMT Val158Met gene variation on circadian preferences, arousal regulation and sleep. Chronobiol Int. 2016;33:893–905.
145. Wang CC, Lung FW. The role of PGC-1 and Apoepsilon4 in insomnia. Psychiatr Genet. 2012;22:82–7.
146. Ziv-Gal A, Flaws JA, Mahoney MM, Miller SR, Zacur HA, Gallicchio L. Genetic polymorphisms in the aryl hydrocarbon receptor-signaling pathway and sleep disturbances in middle-aged women. Sleep Med. 2013;14:883–7.
147. Ban HJ, Kim SC, Seo J, Kang HB, Choi JK. Genetic and metabolic characterization of insomnia. PLoS One. 2011;6:e18455.
148. Byrne EM, Gehrman PR, Medland SE, Nyholt DR, Heath AC, Madden PA, et al. A genome-wide association study of sleep habits and insomnia. Am J Med Genet B Neuropsychiatr Genet. 2013;162B:439–51.
149. Parsons MJ, Lester KJ, Barclay NL, Nolan PM, Eley TC, Gregory AM. Replication of Genome-Wide Association Studies (GWAS) loci for sleep in the British G1219 cohort. Am J Med Genet B Neuropsychiatr Genet. 2013;162B:431–8.
150. Spada J, Scholz M, Kirsten H, Hensch T, Horn K, Jawinski P, et al. Genome-wide association analysis of actigraphic sleep phenotypes in the LIFE Adult Study. J Sleep Res. 2016;25:690–701.
151. Amin N, Allebrandt KV, van der Spek A, Muller-Myhsok B, Hek K, Teder-Laving M, et al. Genetic variants in RBFOX3 are associated with sleep latency. Eur J Hum Genet. 2016;24:1488–95.
152. Gressier F, Calati R, Balestri M, Marsano A, Alberti S, Antypa N, et al. The 5-HTTLPR polymorphism and posttraumatic stress disorder: a meta-analysis. J Trauma Stress. 2013;26:645–53.
153. Risch N, Herrell R, Lehner T, Liang KY, Eaves L, Hoh J, et al. Interaction between the serotonin transporter gene (5-HTTLPR), stressful life events, and risk of depression: a meta-analysis. JAMA. 2009;301:2462–71.
154. van der Werf YD, Altena E, van Dijk KD, Strijers RL, De Rijke W, Stam CJ, et al. Is disturbed intracortical excitability a stable trait of chronic insomnia? A study using transcranial magnetic stimulation before and after multimodal sleep therapy. Biol Psychiatry. 2010;68:950–5.
155. Buysse DJ, Germain A, Hall M, Monk TH, Nofzinger EA. A neurobiological model of insomnia. Drug Discov Today Dis Models. 2011;8:129–37.
156. Drake CL, Friedman NP, Wright KP Jr, Roth T. Sleep reactivity and insomnia: genetic and environmental influences. Sleep. 2011;34:1179–88.
157. Kalmbach DA, Pillai V, Arnedt JT, Drake CL. Identifying at-risk individuals for insomnia using the Ford insomnia response to stress test. Sleep. 2016;39:449–56.
158. Llorens F, Zarranz JJ, Fischer A, Zerr I, Ferrer I. Fatal familial insomnia: clinical aspects and molecular alterations. Curr Neurol Neurosci Rep. 2017;17:30.
159. Medori R, Tritschler HJ, LeBlanc A, Villare F, Manetto V, Chen HY, et al. Fatal familial insomnia, a prion disease with a mutation at codon 178 of the prion protein gene. N Engl J Med. 1992;326:444–9.
160. Medori R, Montagna P, Tritschler HJ, LeBlanc A, Cortelli P, Tinuper P, et al. Fatal familial insomnia: a second kindred with mutation of prion protein gene at codon 178. Neurology. 1992;42:669–70.

161. Goldfarb LG, Petersen RB, Tabaton M, Brown P, LeBlanc AC, Montagna P, et al. Fatal familial insomnia and familial Creutzfeldt-Jakob disease: disease phenotype determined by a DNA polymorphism. Science. 1992;258:806–8.
162. Krasnianski A, Bartl M, Sanchez Juan PJ, Heinemann U, Meissner B, Varges D, et al. Fatal familial insomnia: clinical features and early identification. Ann Neurol. 2008;63:658–61.
163. Krasnianski A, Heinemann U, Ponto C, Kortt J, Kallenberg K, Varges D, et al. Clinical findings and diagnosis in genetic prion diseases in Germany. Eur J Epidemiol. 2016;31:187–96.
164. Montagna P, Gambetti P, Cortelli P, Lugaresi E. Familial and sporadic fatal insomnia. Lancet Neurol. 2003;2:167–76.
165. Cortelli P, Fabbri M, Calandra-Buonaura G, Capellari S, Tinuper P, Parchi P, et al. Gait disorders in fatal familial insomnia. Mov Disord. 2014;29:420–4.
166. Pedroso JL, Pinto WB, Souza PV, Ricarte IF, Landemberger MC, Martins VR, et al. Complex movement disorders in fatal familial insomnia: a clinical and genetic discussion. Neurology. 2013;81:1098–9.
167. Montagna P, Cortelli P, Avoni P, Tinuper P, Plazzi G, Gallassi R, et al. Clinical features of fatal familial insomnia: phenotypic variability in relation to a polymorphism at codon 129 of the prion protein gene. Brain Pathol. 1998;8:515–20.
168. Gambetti P, Lugaresi E. Conclusions of the symposium. Brain Pathol. 1998;8:571–5.
169. Gambetti P, Parchi P, Petersen RB, Chen SG, Lugaresi E. Fatal familial insomnia and familial Creutzfeldt-Jakob disease: clinical, pathological and molecular features. Brain Pathol. 1995;5:43–51.
170. Dimitri D, Jehel L, Durr A, Levy-Soussan M, Andreux V, Laplanche JL, et al. Fatal familial insomnia presenting as psychosis in an 18-year-old man. Neurology. 2006;67:363–4.
171. Parchi P, Castellani R, Cortelli P, Montagna P, Chen SG, Petersen RB, et al. Regional distribution of protease-resistant prion protein in fatal familial insomnia. Ann Neurol. 1995;38:21–9.
172. Parchi P, Petersen RB, Chen SG, Autilio-Gambetti L, Capellari S, Monari L, et al. Molecular pathology of fatal familial insomnia. Brain Pathol. 1998;8:539–48.
173. Capellari S, Strammiello R, Saverioni D, Kretzschmar H, Parchi P. Genetic Creutzfeldt-Jakob disease and fatal familial insomnia: insights into phenotypic variability and disease pathogenesis. Acta Neuropathol. 2011;121:21–37.
174. Krasnianski A, Sanchez Juan P, Ponto C, Bartl M, Heinemann U, Varges D, et al. A proposal of new diagnostic pathway for fatal familial insomnia. J Neurol Neurosurg Psychiatry. 2014;85:654–9.
175. Lee S, Antony L, Hartmann R, Knaus KJ, Surewicz K, Surewicz WK, et al. Conformational diversity in prion protein variants influences intermolecular beta-sheet formation. EMBO J. 2010;29:251–62.
176. Riek R, Wider G, Billeter M, Hornemann S, Glockshuber R, Wuthrich K. Prion protein NMR structure and familial human spongiform encephalopathies. Proc Natl Acad Sci U S A. 1998;95:11667–72.
177. Swietnicki W, Petersen RB, Gambetti P, Surewicz WK. Familial mutations and the thermodynamic stability of the recombinant human prion protein. J Biol Chem. 1998;273:31048–52.
178. Tian C, Liu D, Sun QL, Chen C, Xu Y, Wang H, et al. Comparative analysis of gene expression profiles between cortex and thalamus in Chinese fatal familial insomnia patients. Mol Neurobiol. 2013;48:36–48.
179. Frau-Mendez MA, Fernandez-Vega I, Ansoleaga B, Blanco Tech R, Carmona Tech M, Antonio Del Rio J, et al. Fatal familial insomnia: mitochondrial and protein synthesis machinery decline in the mediodorsal thalamus. Brain Pathol. 2017;27:95–106.
180. Panda S. Circadian physiology of metabolism. Science. 2016;354:1008–15.
181. Jones CR, Campbell SS, Zone SE, Cooper F, DeSano A, Murphy PJ, et al. Familial advanced sleep-phase syndrome: a short-period circadian rhythm variant in humans. Nat Med. 1999;5:1062–5.
182. Toh KL, Jones CR, He Y, Eide EJ, Hinz WA, Virshup DM, et al. An hPer2 phosphorylation site mutation in familial advanced sleep phase syndrome. Science. 2001;291:1040–3.

183. Xu Y, Padiath QS, Shapiro RE, Jones CR, Wu SC, Saigoh N, et al. Functional consequences of a CKIdelta mutation causing familial advanced sleep phase syndrome. Nature. 2005;434:640–4.
184. Vink JM, Groot AS, Kerkhof GA, Boomsma DI. Genetic analysis of morningness and eveningness. Chronobiol Int. 2001;18:809–22.
185. Aguiar GF, da Silva HP, Marques N. Patterns of daily allocation of sleep periods: a case study in an Amazonian riverine community. Chronobiologia. 1991;18:9–19.
186. Carpen JD, Archer SN, Skene DJ, Smits M, von Schantz M. A single-nucleotide polymorphism in the 5′-untranslated region of the hPER2 gene is associated with diurnal preference. J Sleep Res. 2005;14:293–7.
187. Carpen JD, von Schantz M, Smits M, Skene DJ, Archer SN. A silent polymorphism in the PER1 gene associates with extreme diurnal preference in humans. J Hum Genet. 2006;51:1122–5.
188. Katzenberg D, Young T, Finn L, Lin L, King DP, Takahashi JS, et al. A CLOCK polymorphism associated with human diurnal preference. Sleep. 1998;21:569–76.
189. Mishima K, Tozawa T, Satoh K, Saitoh H, Mishima Y. The 3111T/C polymorphism of hClock is associated with evening preference and delayed sleep timing in a Japanese population sample. Am J Med Genet B Neuropsychiatr Genet. 2005;133B:101–4.
190. Parsons MJ, Lester KJ, Barclay NL, Archer SN, Nolan PM, Eley TC, et al. Polymorphisms in the circadian expressed genes PER3 and ARNTL2 are associated with diurnal preference and GNbeta3 with sleep measures. J Sleep Res. 2014;23:595–604.

Chapter 14
Pharmacokinetics, Pharmacodynamics, and Toxicities: What Should We Know About Genetic Factors that Affect the Pharmacotherapy of Pulmonary Diseases?

Takashi Sato

Abstract There have been significant recent advances in the pharmacotherapy of lung diseases, particularly, molecular targeted therapy of lung cancer and idiopathic pulmonary fibrosis. However, there are some limitations inherent to this type of next-generation pharmacotherapy such as adverse drug reactions and nonresponse to therapy. Several factors may underlie the variability in response to therapy, including inherited variants in drug-metabolizing enzymes, transporters, receptors, and the fact that different signaling proteins can elicit different biological responses. Therefore, understanding the genetic factors that affect pharmacodynamics would help physicians determine interindividual differences in the absorption, distribution, metabolism, and excretion of specific drugs. Here, we review representative drugs often prescribed by pulmonologists, with special focus on genetic factors relating to efficacy, toxicity, safety, and responsiveness. An understanding of the genetic variants underlying interindividual differences in drug pharmacokinetics and pharmacodynamics could move us toward personalized precision medicine in which cutting-edge pharmacogenomic analyses are used. In addition, advanced high-throughput technologies such as a multigene panel platform could encourage physicians to optimize therapy with more potent but less toxic drugs and to characterize individual genetic backgrounds.

Keywords Genetic polymorphism · Drug-metabolizing enzyme
Pharmacokinetics · Pharmacodynamics · Pharmacogenomics

T. Sato
Department of Pulmonology, Yokohama City University Graduate School of Medicine, Yokohama, Kanagawa, Japan
e-mail: satotak@yokohama-cu.ac.jp

T. Kaneko (ed.), *Clinical Relevance of Genetic Factors in Pulmonary Diseases*, Respiratory Disease Series: Diagnostic Tools and Disease Managements, https://doi.org/10.1007/978-981-10-8144-6_14

14.1 Introduction

Recently, genome-wide association studies (GWAS) have been conducted for detecting single-nucleotide polymorphisms (SNPs) in the genome. The identification of polymorphisms can help pulmonary scientists understand the abnormal genes responsible for lung diseases as well as those that can be therapeutically targeted. Although the pharmacotherapy of pulmonary diseases has progressed, it is still challenging to elucidate the factors affecting individual variations in drug responses. To this end, we should understand pharmacokinetic and pharmacodynamic drug interactions, particularly when several drugs are administered simultaneously. Drug responses partly depend on ethnicity, age, sex, weight, nutrition, smoking-inherited factors, and comorbidities, especially those affecting liver and renal function (Fig. 14.1). Of these, inherited variants in drug-metabolizing enzymes, transporters, receptors, and signaling molecules are thought to be of critical importance to the drug response. Genetic factors could be responsible for 20–95% of variability in drug disposition [1]. Therefore, understanding genetically determined differences in an individual's capacity to metabolize drugs would improve the benefit–risk profile. To this end, recent developments in genotyping

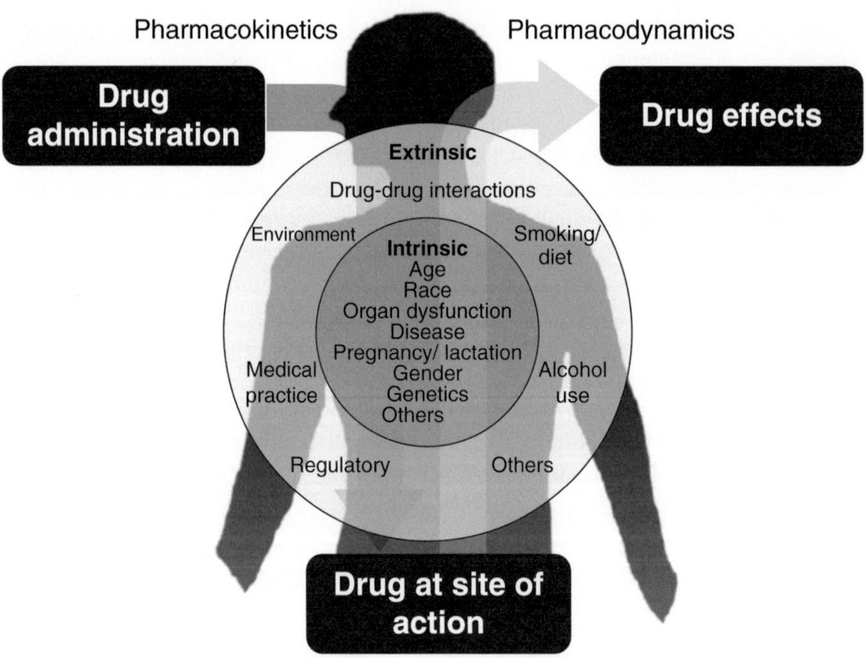

Fig. 14.1 The interindividual differences of response to drug are defined by many intrinsic and extrinsic factors affecting pharmacokinetics and pharmacodynamics processes. These factors influence drug concentration at the site of action and further observed drug effect. Adapted from reference [3] with permission

microarray platforms specifically focusing on drug-metabolizing enzymes and transporters could be useful for drug optimization [2]. This chapter summarizes critical genetic factors affecting the pharmacotherapy of respiratory diseases that pulmonary physicians should be aware of.

14.2 Pharmacokinetics and Pharmacodynamics

Pharmacokinetics is the time-course analysis of drug absorption, distribution, metabolism, and excretion processes. Of these, metabolism and excretion are the important drug elimination steps from the body. Genetic polymorphisms have been identified for many drug-metabolizing enzymes. Genetic variants lead to reduced or increased enzyme activity compared to wild-type alleles. Pharmacodynamics is the analysis of the relationship between drug concentration at the site of action and the resulting effects, including onset, intensity, and duration of the pharmacologic effects, and adverse events. Therefore, pharmacodynamics can be described as "the drug's action on the body." In contrast, pharmacokinetics can be described as "the action of the body on the drug." Understanding the relationship among pharmacokinetics, pharmacodynamics, and factors affecting each process would help physicians optimize medications and dosages for individual patients with enhanced efficacy and decreased toxicity (Fig. 14.1). As depicted in Fig. 14.1, individual variation in drug responses can be attributed to intrinsic ethnic factors (e.g., age, race, and genetics), extrinsic ethnic factors (e.g., environmental and cultural behaviors of diet, alcohol, and smoking), drug-drug interactions, and tolerance [3]. Since many drugs share the same metabolic enzymes and/or target the same receptors, it is also important to know the potential drug-drug interactions of representative drugs for the respiratory system.

14.3 Drug-Metabolizing Enzymes

Drug-metabolizing enzymes have been the focus of recent pharmacogenetic studies. Drug metabolism occurs in two phases (phase I and phase II). Phase I reactions involve formation of a new or modified functional group or cleavage (oxidation, reduction, hydrolysis). These reactions primarily occur in the liver during hepatic circulation secondary to minor reactions occurring in the target organ such as gastrointestinal epithelial (via oral intake), skin (topical application), and lung tissues (inhalation). The most important phase I reaction is "oxidation" via cytochrome P450 (CYP); thus, hepatic CYP is the most critical enzyme in phase I drug metabolism. Phase II reactions, also called conjugation reactions, act as the detoxifying step in drug metabolism. Key phase II enzymes are mainly transferases such as UDP-glucuronosyltransferases (UGTs), N-acetyltransferases (NATs), sulfotransferases, glutathione S-transferases (GSTs), and methyltransferases (mainly

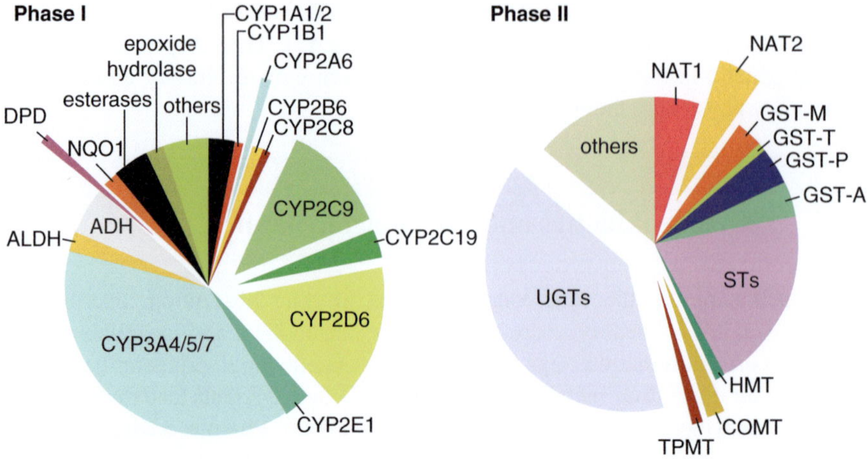

Fig. 14.2 Administering drugs are metabolized by drug-metabolizing enzymes (DMEs) through the processes of oxidation and conjugation. The oxidation process is mediated by phase I (left) DMEs, while conjugation process is mediated by phase II (right) DMEs. The contribution of each phase I and II DME to drug oxidation is indicated by the relative size of the corresponding pie. The majority of these phase I and II DMEs are polymorphic. *ADH* alcohol dehydrogenase, *ALDH* aldehyde dehydrogenase, *CYP* cytochrome P450, *DPD* dihydropyrimidine dehydrogenase, *NQO1* NADPH/quinone oxidoreductase or DT diaphorase, *COMT* catechol *O*-methyltransferase, *GST* glutathione *S*-transferase, *HMT* histamine methyltransferase, *NAT* *N*-acetyltransferase, *STs* sulfotransferases, *TPMT* thiopurine methyltransferase, *UGTs* uridine 5′-triphosphate glucuronosyltransferases. Reprinted from reference [6] with permission

thiopurine S-methyltransferases [TPMTs] and catechol O-methyltransferase). Some of these clinically used drugs are shown in Fig. 14.2 [4]. The majority of these phase I and phase II drug-metabolizing enzymes (DMEs) are polymorphic [5]. Most common polymorphisms in phase II metabolism occur in the NAT, GST, and TPMT enzymes. Polymorphisms in DME genes are the most important factors affecting interindividual differences in drug response and adverse drug reactions [6, 7]. The genetic polymorphisms in DMEs of several major drugs for respiratory diseases are shown in Table 14.1.

14.3.1 CYP Enzymes

CYP enzymes involved in phase I drug metabolism are mainly located in the endoplasmic reticulum of the liver. A total of 57 human CYPs have been identified and classified into 18 families and 43 subfamilies [8]. Indeed, CYP enzymes metabolize more than 80% of drugs used in clinical practice [9]. As shown in Fig. 14.2, CYP3A4/5 is involved in the metabolism of most drugs (30.2%), followed by

Table 14.1 Representative genetic polymorphic drug-metabolizing enzymes affecting drugs for respiratory diseases

Disease	Treatment	Drug-metabolizing enzyme/ common variant alleles	Effect
Bronchial asthma	Theophylline	Cytochrome P450/*CYP1A2*1F*	Increased enzymatic activity
	Fluticasone propionate	Cytochrome P450/*CYP3A4*22, CYP3A5*3*	Decreased enzymatic activity
COPD	Macrolide	Cytochrome P450/*CYP3A4*1B*	Controversial
Idiopathic pulmonary fibrosis	Pirfenidone	Cytochrome P450/*CYP1A2*1F*	Unclear
Lung cancer	S-1	Cytochrome P450/*CYP2A6*4*	Unclear
	Irinotecan	Uridine diphosphate glucuronosyl trasferase/*UGT1A1*28, UGT1A1*6, UGT1A1*27*	Decreased enzymatic activity
Pulmonary mycosis	Voriconazole	Cytochrome P450/*CYP2C19*17*	Increased enzymatic activity
Tuberculosis	Isoniazid	N-acetyltrasferase type 2/ *NAT2*5, NAT2*6, NAT2*7*	Decreased enzymatic activity

CYP2D6 (20%), CYP2C9 (12.8%), CYP1A2 (8.9%), CYP2B6 (7.2%), CYP2C19 (6.8%), CYP2C8 (4.7%), CYP2A6 (3.4%), and CYP2E1 (3%) [10]. Of these, five isoforms of CYP1A2, CYP2C9, CYP2C19, CYP2D6, and CYP3A4 are responsible for nearly all drug-related side effects [11]. Genetic variations in CYP enzymes depend on ethnicity, with variations occurring in 1–30% of populations [12]. Although individual functional polymorphisms may cause the same functional effects in different ethnic populations, there is still ethnic diversity in drug response and drug-drug interactions. Here we review representative CYP polymorphisms that contribute to disease progression and pharmacotherapies of lung disease.

14.3.1.1 CYP1A2

CYP1A2 contributes to theophylline metabolism. The human CYP1A2 gene is located on chromosome 15q24.1 and is known for its impact on blood pressure. Recently, the *CYP1A2*1F* allele was shown to be associated with caffeine intake and reduced hypertension risk among nonsmokers [13]. Several CYP1A2 variants have been reported in Japanese populations, with *CYP1A2*1F* allele (–163C > A) being the most frequently occurring [14]. Theophylline is mostly metabolized by CYP1A2 [15], and the *CYP1A2*1F* (–163C > A) polymorphism increases CYA1A2 activity, resulting in increased theophylline metabolism [16]. Thus, serum theophylline concentration should be monitored and generally maintained at peak concentrations between 10 and 15 μg/mL to achieve the desired benefits. Theophylline has traditionally been classified as a bronchodilator with multifunctional characteristics of anti-inflammatory, immunomodulatory, and bronchoprotective effects and is used as a prophylactic anti-asthma drug and to treat chronic obstructive pulmonary disease [17–20]. Pirfenidone, a newly developed anti-fibrotic agent for idiopathic pulmonary fibrosis, which was approved by the US Food and Drug Administration in 2014, is also mainly metabolized by CYP1A2 [21]. Thus, the *CYP1A2*1F* (−163C > A) polymorphism should be taken into account by pulmonary physicians. Also, it should be noted that the activity of CYP1A2 may be altered by cigarette smoking (inducer) [21] or by co-medications, especially antibiotics such as ciprofloxacin (CYP1A2 inhibitor) and rifampicin (CYP1A2 inducer) [22, 23]. The role of CYP1A2 has been excluded in macrolide-theophylline interactions [24].

14.3.1.2 CYP2A6

The CYP2A6 enzyme is critical in the metabolism of nicotine to inactive metabolite cotinine; thus, the pharmacokinetics of nicotine are influenced by CYP2A6 polymorphisms. In Asian populations, *CYP2A6*4* (whole deletion type of the *CYP2A6* gene), *CYP2A6*7*, and *CYP2A6*9* are major polymorphisms that reduce the activity of CYP2A6, leading to decreased daily cigarette consumption [25]. The combined frequencies of the *CYP2A6* allele are relatively higher in Japanese populations compared with Caucasian populations. Approximately 30% of Japanese individuals have impaired CYP2A6 activity, mainly due to *CYP2A6*4*. Moreover, Japanese individuals have lower expression of CYP2A6 enzymes than Caucasian individuals [26]. Taken together, these data show that CYP2A6 activity is impaired or decreased in many Japanese individuals, which may result in limited lifelong cigarette consumption by smokers, leading to a reduced risk of lung cancer and emphysema [25]. The association between CYP2A6 polymorphisms and lung cancer risk has been assessed but there is no conclusive evidence to date. Although CYP2A6 was not identified as a risk variant for lung cancer by GWAS analysis, a recent study reported that candidate predictive markers of genetic variants have greater CYP2A6 activity, increasing lung cancer risk in smokers [27]. The analysis of causal variants of lung cancer in CYP2A6 among smokers is still being studied. In clinical situations, these three main CYP2A6 polymorphisms should be considered when establishing an individualized smoking cessation program. S-1, a novel oral anticancer drug for non-small cell lung cancer, is a combination of three pharmacological compounds: tegaful, gimeracil, and oteracil potassium. Tegaful is a prodrug of fluorouracil (5-FU) that is converted to 5-FU by the liver enzyme CYP2A6. Japanese patients homozygous for the *CYP2A6*4* allele, which causes decreased CYP2A6 activity, show significantly lower 5-FU levels [28]. CYP2A6 variants are associated with the pharmacokinetic variability of tegaful; however, gimeracil is a key determinant in the pharmacokinetic variability of 5-FU [29]. Therefore, dose adjustments of S-1 in accordance with CYP2A6 polymorphisms have not been recommended [30].

14.3.1.3 CYP2C9

CYP2C9 is involved in the metabolism of many common drugs including warfarin, a mixture of S- and R-warfarin. Because S-warfarin is a fivefold more potent anticoagulant than R-warfarin and is mainly metabolized by CYP2C9, the activity of CYP2C9 influences its antithrombotic effects. The most common variants of *CYP2C9*2* and *CYP2C9*3* are associated with reduced enzyme activity; thus, *CYP2C9* genotypes should be considered if the patient's genotypes are available. A recent study reported that *CYP2C9*3* increased the risk of upper gastrointestinal bleeding associated with nonsteroidal anti-inflammatory drugs when the patient took more than half the average dose [31]. In Japanese individuals, homozygosity for *CYP2C9*3* was not detected; however, the incidence of heterozygous subjects who were intermediate metabolizers was about 5.3% [32]. Pulmonary physicians should note that CYP2C9 is induced by rifampicin, a drug used for the treatment of tuberculosis, thereby reducing the anticoagulant effects of warfarin [33].

14.3.1.4 CYP2C19

CYP2C19 plays a critical role in the metabolism of several important groups of drugs such as antibiotic (e.g., clarithromycin), antifungal (e.g., voriconazole), anticancer (e.g., cyclophosphamide and tamoxifen), antidepressant (e.g., amitriptyline), antiplatelet (e.g., cilostazol and clopidogrel), and antiulcer (e.g., omeplazole and lansoprazole) drugs. The human *CYP1A2* gene is located on chromosome 10 (10q24.1-q24.3), and polymorphisms in this gene such as *CYP2C19*2*, **3*, and **17* have been reported. *CYP2C19*2* and *CYP2C19*3*, which are found in 12–23% of Asians, contribute to this population being poor metabolizers of the CYP2C19 gene, whereas *CYP2C19*17*, a very rare allele found in 0.15–0.44% of Asians, is considered an ultra-rapid metabolizer allele [34]. Both omeprazole and clarithromycin are metabolized by CYP2C19. A previous report revealed that clarithromycin inhibits omeprazole metabolism, leading to elevated serum concentrations of omeprazole irrespective of *CYP2C19* genotypes. Thus, care should be taken when initiating triple therapy with omeprazole, amoxicillin, and clarithromycin for the eradication of *Helicobacter pylori* in patients who are poor metabolizers [35]. Although the *CYP2C19*17* allele is very rare in Japanese individuals, voriconazole, an antifungal with a narrow therapeutic range, is rapidly metabolized by *CYP2C19*17* carriers, causing increased serum concentrations of voriconazole of 6.75 mg/kg compared to 2.57 mg/kg in patients with wild-type CYP2C19 [36].

14.3.1.5 CYP2D6

CYP2D6, a highly polymorphic enzyme, has more than 75 allelic variants [37], of which the most common, *CYP2D6*3*, **4*, **5*, and **6*, are associated with poor metabolism. Although this poor metabolizer phenotype is present in 5–10% of individuals in Europe and the United States, the frequency in Asian populations is less than 1%. In Japanese populations, the *CYP2D6*10* allele is the most common and has been identified as an intermediate metabolizer. In a recent report, 23.7% of Japanese subjects were homozygous for the *CYP2D6*10* allele, which may require appropriate dose adjustment, especially when administering prodrug for improved parenteral administration [32]. Codeine and tramadol are prodrugs that are mainly metabolized by CYP2D6 to its active metabolite morphine and opioid analgesic metabolites (O-demethylation product M1), respectively. In fact, clinical studies have revealed that CYP2D6 poor metabolizers have poor analgesic responses due to reduced conversion to the active form.

14.3.1.6 CYP3A4/5

CYP3A is the most abundant CYP enzyme, and is encoded by four genes located on chromosome 7 (7q21.1): *CYP3A4*, *CYP3A5*, *CYP3A7*, and *CYP3A43*. Of these, CYP3A4 and CYP3A5 are recognized as the major DMEs. Erythromycin and clarithromycin are potential inhibitors of CYP3A4, as these drugs decrease the activity of CYP3A4 in a time-dependent manner [38]. The antifungals itraconazole and ketoconazole are also potent inhibitors of CYP3A4 inhibitors. Gefitinib and erlotinib, epidermal growth factor receptor tyrosine kinase inhibitors, are both primarily metabolized by CYP3A4, and subsequently by CYP2D6 or CYP1A1, respectively [39]. In Japanese patients, gefitinib-induced hepatotoxicity was apparent when CYP3A4 was inhibited by coadministered drugs in patients with the *CYP2D6*10* allele [40]. Erlotinib-induced skin toxicity is often a limiting factor due to its severity in some patients; thus, critical genetic polymorphisms in DMEs are still being studied. In this way, clinically important kinase inhibitors such as afatinib, ceritinib, crizotinib, erlotinib, gefitinib, and nintedanib alter metabolism by CYP3A4 inducers/inhibitors. Rifampicin is a CYP3A inducer that leads to a marked decrease in the plasma concentration of various coadministered drugs. Therefore, in addition to genetic variations in CYP3A, drug-drug interactions caused by CYP3A inhibition/induction are extremely important, and will be summarized later in this chapter. Previous reports showed that there are 22 and 11 types of polymorphisms in CYP3A4 and CYP3A5, respectively [41]. Most CYP3A4/5 polymorphisms have a low incidence, and in particular, polymorphisms in CYP3A4 are rare in Asian populations [32]. *CYP3A4*1B* has been associated with the rapid metabolism of anticancer drugs such as docetaxel and cyclophosphamide; however, this allele has not been detected in Asian populations [42]. *CYP3A4*22*, which alters statin, tacrolimus, and cyclosporine metabolism, has only been found in Caucasian populations [42]. Thus, we focused on polymorphisms in the CYP3A5 enzyme. The *CYP3A5*3* allele, found most frequently in CYP3A5, produces nonfunctional protein, thus leading to poor metabolism. In Japanese populations, homozygosity for the *CYP3A*5* allele was found in as many as 58.4% of subjects [32]. More importantly, CYP3A5 is the predominant CYP in the lung, and CYP3A4 is usually not found in respiratory tissues. Inhaled glucocorticoids such as budesonide and fluticasone propionate are primarily metabolized by airway CYP3A5. Fluticasone propionate is an inactivator of CYP3A5, but budesonide is not [43]. Thus, in addition to the potential factor of gradual inactivation of CYP3A5 by repeated inhalation use of fluticasone propionate, careful consideration should be taken when treating patients who are potentially homozygous for the *CYP3A5*3* allele, a poor metabolizer phenotype, as this drug can cause systematic adverse effects. CYP3A4/5 is profoundly associated with metabolism in more than 30% of clinically important drugs such as tacrolimus and midazolam, which should be considered in potential poor metabolizers, especially in Japanese patients.

14.3.2 Phase II Metabolizing Enzymes

Phase II drug metabolism is the detoxifying step of drug metabolism. Therefore, gene polymorphisms in enzymes involved in phase II reactions may cause serious adverse events. Pulmonary physicians should take note of major phase II enzymes such as NATs and uridine diphosphate glucuronosyltransferases (UGTs).

14.3.2.1 NAT2

NAT2 is a target of genetic polymorphisms and carries at least one wild-type allele (*NAT2*4*) or high-activity variant allele (*NAT2*12*), which results in high NAT2 activity (means rapid acetylator). Isoniazid, a first-line drug for tuberculosis, is metabolized to acetylisoniazid by hepatic NAT2. The occurrence of adverse events also depends on NAT2 activity. For example, low NAT2 activity (having two low-activity variants) leads to risk of hepatic toxicities in 28% of individuals compared to rapid acetylators. Thus, *NAT2* genotyping before initiating antituberculosis therapy including isoniazid could be beneficial [44]. Studies of individual dose adjustment therapy with isoniazid according to *NAT2* genotypes were planned for a tuberculosis patient in Europe (IDANET2) and in Japan; however, IDANET2 was prematurely terminated due to a low recruitment. The planned dosage of isoniazid was 5.0 mg/kg (standard dose) for intermediate acetylators, but patients classified as slow acetylators were randomly divided into 2.5 mg/kg and 5.0 mg/kg regimens. Patients classified as rapid acetylators were also randomly divided into 5.0 mg/kg and 7.5 mg/kg regimens. In enrolled Japanese patients, the incidence of slow acetylator genotypes without *NAT2*4* was 9.3%, and that of rapid acetylator genotypes homozygous for *NAT2*4* was 53.5% [45]. Liver toxicity occurred in 77.8% of slow acetylators receiving standard 5.0 mg/kg regimens, while those receiving 2.5 mg/kg had no liver toxicity with successful treatment. In rapid acetylators, the incidence of liver toxicity was almost the same at 4.2 and 4.5% with standard 5.0 mg/kg and increased 7.5 mg/kg regimens, respectively. More importantly, early treatment failure, defined as persistent positive culture and/or no improvement in chest radiograph at 8 weeks, was significantly lower at 15% in 7.5 mg/kg regimens compared to 38% with standard 5.0 mg/kg regimens in rapid acetylators [45]. Thus, NAT2 genotype-guided dose adjustment therapy could improve pharmacotherapy of many diseases.

14.3.2.2 Uridine Diphosphate Glucuronosyltransferase

Uridine diphosphate glucuronosyltransferase (UGT1A1) contributes to irinotecan metabolism. Irinotecan (also known as CPT-11), an analog of camptothecin, is frequently used for extensive stage small-cell lung cancer in combination with platinum therapy, especially in Japanese patients. Irinotecan is a prodrug that is hydrolyzed to its active form SN-38 and is then detoxified through glucuronidation by UGT1A1. Active SN-38 causes major adverse events such as diarrhea and neutropenia, which limits the use of irinotecan as it can be life-threatening [46]. Irinotecan toxicities are strongly associated with UGT1A1 polymorphisms in the common promoter lesion (*UGT1A1*28*), especially when administered at moderate to high doses (200–350 mg/m^2), leading to variation in UGT1A1 expression [47]. The UGT1A1 enzyme is responsible for hapatic bilirubin glucuronidation. The *UGT1A1*28* allele has been associated with significantly lower UGT1A1 expression, leading to reduced glucuronidation of SN-38. The frequency of the *UGT1A1*28* allele is as low as 15% in the Japanese population [48], which is about one-half or one-third lower than Caucasian, African-American, Hispanic, and African populations (range, 26–45%). In Asian populations, other UGT1A1 polymorphisms such as *UGT1A1*6* (exon1 G71R polymorphism) are also important for irinotecan-induced toxicity. Although Japanese cancer patients with the UGT1A1*6 haplotype alone showed no difference in SN-38 glucuronidation when receiving irinotecan, patients with the two haplotypes *UGT1A1*6* and **28* had significantly lower SN-38 glucuronidation [49]. In Japan, genetic testing for *UGT1A1*6* and **28* polymorphisms has been available and covered by health insurance since November 2008. In a recent report, patients homozygous for UGT1A1 (**28/*28, *6/*6, *28/*6*) receiving an 80% dose of irinotecan in combination with 5-FU and l-leucovorin still had a risk of Grade ≥ 3 neutropenia (28.6%) [50]. Thus, pulmonary physicians and oncologists should note that even heterozygous carriers of **6* and **28* have significant changes in irinotecan metabolism. Actually, Grade ≥ 3 neutropenia occurred in 25.4% of heterozygous carriers compared to 17.3% of wild-type carriers receiving a 100% dose of irinotecan [50]. *UGT1A1*6* and **28* are pharmacogenomic markers of irinotecan toxicity, although other factors such as transporter gene (ABCB1, ABCC2, ABCG2) polymorphisms might affect irinotecan pharmacodynamics.

14.4 Drug Target

The pharmacologic response to a drug could be mediated through the interaction between drugs and specific target proteins such as receptors, enzymes, and signal transduction proteins. There are several genetic polymorphisms in drug target genes that are associated with the response to drugs that are frequently used in respiratory medicine (Table 14.2).

Table 14.2 Representative genetic polymorphisms in drug target genes associated with drugs for respiratory diseases

Drug target gene	Treatment	Effect
β2-Adrenergic receptor (B16 Arg/Arg)	Short-acting β2 agonist	Lose effectiveness
Glucocorticoid receptor NR3C1 (646 C > G)	Glucocorticoid	Lose effectiveness?
Leukotriene C4 syntase	Leukotriene receptor antagonists	Marked amelioration
5-lipoxygenase	Leukotriene receptor antagonists	Marked amelioration

14.4.1 β2-Adrenergic Receptor

Patients with the β2-adrenergic receptor (ADRB2) arginine genotype showed poor asthma control with frequent symptoms and decreased forced expiratory volume in 1 second compared to those with the glycine genotype [51]. Patients with a genetic polymorphism that results in homozygosity for arginine at amino acid 16 of the β2-adrenergic receptor (B16 Arg/Arg) lost effects of the long-term response to short-acting β2-agonist (albuterol/salbutamol), which was not observed in patients homozygous for glycine (B16 Gly/Gly) [52]. This data suggest that pulmonary physicians should avoid using short-acting β2-agonists (albuterol/salbutamol) in patients with the B16 Arg/Arg genotype. With regard to long-acting β2-agonists, some studies have suggested that patients with the B16 Arg/Arg genotype also benefit less from treatment with long-acting β2-agonists plus inhaled corticosteroids compared to those with the B16 Gly/Gly genotype. However, *ADRB2* polymorphisms did not affect the pharmacogenetic response to inhaled corticosteroids plus long-acting β2-agonist in patients with asthma [53, 54]. Because patients treated with long-acting β2-agonists plus inhaled corticosteroids had improved airway function compared with those treated with inhaled corticosteroid alone irrespective of B16 genotype, pulmonary physicians can use these drugs in patients with or without the genetic polymorphism.

14.4.2 Glucocorticoid Receptor

Glucocorticoid receptor gene polymorphisms could lead to resistance to glucocorticoids, resulting in the development of severe bronchial asthma. In particular, NR3C1 (originally determined as nuclear receptor subfamily 3, group C, member 1), which encodes the glucocorticoid receptor has 2571 polymorphisms, with the most common polymorphism being NR3C1 646 C > G [55]. Polymorphisms in NR3C1 may inhibit formation of glucocorticoid/glucocorticoid receptor complexes, resulting in a reduced response to glucocorticoids. Further studies are needed to elucidate the association between NR3C1 gene polymorphisms and resistance to glucocorticoids in patients with asthma.

14.4.3 Leukotriene C4 Synthase

Leukotriene receptor antagonists block leukotriene C4 synthase, resulting in prevention of leukotriene-mediated bronchoconstriction. Polymorphisms in the leukotriene C4 synthase gene may increase asthma prevalence. Higher levels of cysteinyl leukotriene variants in the leukotriene C4 synthase genotype were correlated with asthma severity. Thus, leukotriene modifiers in these patients could be beneficial [56].

14.4.4 5-Lipoxygenase

Leukotriene receptor antagonists block 5-lipoxygenase, which also inhibits leukotriene-mediated bronchoconstriction. Approximately 5% of patients with asthma have the 5-lipoxygenase polymorphism, which is linked to asthma severity. Administering leukotriene antagonists in this population leads to a greater improvement in lung function compared to patients with the normal 5-lipoxygenase genotype.

14.5 Enzyme Induction and Inhibition (Drug-Drug Interaction)

Many drugs for the respiratory system influence on liver metabolic activity. Thus, regardless of favorable or adverse genetic factors in drug metabolism, enzyme induction and inhibition should be considered. Clinically important drugs with a special focus on drug-drug interactions are summarized in Table 14.3. Rifampicin, a first-line regimen for tuberculosis and nontuberculosis mycobacterium infection

Table 14.3 Drug-drug interaction with respect to clinically important drugs for respiratory diseases

	CYP1A2	CYP2C9	CYP2C19	CYP3A
Strong inhibitor				Erythromycin Clarithromycin Itraconazole Voriconazole
Moderate inhibitor			Clarithromycin	
Major inducer	Rifampicin	Rifampicin	Rifampicin	Rifampicin

in some cases, activates CYP3A4 [57]. Rifabutin, another rifamycin that is used as an alternative of rifampicin, is a weak inducer of CYP3A4 compared to rifampicin [58]. Thus, physicians should consider increasing the dose of coadministered drug metabolized by CYP3A4 if rifampicin is used. Macrolide, a clinically relevant drug that interacts with CYP3A4, has variable abilities to bind to and inhibit CYP3A4. Erythromycin strongly binds to and inhibits CYP3A4, while clarithromycin has a lower affinity for this enzyme. The majority of currently approved kinase inhibitors such as gefitinib, erlotinib, afatinib, alectinib, ceritinib, crizotinib, and nintedanib are markedly affected by CYP3A4 inhibitors/inducers. These kinase inhibitors should be closely monitored for tolerability upon the concomitant use of CYP3A4 inhibitors such as macrolides and azole antifungal drugs like itraconazole, a more potent inhibitor of CYP3A4 than fluconazole or voriconazole. Preclinical and clinical drug interaction studies would establish personalized dosing recommendations.

14.6 Genotyping Platform

Recent advances in genotyping microarray platforms for detecting SNPs in DMEs are strong tools for individualized medicine. AmpliChip CYP450 Test (Roche Diagnostics Corporation), which was approved for clinical use by the US Food and Drug Administration in 2005, was first available in Japan in 2009 and detected 33 CYP2D6 alleles and 3 CYP2C19 alleles. CodeLink Uniset Human I Bioarray (GE Healthcare), which covered 32 Human CYP genes including CYP1A1, 2B6, 2C9, 2D6, and 3A5, is no longer used in Japan. Illumina, Inc., produced a genotyping tool for 34 ADME genes using VeraCode technology in 2010. This covers over 95% of the PharmaADME Core list, which includes 184 putative functional genetic variants in 33 significant ADME genes of phase I/II drug-metabolizing enzymes and transporters. The DMET™ (Drug Metabolism Enzymes and Transporters) platform developed by Affymetrix expanded the coverage of 76 phase I enzymes, 62 phase II enzymes, 51 transporters, and 41 other genes. The DMET™ platform, first released in 2007, is currently indicated for research use only; however, it will become a companion diagnostic tool for prospective clinical trials requiring genotyping of ADME genes to determine interindividual variability and therapeutic outcome.

14.7 Conclusions

Although the drug response in subjects is variable due to many intrinsic and extrinsic factors, genetic factors remain constant throughout life. Therefore, if the genotype-response relationship has been elucidated, prospective genetic testing would be beneficial for predicting the drug response. In considering genetic factors, efforts should be made to understand pharmacokinetics, pharmacodynamics, and drug-drug interactions to support personalized medicine.

References

1. Kalow W, Tang BK, Endrenyi L. Hypothesis: comparisons of inter- and intra-individual variations can substitute for twin studies in drug research. Pharmacogenetics. 1998;8(4):283–9.
2. Arbitrio M, Di Martino MT, Scionti F, Agapito G, Guzzi PH, Cannataro M, et al. DMET (Drug Metabolism Enzymes and Transporters): a pharmacogenomic platform for precision medicine. Oncotarget. 2016;7(33):54028–50. https://doi.org/10.18632/oncotarget.9927.
3. Huang SM, Temple R. Is this the drug or dose for you? Impact and consideration of ethnic factors in global drug development, regulatory review, and clinical practice. Clin Pharmacol Ther. 2008;84(3):287–94. https://doi.org/10.1038/clpt.2008.144.
4. Fakunle ES, Loring JF. Ethnically diverse pluripotent stem cells for drug development. Trends Mol Med. 2012;18(12):709–16. https://doi.org/10.1016/j.molmed.2012.10.007.
5. Sim SC, Ingelman-Sundberg M. Pharmacogenomic biomarkers: new tools in current and future drug therapy. Trends Pharmacol Sci. 2011;32(2):72–81. https://doi.org/10.1016/j.tips.2010.11.008.
6. Evans WE, Relling MV. Pharmacogenomics: translating functional genomics into rational therapeutics. Science. 1999;286(5439):487–91.
7. Frueh FW, Amur S, Mummaneni P, Epstein RS, Aubert RE, DeLuca TM, et al. Pharmacogenomic biomarker information in drug labels approved by the United States food and drug administration: prevalence of related drug use. Pharmacotherapy. 2008;28(8):992–8. https://doi.org/10.1592/phco.28.8.992.
8. Ingelman-Sundberg M. The human genome project and novel aspects of cytochrome P450 research. Toxicol Appl Pharmacol. 2005;207(2 Suppl):52–6. https://doi.org/10.1016/j.taap.2005.01.030.
9. Nebert DW, Russell DW. Clinical importance of the cytochromes P450. Lancet. 2002;360(9340):1155–62. https://doi.org/10.1016/S0140-6736(02)11203-7.
10. Zanger UM, Schwab M. Cytochrome P450 enzymes in drug metabolism: regulation of gene expression, enzyme activities, and impact of genetic variation. Pharmacol Ther. 2013;138(1):103–41. https://doi.org/10.1016/j.pharmthera.2012.12.007.
11. Slaughter RL, Edwards DJ. Recent advances: the cytochrome P450 enzymes. Ann Pharmacother. 1995;29(6):619–24. https://doi.org/10.1177/106002809502900612.
12. Rostami-Hodjegan A, Tucker GT. Simulation and prediction of in vivo drug metabolism in human populations from in vitro data. Nat Rev Drug Discov. 2007;6(2):140–8. https://doi.org/10.1038/nrd2173.
13. Guessous I, Dobrinas M, Kutalik Z, Pruijm M, Ehret G, Maillard M, et al. Caffeine intake and CYP1A2 variants associated with high caffeine intake protect non-smokers from hypertension. Hum Mol Genet. 2012;21(14):3283–92. https://doi.org/10.1093/hmg/dds137.
14. Soyama A, Saito Y, Hanioka N, Maekawa K, Komamura K, Kamakura S, et al. Single nucleotide polymorphisms and haplotypes of CYP1A2 in a Japanese population. Drug Metab Pharmacokinet. 2005;20(1):24–33.
15. Yim EY, Kang HR, Jung JW, Sohn SW, Cho SH. CYP1A2 polymorphism and theophylline clearance in Korean non-smoking asthmatics. Asia Pac Allergy. 2013;3(4):231–40. https://doi.org/10.5415/apallergy.2013.3.4.231.
16. Zhou SF, Yang LP, Zhou ZW, Liu YH, Chan E. Insights into the substrate specificity, inhibitors, regulation, and polymorphisms and the clinical impact of human cytochrome P450 1A2. AAPS J. 2009;11(3):481–94. https://doi.org/10.1208/s12248-009-9127-y.
17. Barnes PJ. Theophylline: new perspectives for an old drug. Am J Respir Crit Care Med. 2003;167(6):813–8. https://doi.org/10.1164/rccm.200210-1142PP.
18. Culpitt SV, de Matos C, Russell RE, Donnelly LE, Rogers DF, Barnes PJ. Effect of theophylline on induced sputum inflammatory indices and neutrophil chemotaxis in chronic obstructive pulmonary disease. Am J Respir Crit Care Med. 2002;165(10):1371–6.

19. Hirano T, Yamagata T, Gohda M, Yamagata Y, Ichikawa T, Yanagisawa S, et al. Inhibition of reactive nitrogen species production in COPD airways: comparison of inhaled corticosteroid and oral theophylline. Thorax. 2006;61(9):761–6. https://doi.org/10.1136/thx.200X.058156.
20. Kobayashi M, Nasuhara Y, Betsuyaku T, Shibuya E, Tanino Y, Tanino M, et al. Effect of low-dose theophylline on airway inflammation in COPD. Respirology. 2004;9(2):249–54. https://doi.org/10.1111/j.1440-1843.2004.00573.x.
21. Yu J, Ritchie TK, Zhou Z, Ragueneau-Majlessi I. Key findings from preclinical and clinical drug interaction studies presented in new drug and biological license applications approved by the Food and Drug Administration in 2014. Drug Metab Dispos. 2016;44(1):83–101. https://doi.org/10.1124/dmd.115.066720.
22. Backman JT, Granfors MT, Neuvonen PJ. Rifampicin is only a weak inducer of CYP1A2-mediated presystemic and systemic metabolism: studies with tizanidine and caffeine. Eur J Clin Pharmacol. 2006;62(6):451–61. https://doi.org/10.1007/s00228-006-0127-x.
23. Granfors MT, Backman JT, Neuvonen M, Neuvonen PJ. Ciprofloxacin greatly increases concentrations and hypotensive effect of tizanidine by inhibiting its cytochrome P450 1A2-mediated presystemic metabolism. Clin Pharmacol Ther. 2004;76(6):598–606. https://doi.org/10.1016/j.clpt.2004.08.018.
24. Polasek TM, Miners JO. Macrolide-theophylline interactions: no role for the inhibition of cytochrome P4501A2. Br J Clin Pharmacol. 2008;66(6):898–900. https://doi.org/10.1111/j.1365-2125.2008.03299.x.
25. Minematsu N, Nakamura H, Furuuchi M, Nakajima T, Takahashi S, Tateno H, et al. Limitation of cigarette consumption by CYP2A6*4, *7 and *9 polymorphisms. Eur Respir J. 2006;27(2):289–92. https://doi.org/10.1183/09031936.06.00056305.
26. Shimada T, Yamazaki H, Guengerich FP. Ethnic-related differences in coumarin 7-hydroxylation activities catalyzed by cytochrome P4502A6 in liver microsomes of Japanese and Caucasian populations. Xenobiotica. 1996;26(4):395–403.
27. Patel YM, Park SL, Han Y, Wilkens LR, Bickeboller H, Rosenberger A, et al. Novel association of genetic markers affecting CYP2A6 activity and lung cancer risk. Cancer Res. 2016;76(19):5768–76. https://doi.org/10.1158/0008-5472.CAN-16-0446.
28. Kaida Y, Inui N, Suda T, Nakamura H, Watanabe H, Chida K. The CYP2A6*4 allele is determinant of S-1 pharmacokinetics in Japanese patients with non-small-cell lung cancer. Clin Pharmacol Ther. 2008;83(4):589–94. https://doi.org/10.1038/sj.clpt.6100484.
29. Hirose T, Fujita K, Nishimura K, Ishida H, Yamashita K, Sunakawa Y, et al. Pharmacokinetics of S-1 and CYP2A6 genotype in Japanese patients with advanced cancer. Oncol Rep. 2010;24(2):529–36.
30. Kobayakawa M, Kojima Y. Tegafur/gimeracil/oteracil (S-1) approved for the treatment of advanced gastric cancer in adults when given in combination with cisplatin: a review comparing it with other fluoropyrimidine-based therapies. Onco Targets Ther. 2011;4:193–201. https://doi.org/10.2147/OTT.S19059.
31. Figueiras A, Estany-Gestal A, Aguirre C, Ruiz B, Vidal X, Carvajal A, et al. CYP2C9 variants as a risk modifier of NSAID-related gastrointestinal bleeding: a case-control study. Pharmacogenet Genomics. 2016;26(2):66–73. https://doi.org/10.1097/FPC.0000000000000186.
32. Ota T, Kamada Y, Hayashida M, Iwao-Koizumi K, Murata S, Kinoshita K. Combination analysis in genetic polymorphisms of drug-metabolizing enzymes CYP1A2, CYP2C9, CYP2C19, CYP2D6 and CYP3A5 in the Japanese population. Int J Med Sci. 2015;12(1):78–82. https://doi.org/10.7150/ijms.10263.
33. Chen J, Raymond K. Roles of rifampicin in drug-drug interactions: underlying molecular mechanisms involving the nuclear pregnane X receptor. Ann Clin Microbiol Antimicrob. 2006;5:3. https://doi.org/10.1186/1476-0711-5-3.
34. Hirota T, Eguchi S, Ieiri I. Impact of genetic polymorphisms in CYP2C9 and CYP2C19 on the pharmacokinetics of clinically used drugs. Drug Metab Pharmacokinet. 2013;28(1):28–37.

35. Furuta T, Ohashi K, Kobayashi K, Iida I, Yoshida H, Shirai N, et al. Effects of clarithromycin on the metabolism of omeprazole in relation to CYP2C19 genotype status in humans. Clin Pharmacol Ther. 1999;66(3):265–74. https://doi.org/10.1016/S0009-9236(99)70034-2.
36. Lamoureux F, Duflot T, Woillard JB, Metsu D, Pereira T, Compagnon P, et al. Impact of CYP2C19 genetic polymorphisms on voriconazole dosing and exposure in adult patients with invasive fungal infections. Int J Antimicrob Agents. 2016;47(2):124–31. https://doi.org/10.1016/j.ijantimicag.2015.12.003.
37. Belle DJ, Singh H. Genetic factors in drug metabolism. Am Fam Physician. 2008;77(11):1553–60.
38. Akiyoshi T, Ito M, Murase S, Miyazaki M, Guengerich FP, Nakamura K, et al. Mechanism-based inhibition profiles of erythromycin and clarithromycin with cytochrome P450 3A4 genetic variants. Drug Metab Pharmacokinet. 2013;28(5):411–5.
39. Li J, Zhao M, He P, Hidalgo M, Baker SD. Differential metabolism of gefitinib and erlotinib by human cytochrome P450 enzymes. Clin Cancer Res. 2007;13(12):3731–7. https://doi.org/10.1158/1078-0432.CCR-07-0088.
40. Takimoto T, Kijima T, Otani Y, Nonen S, Namba Y, Mori M, et al. Polymorphisms of CYP2D6 gene and gefitinib-induced hepatotoxicity. Clin Lung Cancer. 2013;14(5):502–7. https://doi.org/10.1016/j.cllc.2013.03.003.
41. Elens L, van Gelder T, Hesselink DA, Haufroid V, van Schaik RH. CYP3A4*22: promising newly identified CYP3A4 variant allele for personalizing pharmacotherapy. Pharmacogenomics. 2013;14(1):47–62. https://doi.org/10.2217/pgs.12.187.
42. Lee JS, Cheong HS, Kim LH, Kim JO, Seo DW, Kim YH, et al. Screening of genetic polymorphisms of CYP3A4 and CYP3A5 genes. Korean J Physiol Pharmacol. 2013;17(6):479–84. https://doi.org/10.4196/kjpp.2013.17.6.479.
43. Murai T, Reilly CA, Ward RM, Yost GS. The inhaled glucocorticoid fluticasone propionate efficiently inactivates cytochrome P450 3A5, a predominant lung P450 enzyme. Chem Res Toxicol. 2010;23(8):1356–64. https://doi.org/10.1021/tx100124k.
44. Ohno M, Yamaguchi I, Yamamoto I, Fukuda T, Yokota S, Maekura R, et al. Slow N-acetyltransferase 2 genotype affects the incidence of isoniazid and rifampicin-induced hepatotoxicity. Int J Tuberc Lung Dis. 2000;4(3):256–61.
45. Azuma J, Ohno M, Kubota R, Yokota S, Nagai T, Tsuyuguchi K, et al. NAT2 genotype guided regimen reduces isoniazid-induced liver injury and early treatment failure in the 6-month four-drug standard treatment of tuberculosis: a randomized controlled trial for pharmacogenetics-based therapy. Eur J Clin Pharmacol. 2013;69(5):1091–101. https://doi.org/10.1007/s00228-012-1429-9.
46. Fuchs CS, Moore MR, Harker G, Villa L, Rinaldi D, Hecht JR. Phase III comparison of two irinotecan dosing regimens in second-line therapy of metastatic colorectal cancer. J Clin Oncol. 2003;21(5):807–14. https://doi.org/10.1200/JCO.2003.08.058.
47. Hoskins JM, Goldberg RM, Qu P, Ibrahim JG, McLeod HL. UGT1A1*28 genotype and irinotecan-induced neutropenia: dose matters. J Natl Cancer Inst. 2007;99(17):1290–5. https://doi.org/10.1093/jnci/djm115.
48. Ando Y, Saka H, Ando M, Sawa T, Muro K, Ueoka H, et al. Polymorphisms of UDP-glucuronosyltransferase gene and irinotecan toxicity: a pharmacogenetic analysis. Cancer Res. 2000;60(24):6921–6.
49. Sai K, Saeki M, Saito Y, Ozawa S, Katori N, Jinno H, et al. UGT1A1 haplotypes associated with reduced glucuronidation and increased serum bilirubin in irinotecan-administered Japanese patients with cancer. Clin Pharmacol Ther. 2004;75(6):501–15. https://doi.org/10.1016/j.clpt.2004.01.010.
50. Miyata Y, Touyama T, Kusumi T, Morita Y, Mizunuma N, Taniguchi F, et al. UDP-glucuronosyltransferase 1A1*6 and *28 polymorphisms as indicators of initial dose level of irinotecan to reduce risk of neutropenia in patients receiving FOLFIRI for colorectal cancer. Int J Clin Oncol. 2016;21(4):696–703. https://doi.org/10.1007/s10147-015-0937-x.

51. Tan S, Hall IP, Dewar J, Dow E, Lipworth B. Association between beta 2-adrenoceptor polymorphism and susceptibility to bronchodilator desensitisation in moderately severe stable asthmatics. Lancet. 1997;350(9083):995–9. https://doi.org/10.1016/S0140-6736(97)03211-X.
52. Israel E, Chinchilli VM, Ford JG, Boushey HA, Cherniack R, Craig TJ, et al. Use of regularly scheduled albuterol treatment in asthma: genotype-stratified, randomised, placebo-controlled cross-over trial. Lancet. 2004;364(9444):1505–12. https://doi.org/10.1016/S0140-6736(04)17273-5.
53. Bleecker ER, Postma DS, Lawrance RM, Meyers DA, Ambrose HJ, Goldman M. Effect of ADRB2 polymorphisms on response to longacting beta2-agonist therapy: a pharmacogenetic analysis of two randomised studies. Lancet. 2007;370(9605):2118–25. https://doi.org/10.1016/S0140-6736(07)61906-0.
54. Wechsler ME, Kunselman SJ, Chinchilli VM, Bleecker E, Boushey HA, Calhoun WJ, et al. Effect of beta2-adrenergic receptor polymorphism on response to longacting beta2 agonist in asthma (LARGE trial): a genotype-stratified, randomised, placebo-controlled, crossover trial. Lancet. 2009;374(9703):1754–64. https://doi.org/10.1016/S0140-6736(09)61492-6.
55. Mohamed NA, Abdel-Rehim AS, Farres MN, Muhammed HS. Influence of glucocorticoid receptor gene NR3C1 646 C>G polymorphism on glucocorticoid resistance in asthmatics: a preliminary study. Cent Eur J Immunol. 2015;40(3):325–30. https://doi.org/10.5114/ceji.2015.54594.
56. Asano K, Shiomi T, Hasegawa N, Nakamura H, Kudo H, Matsuzaki T, et al. Leukotriene C4 synthase gene a(−444)C polymorphism and clinical response to a CYS-LT(1) antagonist, pranlukast, in Japanese patients with moderate asthma. Pharmacogenetics. 2002;12(7):565–70.
57. Finch CK, Chrisman CR, Baciewicz AM, Self TH. Rifampin and rifabutin drug interactions: an update. Arch Intern Med. 2002;162(9):985–92.
58. Reinach B, de Sousa G, Dostert P, Ings R, Gugenheim J, Rahmani R. Comparative effects of rifabutin and rifampicin on cytochromes P450 and UDP-glucuronosyl-transferases expression in fresh and cryopreserved human hepatocytes. Chem Biol Interact. 1999;121(1):37–48.

Part III
Oncogenic Driver Mutation (Somatic Mutations) in Lung Cancer

Chapter 15
EGFR: How Important Is EGFR Mutation Status in the Management of Lung Cancer?

Mizuki Haraguchi and Kazuhisa Takahashi

Abstract The underlying basis of the cancer phenotype is caused by the alteration of genes that regulate cell growth, differentiation, proliferation, and programmed cell death. Along with the molecular biology of the cell, over the last several decades, numerous other important factors that contribute to cell growth, differentiation, and proliferation processes have been found. In contrast to normal cells, cancer cells have the capacity to proliferate without external stimuli, usually as a consequence of gene mutations. The human epidermal growth factor receptor (EGFR) is overexpressed or dysfunctional in many human malignancies. EGFR is one of the human epidermal growth factor receptor (HER) family proteins, and signaling intermediated by EGFR has received intense focus, resulting in the emergence of attractive candidates for anticancer therapy, especially in lung cancer. In this section, we focus on the signaling cascade via EGFR and overview the therapeutic approach against EGFR.

Keywords Epidermal growth factor receptor (EGFR) · Driver mutation EGFR-tyrosine kinase inhibitor · Resistance

15.1 Molecular Mechanism of EGFR

The underlying bases of the cancer phenotype are referred to as cancer hallmarks and include deregulated cell growth, local invasiveness, and the ability to form distant metastases, which stem from genomic alterations that change the expression and function of key genes and thereby impart a malignant phenotype [1]. There are

M. Haraguchi · K. Takahashi (✉)
Department of Respiratory Medicine, Graduate School of Medicine, Juntendo University, Bukyo-ku, Tokyo, Japan
e-mail: kztakaha@juntendo.ac.jp

T. Kaneko (ed.), *Clinical Relevance of Genetic Factors in Pulmonary Diseases*, Respiratory Disease Series: Diagnostic Tools and Disease Managements, https://doi.org/10.1007/978-981-10-8144-6_15

two types of gene whose products influence cells acquiring neoplasmic characteristics in the course of independent cell growth. Genes that promote autonomous cell growth in cancer cells are called oncogenes, and proto-oncogenes are their cellular counterparts without the mutations. Oncogenes are created by mutations in proto-oncogenes and gain the activity of the protein product from proto-oncogene that can promote cell growth in the absence of normal growth-promoting signals. While oncogenes drive the proliferation of cells, the products of most tumor suppressor genes apply brakes to cell proliferation, and abnormalities in these genes lead to the failure of growth inhibition, another fundamental hallmark of carcinogenesis. In a cancer cell, aggregations of oncogenes and tumor suppressor genes lead to widespread changes in the cell's gene expression profile and free the cell from the normal checkpoints and controls that are tightly controlled in normal cells, subsequently resulting in excessive proliferation. Therefore, tumors are known to sometimes harbor these aberrant mutations [2]. The binding of a ligand to its specific receptor is one of several cell communication tools. In response to this binding, the activation of internal receptors triggers a cascade of intracellular events, culminating in the desired cellular response that includes any of a number of different cellular processes, including the cell growth, proliferation, survival and invasion. In normal cells, these processes are strictly controlled, but the investigation of the signal transduction pathways that regulate normal cellular functions has revealed that key components of these networks are commonly constitutively activated or suppressed in cancer cells by mutations, amplification/deletion, chromosomal translocation, overexpression, or epigenetic silencing [3]. A subset of cancers is dependent on genomic alterations in oncogenes or tumor suppressor genes for their growth and survival, so molecules that inhibit these oncogenes directly lead to cancer cell apoptosis, a phenomenon known as "oncogene addiction [4, 5]." This fact has spurred a number of studies, leading to the development of drugs that selectively inhibit altered proteins that are critical for the maintenance of the transformed phenotype. These agents have shown unprecedented clinical activity in genetically defined subsets of cancers. Imatinib is a first-generation molecular-targeted drug approved by FDA in 2001. Imatinib has provided the first proof that tyrosine kinase modulation, through tyrosine kinase inhibitors (TKIs), can result in improved clinical outcomes in cancer therapy. The impressive clinical benefits of imatinib in hematological malignancies with BCR-ABL overexpression have attracted attention. For example, the treatment of chronic myeloid leukemia (CML) harboring BCL-ABL with imatinib prolonged the overall survival. This success has demonstrated the effectiveness of targeting the critical genetic region that promotes proliferative signals in cancer cells [6]. Over the past several years, it has become evident that HER/ERBB family members play a prominent role in the initiation and maintenance of several solid tumors. This has led to the development and widespread implementation of specific HER/ERBB inhibitors as cancer therapies. HER/ERBB family members have been of much attention for the molecular targeting of cancer therapeutics owing to their abnormal overexpression or activation in many epithelial tumors and their influence on the growth and survival in malignant states [7, 8]. Since EGFR is crucial target especially in lung cancer, investigation of EGFR-mediated signaling is essential to understand EGFR-targeted therapy [9]. EGFR-mediated signal transduction involves several steps, as follows: (1) the ligand binds to EGFR, (2) homo-/heterodimers are formed, and autophosphorylation occurs, and (3) various intracellular pathways are stimulated. In this section, we first overview the structure of EGFR and signal transduction through EGFR.

15.1.1 The Ligand Binds to EGFR *(Fig. 15.1a)*

The signaling cascade mediated by EGFR is initiated on binding of the EGFR ligands to the extracellular domain of EGFR. One of the EGFR ligands is EGF, which was initially purified from mouse submaxillary glands in 1962 by Cohen et al. Those

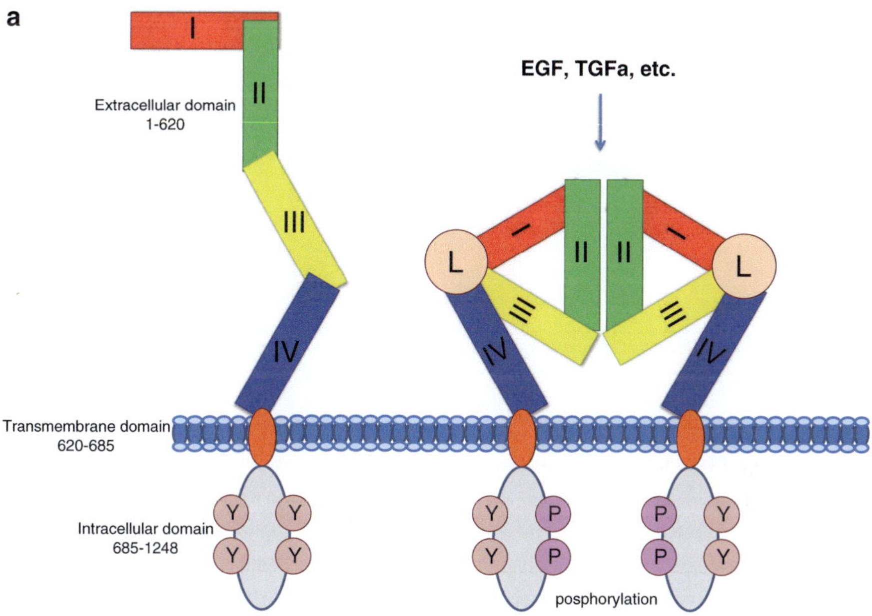

Fig. 15.1 The ErbB family receptors consist of an extracellular domain, transmembrane domain, and intracellular domain. The extracellular domain of each ErbB receptor consists of four domains (I–IV). In the diagram of the ectdomain, DI is colored red, DII green, DIIII yellow, and DIV blue. Left: before ligand binding, ErbB receptors assume a tethered structure. Right: binding of ligands to the extracellular domain of ErbB receptors results in receptor dimerization, tyrosine kinase activation, and autophosphorylation (**a**). Activation of ErbB family receptors and downstream signaling pathways. Activated ErbB family receptors form homo- or heterodimers with other family members, resulting in activation of downstream signaling pathways, along with some of the key constituent signaling molecules are shown. The signaling cascade mediated by activated ErbB family receptors includes two broad categories of pathways, the RAS/RAF/MEK/ERK pathway is shown on the right, and the PI3K/Akt/mTOR pathway is shown on the left. The activation of downstream signaling pathways leads to the cell proliferation, angiogenesis, anti-apoptosis, migration, adhesion, and invasion (**b**)

b

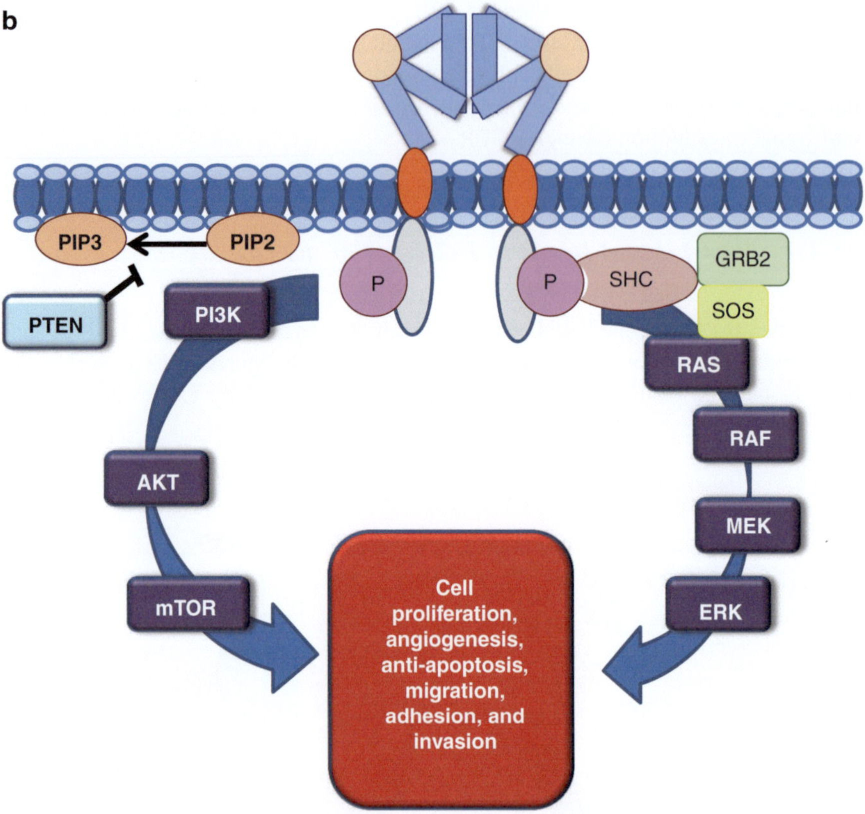

Fig. 15.1 (continued)

authors found that EGF promotes premature eyelid opening and incisor eruption. In 1978, EGFR was identified as the cell surface receptor for EGF [3]. EGFR was later learned to be a 486-amino-acid receptor protein of 170 kDa with one transmembrane sequence between four extracellular and three intracellular domains [10]. EGFR belongs to the ERBB family of receptor tyrosine kinases originally named because of their homology to the erythroblastoma viral gene product, v-erbB [11]. The ERBB protein receptor family comprises four receptors: EGFR/ERBB1, HER2/ERBB2, HER3/ERBB3, and HER4/ERBB4. All four members of the HER/ERBB family are receptor tyrosine kinases (RTKs) with an analogous structure, consisting of an extracellular ligand-binding domain, a single hydrophobic transmembrane domain, and an intracellular domain that contains a conserved tyrosine kinase domain [11]. These receptors interact with a family of 13 polypeptide growth factors, which contain a conserved EGF domain, including EGF, transforming growth factor (TGF)-α, heparin-binding (HB) EGF, amphiregulin, betacellulin, and epiregulin [11]. These ligands can bind all ERBB family receptors except HER2/ERBB2 but have different binding affinities for each receptor. The EGF family of ligands can be divided into three groups: the first group binds specifically to EGFR, and the second group shows dual specificity, binding both EGFR and ERBB4. The third group forms two subgroups based on their capacity to bind ERBB3 and ERBB4 or only ERBB4 [12]. The binding of a ligand to the ERBB family receptor initiates signaling cascades through converting extracellular signals to intracellular ones. The structure of the ERBB family receptor is divided into three domains: an extracellular domain which binds to the ligand, a transmembrane domain, and an intracellular domain, which has tyrosine kinase activity. Interestingly, no ligand has been confirmed to bind to HER2, and the intrinsic tyrosine kinase is defective in the cytoplasmic domain of HER3 [9]. These receptors are thought to contribute to the modulation of intracellular signals. The extracellular domain of the ERBB family receptors is important for ligand binding and dimerization and is divided into four domains: DI, DII, DIII, and DIV [13]. It has been shown that the DI and DIII domains are important for ligand binding, and there is a direct receptor-receptor interaction promoted by the DII dimerization arm. Before the conformational change occurs, the extracellular domain of the ERBB family assumes the so-called tethered structure, in which the DII dimerization interface is blocked by intramolecular interactions between DII and DIV. When the ligand binds to the extracellular domain, the ligand is pinched by DI and DIII, and EGFR is stabilized in an extended conformation, exposing the DII dimerization arm and other residues. As mentioned before, ERBB2 lacks the capacity to bind a growth factor ligand. Despite having no soluble ligand, ERBB2 is important because it is the preferred heterodimerization partner of the other ligand-bound family members. The ERBB2 has a fixed conformation that resembles the ligand-activated state of other member of the family, and because DII is exposed, ERBB2 interacts with other family members easily [12]. The binding of growth factors results in the dimerization of ERBB family receptors with itself or others and promotes receptor autophosphorylation [13, 14].

15.1.2 Homo-/Heterodimers Are Formed, and Autophosphorylation Occurs (Fig. 15.1a)

In this step, the intracellular domain of EGFR, which contains tyrosine residues and activity domains of tyrosine kinase, has an important role. The binding of ligands to the extracellular domain of ERBB family receptors induces the formation of receptor homo- or heterodimers, allowing for the activation of the intrinsic tyrosine kinase domain and phosphorylation of the tyrosine residues in the dimer partner [15]. Approximately, ten EGFR tyrosine residues are phosphorylated following receptor dimerization, and different ligands cause the phosphorylation of distinct sets of EGFR tyrosine residues. However, the mechanism is still unclear [16]. Phosphorylated tyrosine residues in ERBB receptors serve as docking sites for a series of cytosolic proteins containing Src homology 2 (SH2) domains, called adaptor proteins, or phospho-tyrosine-binding (PTB) motifs, called docking proteins. More than 117 SH2 domains have been characterized that recognize the unique profile of phosphorylated tyrosine residues plus a specific amino acid sequence motif around the tyrosine residues within their intracellular domains. Adaptor proteins play a pivotal role in mediating interaction RTKs with specific downstream signaling cascades. In contrast, docking proteins have many tyrosine residues, and activated RTKs phosphorylate these residues. Increasing the number of phosphorylated tyrosine residues can promote the assembly of signal transduction. Ligand binding to EGFR results in activation of number of intracellular signaling pathways via adaptor proteins and docking proteins [3, 7].

15.1.3 Various Intracellular Pathways Are Stimulated (Fig. 15.1b)

Autophosphorylation and transphosphorylation of the receptors through their tyrosine kinase domains lead to the recruitment of downstream effectors and the stimulation of proliferative and cell survival signals. The signaling cascade mediated by activated EGFR includes two broad categories of pathways: the RAS/RAF/MEK/ERK pathway and the PI3K/AKT/mTOR pathway, which lead to the cell proliferation, angiogenesis, migration, survival, and adhesion.

15.1.3.1 RAS/RAF/MEK/ERK Pathway [17–20]

RAS proteins are guanine nucleotide-binding proteins. The *RAS* genes encode several highly homologous 21-kDa membrane-bound proteins, including KRAS, HRAS, and NRAS. *KRAS* mutations are frequently reported in lung cancer, but *HRAS* and *NRAS* mutations are only occasionally documented. RAS proteins have intrinsic GTPase activity and exist in two states, cycling between each state: an inactive GDP-bound state and active GTP-bound state. GDP/GTP exchange thus allows RAS proteins to function as binary molecular switches. To activate GDP-bound state RAS proteins, guanine nucleotide exchange factors (GEFs) play important role. They promote RAS activation by binding to GDP-bound RAS and facilitating the release of GDP and the binding of GTP. SOS is one of the mostly highly characterized RAS-GEF. Ligand binding to ERBB family receptors induces receptor dimerization and autophosphorylation of the tyrosine residues in the receptor cytoplasmic tail. SHC, a docking protein, recognizes phosphorylated ERBB family receptor tyrosine residues and acts as a scaffold protein. The adaptor protein GRB2 is recruited to SHC because the SH2 domain of GRB2 recognizes the SHC docking sites. In turn, GRB2 recruits SOS via its SH3 domain. SOS is located close to RAS, thereby positioning SOS near membrane-anchored RAS and resulting in the loading of RAS with GTP. RAS inactivation is catalyzed by GTPase-activating proteins (GAPs), which enhance the intrinsic GTPase activity of RAS proteins by 100,000-fold. The function of RAS as a binary molecular switch is adjusted by GEFs and GAPs. RAS directly interacts with more than 20 effector proteins, and

RAF kinase is the a direct effector of activated RAS. Activated RAF is responsible for the serine/threonine phosphorylation of MEK. Activated MEK serves as a threonine/tyrosine kinase, which in turn phosphorylates ERK. There are many targets of ERK, including cytosol proteins (e.g., p90RSK) and nucleus proteins (e.g., transcription factors Elk1, Ets2, Fos, Jun, ATF2, AP1, Myc, and CREB1), which promote the proliferation and survival.

15.1.3.2 PI3K/AKT/mTOR Pathway [10, 21–23]

A second key intracellular signaling pathway is controlled by the lipid kinase PI3K. The PI3K/AKT/mTOR pathway is downstream of the activated ERBB receptors. ERBB family members can activate this pathway via PLC-γ, and RAS can also promote signaling through this pathway. Activated PI3K phosphorylates the 3-OH group of the inositol ring of phosphatidylinositol, resulting in the generation of PIP3 from PIP2. PIP3 then binds to multiple proteins, such as AKT, that have the PH domain, facilitating their recruitment to the plasma membrane and conformational change and thus regulating their function. The activity of PI3K is regulated by its regulatory subunit. This regulatory subunit associates with phosphorylated tyrosine residues located on the intracellular domains of ERBB family receptors through an SH2 domain, resulting in the allosteric activation of the catalytic subunit of PI3K. The PI3K/AKT/mTOR pathway activity is negatively regulated by the lipid phosphatase PTEN, which degrades PIP3 to PIP2. Finally, serine/threonine kinase mTOR, a downstream effector of AKT, is an important intracellular signaling enzyme in the regulation of the cell growth, motility, and survival of tumor cells. Other signaling pathways in addition to these two signaling pathways, such as the JAK/STAT pathway, have also been reported [24]. These pathways interact with each other and constitute the complicated intracellular signal network for controlling the cell proliferation and/or survival [25].

15.2 Driver Mutations and Molecular Target Drugs

Cancer is a genetic disease caused by genomic abnormalities. Genomic primary structural abnormalities include gene amplification/deletion, point mutation, and rearrangements associated with chromosomal translocations. Cancer is diagnosed according to the state of the cumulative effect of many of these genetic mutations. Among these, in particular, genetic mutations involving in cancer cell development/proliferation or maintaining survival are called driver mutations. On the other hand, mutations only accidentally occurring due to genetic instability or in the process of cell division, which have less effect on carcinogenesis/proliferation, are called passenger mutations. The state in which cell proliferation or maintaining survival strongly depends on a specific driver mutation is expressed as oncogene addiction. Among molecular target drugs targeting such driver mutations, some drugs exhibit

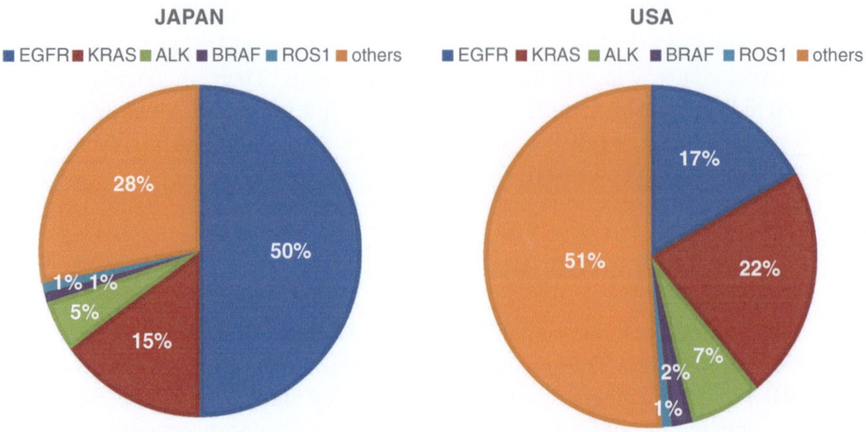

Fig. 15.2 Difference in *EGFR* mutation frequency in patients with non-small cell lung cancer, adenocarcinoma histology between Japan and the USA (left panel, Japan; right panel, the USA) [26]

higher antitumor activity than conventional cytotoxic anticancer drugs and are widely used in lung cancer therapy. Among many driver mutations, epidermal growth factor receptor (EGFR) genetic mutations have been reported to date, the profiles of which are known to significantly vary between Japan and the West (Fig. 15.2) [26].

15.3 EGFR Genetic Mutations and EGFR-TKI

15.3.1 EGFR Genetic Mutations (Fig. 15.3) [27]

EGFR genetic mutations are the driver mutations most frequently occurring in patients with lung cancer in Japan, observed in 35–53% of cases involving pulmonary adenocarcinoma [28, 29]. On the other hand, EGFR genetic mutations occur less in Westerners, particularly Caucasians, observed in less than 20% (Fig. 15.2) [26]. EGFR is a receptor tyrosine kinase which is present in all epithelial cells, and when ligands such as EGF and TGF-α bind together to form dimers, the intrinsic tyrosine kinase of the EGFR is activated, causing autophosphorylation of the tyrosine residues in the intracellular domain, followed by the initiation of multiple signal transductions including RAS/MAP kinase, PI3K/AKT, and STAT routes, leading to cell proliferation or suppression of apoptosis. Consequently, EGFR plays an important role in the control of differentiation, development, proliferation, and maintenance of cells in normal tissues. In cancer cells, mutations occur in exons 18–21, which are the first four exons among the exons encoding tyrosine kinase of EGFR proteins, causing the continuous activation of EGFR which is not dependent on ligands, resulting in carcinogenesis. Among Japanese individuals, EGFR genetic

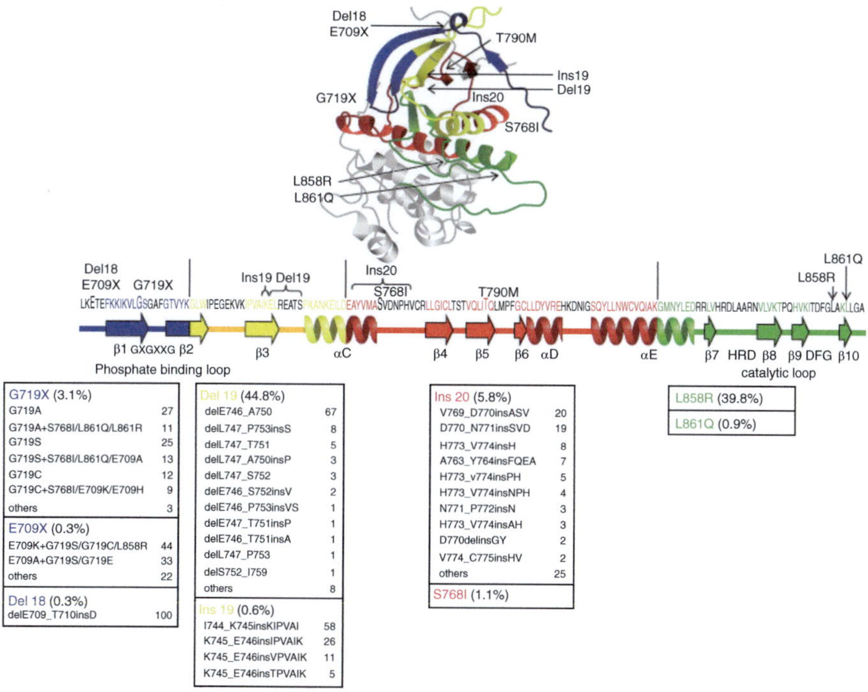

Fig. 15.3 Structure of the epidermal growth factor receptor (EGFR) protein and frequency of EGFR mutations in lung cancer by a compilation of recent large studies. Each codon of representative mutations was mapped on the protein sequence of the EGFR kinase domain. Codons in exon 18, 19, 20, and 21 are shown in blue, yellow, red, and green, respectively. Spiral structures represent alpha-helixes. Thick arrows indicate beta-sheet (Ref. [27])

mutations are observed in approximately 50% of cases involving lung adenocarcinoma (Fig. 15.2), which is the therapeutic target.

15.3.2 EGFR *Genetic Mutation Testing*

Detection methods have been successively reported since the discovery of EGFR genetic mutations. Moreover, recently, multiplex testing using the next-generation sequence (NGS) method, etc. has become available and is increasingly used for laboratory developed tests (LDT) in medical institutions and examination centers with CLIA/CAP certification in the USA (Table 15.1) [30–41]. Generally, the detection sensitivity required in EGFR mutation examinations using tumor tissues is said to be approximately 1–5%. This examination was originally conducted by major examination centers in which a quality guarantee system was maintained using an examination method equivalent to the abovementioned LDT method (LDT equivalent method). Subsequently, an examination method approved for in vitro

Table 15.1 EGFR genetic mutation testing

Class (in tissue)		Technique	Sensitivity (% Mutant DNA)	Mutations Identified	Detection of Co-mutations	Potential Applications	Ref(s)
IVD	JP US EU	Cobas	3%–5%	Known only	No	Tissue, Plasma	[30]
		Therascreen	1%–10%	Known only	No	Tissue, Plasma	[30]
	EU only	MassARRAY Dx Lung Panel	1%–10%	Known only	Yes (hotspots)	Tissue	[31] [32]
		Oncomine™ Solid Tumour DNA Kit	1%–10%	Known and new	Yes	Tissue	–
RUO		Direct sequencing	10%–25%	Known and new	No	Tissue	MS
		Pyrosequencing	5%–10%	Known only	No	Tissue	[33]
		Multiplex PCR (Snapshot)	5%	Known only	Yes (hotspots)	Tissue	[34]
		WAVE-surveyor	2%	Known only	No	Tissue, Plasma	[35]
		High-depth NGS (at least 1000× depth)	1%–10%	Known and new	Yes	Tissue, Plasma	[36]
		Scorpion ARMS	1%	Known only	No	Tissue, Plasma	–
		Locked nucleic acid clamp	1%	known only	No	Tissue, Plasma	[37]
		TAm-Seq	2%	Known and new	Yes	Tissue, Plasma	[38]
		BEAMing	<0.1%	Known only	No	Tissue, Plasma	[39]
		Digital droplet PCR	<0.1 %	Known only	No	Tissue, Plasma	[40]
		CAPP-Seq	~0.02%	Known and new	Yes	Plasma	[41]

EGFR epidermal growth factor receptor gene, *PCR* Polymerase Chain reaction, *NGS* next-generation sequencing, *ARMS* amplification refractory mutation system, *CAPP* cancer personalized profiling by deep sequencing, *RUO* research use only, *IVD* in v'itïo diagnostics, *MS* multiple studies

diagnostics (IVD) was put on the market in 2012; furthermore, an examination method approved for IVD companion diagnostics, which was the first method for EGFR mutation examinations in Japan, became available in 2016, resulting in a rapid rise in the use of the IVD method. Because 90% of EGFR mutations are either exon 21 L858R mutations or exon 19 deletion mutations, it is possible to conduct searches targeting specific mutations. Since this examination came to be covered by insurance in 2007, three LDT equivalent methods including the PNA LNA

PCR-Clamp method, PCR-Invader method, and Cycleave method, which have been adopted in major examination centers, became mainstream examination methods in Japan. Subsequently, the real-time PCR method using the Scorpion ARMS method (therascreen® EGFR mutation detection kit; QIAGEN) and the real-time PCR method using the TaqMan probe method (cobas® EGFR mutation detection kit; Roche Diagnostics) were, respectively, approved for IVD in February 2012 and January 2014. Mutations to be targeted by searches in the initial examination prior to EGFR-TKI administration include, when the IVD method is used, the rare G719X mutation, L861Q mutation, exon 20 insertion mutation, and S768I mutation as well as the major L858R mutation, exon 19 deletion mutation, and T790M mutation. Integrated analysis of LUX-Lung2, LUX-Lung3, and LUX-Lung6 revealed that, among rare mutations which can be searched for using the IVD method, the G719X mutation, L861Q mutation, and S768I mutation exhibited sensitivity to afatinib [48]. Moreover, regarding the exon 20 insertion mutation, poor effect on first- and second-generation EGFR-TKIs has been reported [42–48]. The cobas® EGFR gene mutation detection kit ver.2 (Roche Diagnostics®) has been approved in November 2015 in the USA and March 2016 in Japan, respectively, as IVD companion diagnostic kit to detect secondary T790M mutation, which is heavily involved in 2nd generation of EGFR-TKI. The samples to be analyzed in this kit is genome DNA extracted from formalin-fixed paraffin embedded (FFPE). This kit is only one approved companion diagnostic kit for osimertinib, third-generation EGFR-TKI. The concordance between this kit and other approved IVD tests and NGS is 95.6% and 91%, respectively.

15.3.3 EGFR-TKI

EGFR-tyrosine kinase inhibitor (TKI) is a drug which inhibits signal transduction downstream by binding to ATP binding sites of tyrosine kinase present in the EGFR intracellular domain and exerts an antitumor effect. In the abovementioned *EGFR* genetic mutations, particularly in non-small cell lung cancers with the exon 19 deletion mutation and exon 21 point mutation (L858R), the affinity of EGFR-TKI is known to be high. High-frequency adverse effects include exanthema and diarrhea which are associated with inhibiting wild-type EGFR, the control of which is important for long-term administration. Moreover, as a fatal adverse event, attention must be paid to interstitial pneumonia.

15.3.3.1 First-Generation EGFR-TKI

In Japan, gefitinib (Iressa®) and erlotinib (Tarceva®) are approved for medical insurance. Both drugs exhibited effects significantly exceeding standard platinum combination chemotherapy in multiple phase III studies for untreated advanced *EGFR* genetic mutation-positive non-small cell lung cancer (Table 15.2) [49–52] and have

Table 15.2 Randomized phase III studies comparing 1st and 2nd generation of EGFR-TKI with chemotherapy in patients with non-small cell lung cancer harboring with EGFR activation mutations

Study	Regimen	Case (n)	mPFS	HR (95%CI)
NEJ002 [49]	Gefitinib	99	10.8m	0.30 (0.22–0.41) $p < 0.001$
	CBDCA+PTX	101	5.4m	
WJTOG3405 [50]	Gefitinib	88	9.2m	0.489 (0.336–0.710) $p < 0.001$
	CDDP+DTX	88	6.3m	
OPTIMAL [51]	Erlotinib	82	13.1m	0.16 (0.10–0.26) $p < 0.0001$
	CBDCA+GEM	72	4.6m	
EURTAC [52]	Erlotinib	86	9.7m	0.37 (0.25–0.54) $p < 0.0001$
	Platinum doublet	87	5.2m	

CBDCA carboplatin, *PTX* pactlitaxel, *CDDP* cisplatin, *DTX* doxetaxel, *GEM* gemcitabine

Table 15.3 Frequency of toxicity induced by EGFR-TKI

		Gefitinib	Erlotinib	Afatinib	Osimertinib
Skin toxicity	Any grade	71.1%–85.1%	66.7%–73.5%	80.8%–89.1%	21.4%–33.7%
	Grade 3, 4, or 5	2.3%–5.3%	2.4%–13.1%	9.4%–16.2%	0.0%–0.7%
Diarrhea	Any grade	34.2%–61.0%	25.3%–52.4%	88.3%–95.2%	36.5%–40.5%
	Grade 3, 4, or 5	0.9%–1.3%	1.2%–4.8%	5.4%–14.4%	0.5%–1.1%
Hepatic toxicity	Any grade	23.9%–70.1%	3.6%–37.3%	9.4%–20.1%	4.9%–6.5%
	Grade 3, 4, or 5	7.5%–27.6%	2.4%–3.6%	0.0%–1.7%	0.7%–1.1%
Interstitial pneumonia	Any grade	2.3%–5.3%	0.0%–1.2%	0.0%–1.3%	2.7%–3.6%

been assessed as one of the standard initial treatments for *EGFR* genetic mutation-positive non-small cell lung cancer. Although differences in the effects of gefitinib and erlotinib have been examined in some prospective clinical trials, no clear difference in effect has been shown [53, 54]. Regarding adverse events, while a highly frequent/severe tendency for diarrhea, exanthema, etc. has been observed with erlotinib, liver dysfunction tends to be frequent with gefitinib (Table 15.3). On the other hand, erlotinib has better cerebrospinal fluid transitivity and greater effect on brain metastasis carcinomatous meningitis than gefitinib.

15.3.3.2 Second-Generation EGFR-TKI

Afatinib (Giotrif®) is a TKI which irreversibly inhibits not only EGFR but also ERBB2 and ERBB4 having the same HER family molecules as EGFR and is called second-generation EGFR-TKI. As with first-generation EGFR-TKI, afatinib also exhibited effects exceeding standard platinum combination chemotherapy in multiple phase III studies in the initial treatment for advanced *EGFR* genetic mutation-positive non-small cell lung cancer [55, 56] and has also been assessed as one of the standard initial treatments for *EGFR* genetic mutation-positive non-small cell lung cancer. In the LUX-Lung 7 study, which is a phase IIB study, differences in the

Table 15.4 Comparison of EGFR-TKI

	Gefitinib Iressa®	Erlotinib Tarceva®	Afatinib Giotrif®
Structure	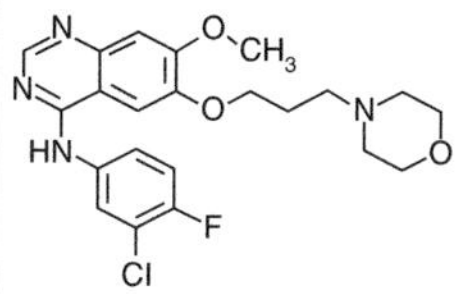 D01977	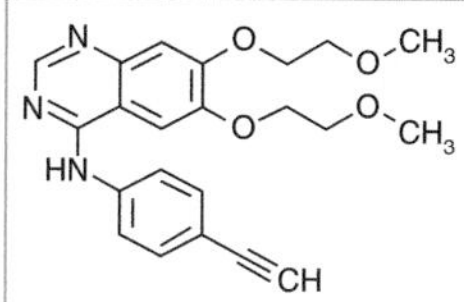 D07907	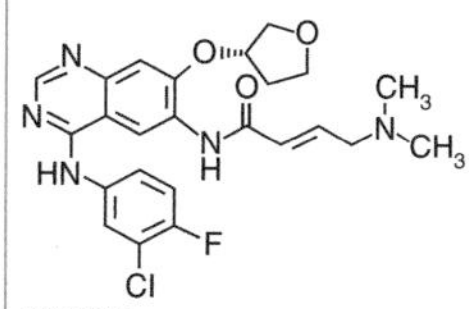 D09724
Target	EGFR	EGFR	EGFR/ERBB2/ERBB4
Mechanism	Reversible	Reversible	Irreversible
Approved	July 2002	October 2007	April 2014
T 1/2	48 h	32 h	33.9 h
MTD	700 mg	150 mg	50 mg
RD	250 mg	150 mg	40 mg

effects of afatinib and gefitinib of first-generation EGFR-TKI were examined regarding EGFR gene-positive non-small cell lung cancer. Regarding progression-free survival (PFS), which is one of the primary endpoints, the median values were 11.0 months with afatinib and 10.9 months with gefitinib ($p = 0.0178$), indicating that afatinib had significantly good results; however, regarding the overall survival (OS), which is another primary endpoint, no significant difference was observed (27.9 months vs. 24.5 months, $p = 0.258$) [57]. On the other hand, afatinib had a more frequent/severe tendency for diarrhea and skin disorders than gefitinib (Table 15.3). As of yet, there is no clear standard regarding the different use of first and second generations, and even in the 2016 guidelines by the Japan Lung Cancer Society, there is no difference in the recommended grades of both. There are differences in the side effects between first- and second-generation EGFR-TKIs, which can currently be used in Japan [58]. In both first- and second-generation EGFR-TKIs, it is known that interstitial pneumonia is more often observed as a side effect compared with Western and Chinese individuals, and regarding the mechanism thereof, prospective clinical trials are currently ongoing. Table 15.4 lists EGFR-TKIs which can be used in practical medical examinations to date.

15.3.3.3 Combination Therapy of First- and Second-Generation EGFR-TKIs

In many cases, first-/second-generation EGFR-TKIs are known to become resistant from 9 to 14 months after administration. Multiple studies regarding combination therapies including EGFR-TKI and other antineoplastic drugs have been conducted to further extend the effect of EGFR-TKI and enhance the effect thereof (Table 15.5). Regarding the phase III controlled studies which have been reported to date, there was only one report from Hong Kong mentioning that PFS was significantly

Table 15.5 Combination treatment with EGFR-TKI in non-small cell lung cancer

Study	Phase	Regimen	N	mPFS	HR (95% CI)	MST	HR (95% CI)
Cheng. IASLC2015	2	Gefitinib	65	10.9m	0.68 (0.48–0.96) $p = 0.029$	NR	–
		Gefitinib+PEM	126	15.8m		NR	
Yoshimura. Lung Cancer 2015	2	Gefitinib+PEM	26	18.0m	–	32.0m	–
NEJ005 [60]	2	Gefitinib+ CBDCA+ PEM sequential	39	15.3m	0.71 (0.42–1.20) $p = 0.20$	30.7m	0.51 (0.26–0.99) $p = 0.042$
		Gefitinib+ CBDCA+ PEM concurrent	41	18.3m		41.9m	
FASTACT-2 [59] (EGFR mt subset)	3	Platinum+GEM	48	6.9m	0.25 (0.16–0.39) $p < 0.001$	20.6m	0.48 (0.27–0.84) $p = 0.0092$
		Erlotinib+ platinum+GEM	49	16.8m		31.4m	
OLCSGT 1001	2	Gefitinib+ bevacizumab	42	14.4m	–	NR	–
JO25567 [61]	2	Erlotinib	75	9.7m	0.54 (0.36–0.79) $p = 0.0015$	NR	–
		Erlotinib+ bevacizumab	77	16.0m		NR	

extended by adding platinum + gemcitabine to gefitinib; however, no significant difference was observed in OS [59]. Other reports involved single arm phase II studies or control phase II studies. The NEJ005 study was a phase II study in which two groups combining gefitinib and CBDCA+PEM sequentially or concurrently were compared. Although PFS was good for both groups at more than 15 months, no significant difference was observed [60]. JO25567 was a randomized controlled phase II study in which an erlotinib group and a group in which bevacizumab, which is an angiogenesis inhibitor, was combined with erlotinib were compared regarding EGFR genetic mutation-positive non-small cell lung cancer, with the result that the combination group significantly extended PFS compared with erlotinib single drug(16.0 M vs. 9.7 M, HR: 0.54 (0.36–0.74), p = 0.0015 [61]. Based on these results, the NEJ026 study, which has a similar design and is a phase III study, is ongoing, and the case registration has just completed. Moreover, regarding EGFR genetic mutation-positive non-small cell lung cancer, a controlled phase III study is ongoing in which gefitinib single drug and the so-called sandwich treatment, in which gefitinib and CDDP+PEM are alternately administered, are compared. Therapies combining other antineoplastic drugs with EGFR-TKI are not standard therapies as of yet. Going forward, the results of these phase III studies are warranted.

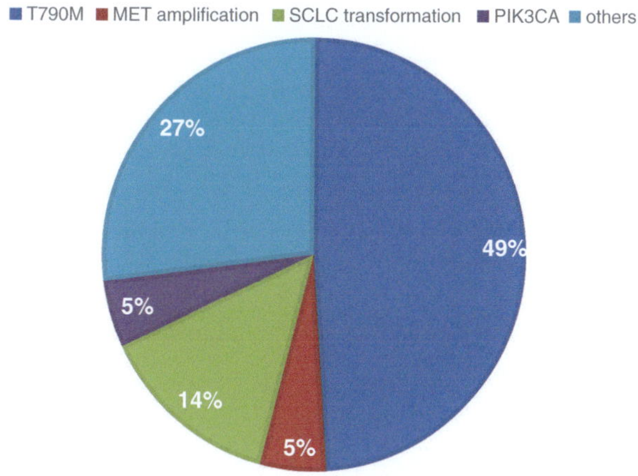

Fig. 15.4 Resistant mechanism for 1st and 2nd generation of EGFR-TKI [62, 63]

15.3.3.4 Resistance to First-/Second-Generation EGFR-TKIs

When first-/second-generation EGFR-TKI is administered for over 1 year, exacerbation is caused in many cases, clinically leading to the occurrence of EGFR-TKI resistance. As the resistance mechanism, the acquisition of second mutations such as exon 20 T790M, bypass signals due to MET/HER2, activation downstream due to PTEN deletion, and transformation to small cell cancer, etc. have been reported; however, among these, resistance due to second mutations such as exon 20 T790M occurs most frequently, accounting for approximately half (Fig. 15.4) [62, 63]. For resistance cases which occurred approximately 1 year following the administration of first-/second-generation EGFR-TKI, clinical trials involving, for example, a shift to chemotherapy on a continuing basis or beyond PD therapy, which combines chemotherapy with the continuous administration of first-/second-generation EGFR-TKI, were conducted; however, no prolonged survival effect was observed.

15.3.3.5 Third-Generation EGFR-TKI

Osimertinib (Tagrisso®) is an EGFR-TKI which irreversibly inhibits exon20 T790M, which is a resistant mutation, as a target in addition to EGFR-TKI sensitivity mutations. In the phase III study (AURA3 study), in which osimertinib and platinum combination chemotherapy were compared, regarding *EGFR* genetic mutation-positive non-small cell lung cancer, in which resistance is caused upon the administration of EGFR-TKI as the first-line treatment and T790M is observed by re-biopsy, osimertinib exhibited significantly good results with a median value of 10.1 months in the PFS of the primary endpoint compared with 4.4 months with platinum combination chemotherapy [64] and has been assessed as one of the standard treatments for *EGFR* T790M-positive non-small cell lung cancer. Low inhibitory activity against wild-type *EGFR* is also one of the characteristics of osimertinib, resulting in the problematic adverse events in conventional EGFR-TKI such as diarrhea and exanthema being relatively mild (Table 15.3). On the other hand, attention must be paid to the incidence of interstitial pneumonia in Japanese patients which is moderately high at 6.3% as well as toxic effects such as QTc prolongation by electrocardiogram. A phase III study (FLAURA study) directly comparing osimertinib and gefitinib for untreated advanced *EGFR* genetic mutation-positive non-small cell lung cancer is currently ongoing, with the potential to lead to drastic changes in the standing of osimertinib depending on the results. Although the *T790M* mutant allele is confirmed by re-biopsy of the tumor tissue, a liquid biopsy using the plasma is also available.

References

1. Vinay K, Abul KA, Jon CA. Neoplasia. In: Robbins and cotran pathologic basis of disease. 9th ed. Philadelphia: Saunders, An Imprint of Elsevier Inc; 2015. p. 265–340.
2. Oxnard GR, Binder A, Jänne PA. New targetable oncogenes in non-small-cell lung cancer. J Clin Oncol. 2013;31(8):1097–104.
3. Aphrothiti H, Gopa L, David S. Intracellular signaling. In: John EN, James OA, Joel ET, editors. Abeloff's clinical oncology. 5th ed. Philadelphia: Elsevier; 2014. p. 22–39.
4. Weinstein IB. Cancer. Addiction to oncogenes-the Achilles heal of cancer. Science. 2002;297(5578):63–4.
5. Sharma SV, Bell DW, Haber DA, et al. Epidermal growth factor receptor mutations in lung cancer. Nat Rev Cancer. 2007;7(3):169–81.
6. Krause DS, Van Etten RA. Tyrosine kinases as targets for cancer therapy. N Engl J Med. 2005;353(2):172–87.
7. Normanno N, De Luca A, Salomon DS, et al. Epidermal growth factor receptor (EGFR) signaling in cancer. Gene. 2006;366(1):2–16.
8. Linardou H, Dahabreh IJ, Murray S, et al. Somatic EGFR mutations and efficacy of tyrosine kinase inhibitors in NSCLC. Nat Rev Clin Oncol. 2009;6(6):352–66.
9. Arteaga CL, Engelman JA. ERBB receptors: from oncogene discovery to basic science to mechanism-based cancer therapeutics. Cancer Cell. 2014;25(3):282–303.
10. Siegelin MD, Borczuk AC. Epidermal growth factor receptor mutations in lung adenocarcinoma. Lab Investig. 2014;94(2):129–37.
11. Citri A, Yarden Y. EGF-ERBB signalling: towards the systems level. Nat Rev Mol Cell Biol. 2006;7(7):505–16.
12. Hynes NE, Lane HA. ERBB receptors and cancer: the complexity of targeted inhibitors. Nat Rev Cancer. 2005;5(5):341–54.
13. Yewale C, Baradia D, Misra A, et al. Epidermal growth factor receptor targeting in cancer: a review of trends and strategies. Biomaterials. 2013;34(34):8690–707.
14. Bublil EM, Yarden Y. The EGF receptor family: spearheading a merger of signaling and therapeutics. Curr Opin Cell Biol. 2007;19(2):124–34.
15. Tebbutt N, Pedersen MW, Johns TG. Targeting the ERBB family in cancer: couples therapy. Nat Rev Cancer. 2013;13(9):663–73.
16. Olayioye MA, Neve RM, Hynes NE, et al. The ErbB signaling network: receptor heterodimerization in development and cancer. EMBO J. 2000;19(13):3159–67.
17. Chang L, Karin M. Mammalian MAP kinase signalling cascades. Nature. 2001;410(6824):37–40.

18. Malumbres M, Barbacid M. RAS oncogenes: the first 30 years. Nat Rev Cancer. 2003;3(6):459–65.
19. Downward J. Targeting RAS signalling pathways in cancer therapy. Nat Rev Cancer. 2003;3(1):11–22.
20. Karnoub AE, Weinberg RA. Ras oncogenes: split personalities. Nat Rev Mol Cell Biol. 2008;9(7):517–31.
21. Vivanco I, Sawyers CL. The phosphatidylinositol 3-kinase AKT pathway in human cancer. Nat Rev Cancer. 2002;2(7):489–501.
22. Sabatini DM. mTOR and cancer: insights into a complex relationship. Nat Rev Cancer. 2006;6(9):729–34.
23. Vanhaesebroeck B, Stephens L, Hawkins P. PI3K signalling: the path to discovery and understanding. Nat Rev Mol Cell Biol. 2012;13(3):195–203.
24. Gschwind A, Fischer OM, Ullrich A. The discovery of receptor tyrosine kinases: targets for cancer therapy. Nat Rev Cancer. 2004;4(5):361–70.
25. Yarden Y, Pines G. The ERBB network: at last, cancer therapy meets systems biology. Nat Rev Cancer. 2012;12(8):553–63.
26. Midha A, Dearden S, McCormack R, et al. *EGFR* mutation incidence in non-small-cell lung cancer of adenocarcinoma histology: a systematic review and global map by ethnicity (mutMapII). Am J Cancer Res. 2015;5(9):2892–911.
27. Kobayashi Y, Mitsudomi T. Not all epidermal growth factor receptor mutations in lung cancer are created equal: perspectives for individualized treatment strategy. Cancer Sci. 2016;107(9):1179–86.
28. Kohno T, et al. KIF5B-RET fusions in lung adenocarcinoma. Nat Med. 2012;18:375–7.
29. Serizawa M, et al. Assessment of mutational profile of Japanese lung adenocarcinoma patients by multitarget assays. Cancer. 2014;120:1471–81.
30. Lopez-Rios F, Angulo B, Gomez B, Mair D, et al. Comparison of molecular testing methods for the detection of EGFR mutations in formalin-fixed paraffin-embedded tissue specimens of non-small cell lung cancer. J Clin Pathol. 2013;66(5):381–5.
31. Arcila ME, Oxnard GR, Nafa K, et al. Rebiopsy of lung cancer patients with acquired resistance to EGFR inhibitors and enhanced detection of the T790M mutation using a locked nucleic acid-based assay. Clin Cancer Res. 2011;17(5):1169–80.
32. Sherwood JL, Müller S, Orr MC, et al. Panel based MALDI-TOF tumour profiling is a sensitive method for detecting mutations in clinical non small cell lung cancer tumour. PLoS One. 2014;9(6):e100566.
33. Young EC, Owens MM, Adebiyi I, et al. A comparison of methods for EGFR mutation testing in non-small cell lung cancer. Diagn Mol Pathol. 2013;22(4):190–5.
34. Dias-Santagata D, Akhavanfard S, David SS, et al. Rapid targeted mutational analysis of human tumours: a clinical platform to guide personalized cancer medicine. EMBO Mol Med. 2010;2(5):146–58.
35. Jänne PA, Borras AM, Kuang Y, et al. A rapid and sensitive enzymatic method for epidermal growth factor receptor mutation screening. Clin Cancer Res. 2006;12(3 Pt 1):751–8.
36. Uchida J, Kato K, Kukita Y, et al. Diagnostic accuracy of noninvasive genotyping of EGFR in lung cancer patients by deep sequencing of plasma cell-free DNA. Clin Chem. 2015;61(9):1191–6.
37. Costa C, Molina MA, Drozdowskyj A, et al. The impact of EGFR T790M mutations and BIM mRNA expression on outcome in patients with EGFR-mutant NSCLC treated with erlotinib or chemotherapy in the randomized phase III EURTAC trial. Clin Cancer Res. 2014;20(7):2001–10.
38. Forshew T, Murtaza M, Parkinson C, et al. Noninvasive identification and monitoring of cancer mutations by targeted deep sequencing of plasma DNA. Sci Transl Med. 2012;4(136):136ra68.
39. Taniguchi K, Uchida J, Nishino K, et al. Quantitative detection of EGFR mutations in circulating tumor DNA derived from lung adenocarcinomas. Clin Cancer Res. 2011;17(24):7808–15.

40. Watanabe M, Kawaguchi T, Isa S, et al. Ultra-sensitive detection of the pretreatment EGFR T790M mutation in non-small cell lung cancer patients with an EGFR-activating mutation using droplet digital PCR. Clin Cancer Res. 2015;21(15):3552–60.
41. Newman AM, Bratman SV, To J, et al. An ultrasensitive method for quantitating circulating tumor DNA with broad patient coverage. Nat Med. 2014;20(5):548–54.
42. Beau-Faller M, Prim N, Ruppert AM, Nanni-Metéllus I, et al. Rare EGFR exon 18 and exon 20 mutations in non-small-cell lung cancer on 10 117 patients: a multicentre observational study by the French ERMETIC-IFCT network. Ann Oncol. 2014;25(1):126–31.
43. Naidoo J, Sima CS, Rodriguez K, et al. Epidermal growth factor receptor exon 20 insertions in advanced lung adenocarcinomas: clinical outcomes and response to erlotinib. Cancer. 2015;121(18):3212–20.
44. Yasuda H, Park E, Yun CH, Sng NJ, et al. Structural, biochemical, and clinical characterization of epidermal growth factor receptor (EGFR) exon 20 insertion mutations in lung cancer. Sci Transl Med. 2013;5(216):216ra177.
45. Voon PJ, Tsui DW, Rosenfeld N, et al. EGFR exon 20 insertion A763-Y764insFQEA and response to erlotinib—letter. Mol Cancer Ther. 2013;12(11):2614–5.
46. Woo HS, Ahn HK, Lee HY, et al. Epidermal growth factor receptor (EGFR) exon 20 mutations in non-small-cell lung cancer and resistance to EGFR-tyrosine kinase inhibitors. Investig New Drugs. 2014;32(6):1311–5.
47. Yasuda H, Kobayashi S, Costa DB, et al. EGFR exon 20 insertion mutations in non-small-cell lung cancer: preclinical data and clinical implications. Lancet Oncol. 2012;13(1):e23–31.
48. Yang JC, Sequist LV, Geater SL, et al. Clinical activity of afatinib in patients with advanced non-small-cell lung cancer harbouring uncommon EGFR mutations: a combined post-hoc analysis of LUX-Lung 2, LUX-Lung 3, and LUX-Lung 6. Lancet Oncol. 2015;16(7):830–8.
49. Maemondo M, et al. Gefitinib or chemotherapy for non-small cell lung cancer with mutated EGFR. N Engl J Med. 2010;362:2380–8.
50. Mitsudomi T, et al. Gefitinib versus cisplatin plus docetaxel in patients with non-small cell lung cancer harbouring mutations of the epidermal growth factor receptor (WJTOG3405): an open label, randomised phase 3 trial. Lancet Oncol. 2010;11:121–8.
51. Zhou C, et al. Erlotinib versus chemotherapy as first-line treatment for patients with advanced EGFR mutation-positive non-small-cell lung cancer (OPTIMAL, CTONG0802): a multicentre, open-label, randomised, phase 3 study. Lancet Oncol. 2011;12:735–42.
52. Rosell R, et al. Erlotinib versus standard chemotherapy as first-line treatment for European patients with advanced EGFR mutation-positive non-small-cell lung cancer (EURTAC): a multicentre, open-label, randomised phase 3 trial. Lancet Oncol. 2010;13:239–46.
53. Urata Y, et al. Randomized phase III study comparing gefitinib with erlotinib in patients with previously treated advanced lung adenocarcinoma: WJOG5108L. J Clin Oncol. 2016;34:3248–57.
54. Yang JJ, et al. A randomized controlled trial of erlotinib versus gefitinib in advanced non-small-cell lung cancer harboring EGFR mutations (CTONG0901). J Thorac Oncol. 2015;10:S321(abstr).
55. Sequist LV, et al. Phase III study of afatinib of cisplatin plus pemetrexed in patients with metastatic lung adenocarcinoma with EGFR mutations. J Clin Oncol. 2013;31:3327–34.
56. Wu YL, et al. Afatinib versus cisplatin plus gemcitabine for first-line treatment of Asian patients with advanced non-small-cell lung cancer harbouring EGFR mutations (LUX-lung 6): an open-label, randomised phase 3 trial. Lancet Oncol. 2014;15:213–22.
57. Paz-Ares L, et al. Afatinib versus gefitinib in patients with EGFR mutation-positive advanced non-small-cell lung cancer: overall survival data from the phase IIb LUX-Lung 7 trial. Ann Oncol. 2017;28:270–7.
58. Takeda M, Okamoto I, Nakagawa K. Pooled safety analysis of EGFR-TKI treatment for EGFR mutation-positive non-small cell lung cancer. Lung Cancer. 2015;88(1):74–9.
59. Wu YL, Lee JS, Thongprasert S, et al. Intercalated combination of chemotherapy and erlotinib for patients with advanced stage non-small-cell lung cancer (FASTACT-2): a randomised, double-blind trial. Lancet Oncol. 2013;14(8):777–86.

60. Sugawara S, Oizumi S, Minato K, et al. Randomized phase II study of concurrent versus sequential alternating gefitinib and chemotherapy in previously untreated non-small cell lung cancer with sensitive EGFR mutations: NEJ005/TCOG0902. Ann Oncol. 2015;26(5):888–94.
61. Seto T, Kato T, Nishio M, et al. Erlotinib alone or with bevacizumab as first-line therapy in patients with advanced non-squamous non-small-cell lung cancer harbouring EGFR mutations (JO25567): an open-label, randomised, multicentre, phase 2 study. Lancet Oncol. 2014;15(11):1236–44.
62. Sequist LV, Waltman BA, Dias-Santagata D, et al. Genotypic and histological evolution of lung cancers acquiring resistance to EGFR inhibitors. Sci Transl Med. 2011;3(75):75ra26.
63. Yu HA, Maria E, Arcila ME, Rekhtman N, et al. Analysis of tumor specimens at the time of acquired resistance to EGFR TKI therapy in 155 patients with *EGFR* mutant lung cancers. Clin Cancer Res. 2013;19(8):2240–7.
64. Mok TS, et al. Osimertinib or platinum-pemetrexed in EGFR T790M-positive lung cancer. N Engl J Med. 2017;376:629–40.

Chapter 16
ALK and Others: How Important Are ALK and Other Mutations in the Management of Lung Cancer?

Hisatsugu Goto and Yasuhiko Nishioka

Abstract The discovery of gene aberrations that drive cancer progression has led to new ways in classifying lung cancer and to the development of various molecular-targeted agents. Over the last decade, treatment strategies for non-small cell lung cancer (NSCLC) patients have rapidly evolved beyond conventional chemotherapy with molecular-targeted agents. Gene aberration in *epidermal growth factor receptor* (*EGFR*) or *anaplastic lymphoma kinase* (*ALK*) has successfully being targeted, and the corresponding tyrosine kinase inhibitors revolutionarily improved the survival of a subset of NSCLC patients. In addition to *EGFR* and *ALK*, other oncogenic driver mutations such as *ROS*, *RET*, *MET*, and *BRAF* have also been identified as minor mutations, and some corresponding inhibitors are in development with success in clinical trials. In the near future, lung cancer is expected to be routinely fractionated into minor populations based on their gene aberration status. This chapter reviews oncogenic mechanisms of minor gene aberrations in NSCLC and discusses the corresponding treatment strategies, mechanism of resistance, and how they are important in the treatment of NSCLC, with particular emphasis on *ALK* rearrangement.

Keywords Non-small cell lung cancer · ALK · Minor mutation

H. Goto (✉) · Y. Nishioka
Department of Respiratory Medicine and Rheumatology, Graduate School of Biomedical Sciences, Tokushima University, Tokushima, Tokushima, Japan
e-mail: hgoto@tokushima-u.ac.jp

T. Kaneko (ed.), *Clinical Relevance of Genetic Factors in Pulmonary Diseases*, Respiratory Disease Series: Diagnostic Tools and Disease Managements,
https://doi.org/10.1007/978-981-10-8144-6_16

16.1 Introduction

Lung cancer is one of the leading causes of cancer death worldwide [1], and non-small cell lung cancer (NSCLC) accounts for 80–90% of cases. The majority of patients are diagnosed when the disease is locally advanced or metastatic, with an estimated 5-year survival of only 15% approximately. Over the past decades, with the development of molecular approach, several genetic alterations vulnerable to targeted inhibition have been identified in NSCLC. The first notable success to opening the gate to a new era of precision medicine in NSCLC was the identification of activating mutations in the *EGFR* gene in 2004 leading to dramatic responses to EGFR tyrosine kinase inhibitors (TKIs) such as gefitinib, erlotinib, and afatinib. Following this success, the discovery of the *EML4-ALK* fusion gene also provided a significant change in the therapeutic strategies for NSCLC patients harboring this *EML4-ALK* rearrangement [2]. Currently, in the era of "genome-wide medicine," multiple nationwide cancer genome screening projects are running, and several other genetic alterations in NSCLC are identified, leading to the active clinical studies accessing the drugs that target those genes. In addition, the development of molecular technology enabled us to deeply sequence the target gene and to identify the resistant mechanism of molecular-targeted agents. In this chapter, recent advances in *ALK*-rearranged NSCLC as well as NSCLC with other minor mutations are described, and we would like to discuss how these minor gene alterations are important in the treatment of NSCLC to develop precision medicine.

16.2 *ALK* Rearrangement in Lung Cancer

ALK is a receptor tyrosine kinase, a member of the insulin RTK family [3], encoded by the *ALK* gene on chromosome 2p23. In 1994, the first translocation of *ALK* with the gene encoding for nucleophosmin was identified in patients with anaplastic large cell lymphoma (ALCL) [4]. Subsequently, *ALK* rearrangements were identified in various malignancies such as inflammatory myofibroblastic tumor (IMT), colorectal cancer, and diffuse large B-cell lymphoma, with the different partner such as *kinesin family member-5B* (*KIF5B*), *cysteine-rich transmembrane BMP regulator 1* (*CRIM1*), and *huntingtin-interacting protein 1* [5]. NSCLC was the second solid tumor in which oncogenic *ALK* fusion with echinoderm microtubule-associated protein-like 4 (EML4) was detected by Soda and colleagues [6]. After dimerization, EML4-ALK transcript constitutively triggers mitogen-activated protein kinase (MAPK), Janus kinase with signal transducer and activator of transcription (JAK-STAT), and phosphoinositide 3-kinase with v-akt murine thymoma viral oncogene homolog (PI3K-AKT), leading to an increase in proliferation and survival of cancer cells [7]. Subsequent retrospective analyses revealed that *ALK* fusions were detected in 3–7% of NSCLCs and were associated with absence of smoking, younger age, and adenocarcinoma histology [8]. Even though the relative proportion of NSCLCs harboring an *ALK* rearrangement is significantly lower than that of ALCL or IMT, patients with NSCLC constitute the largest subset of patients with an *ALK*-rearranged cancer due to the high incidence of lung cancer worldwide [1, 5]. Additionally, studies in NSCLC have identified several other fusion partners with *ALK*, such as *KIF5B*, *CRIM1*, *translocated promoter region, nuclear basket protein* (*TPR*), and *kinesin light chain 1* (*KLC1*) [5], which occur less frequently than *EML4–ALK*. Furthermore, a number of breakpoint variants may be seen for the fusion protein, for example, more than ten distinct variants were detected in *EML4-ALK* [9].

16.3 Targeting Oncogenic ALK

In response to the discovery of EML4-ALK in lung cancer, a large number of ALK inhibitors are currently under development, and some of them are already approved. Only 4 years after the discovery of EML4-ALK in lung cancer, crizotinib, the first ALK TKI, was approved by US FDA.

16.3.1 First-Generation ALK Inhibitor: Crizotinib

Crizotinib, an orally bioavailable small molecule, is the first ALK TKI evaluated and approved for the treatment of patients with ALK-positive NSCLC. The phase I PROFILE 1001 trial evaluated the pharmacokinetic profile and efficacy of crizotinib in patients with ALK-positive NSCLC [10]. Crizotinib was well tolerated at a dose of 250 mg twice daily, and the overall response rate (ORR) was 61%, with the median progression-free survival (PFS) of 9.7 months (Table 16.1). The results were confirmed in the phase II PROFILE 1005 study that enrolled patients with advanced previously treated ALK-positive NSCLC and obtained ORR of 60% and median PFS of 8.1 months [2]. Two phase III clinical trials comparing crizotinib with standard chemotherapy in the first- and second-line settings have been conducted. In the PROFILE 1014 study, patients with ALK-positive non-squamous NSCLC were randomly assigned to receive first-line crizotinib or a platinum-based regimen with pemetrexed [11]. The results confirmed the high efficacy of crizotinib, with a PFS of 10.9 months compared with 7 months with chemotherapy. The ORR was 74% with crizotinib and 45% with chemotherapy. In the PROFILE 1007 trial, patients with advanced or metastatic ALK-positive NSCLC, previously treated with a platinum-based chemotherapy, were enrolled and randomized to receive crizotinib or standard chemotherapy [12]. Better median PFS was obtained with crizotinib (7.7 months vs. 3 months). Collectively, the results from these clinical studies suggested that crizotinib is effective and well-tolerated treatment in NSCLC, and thus crizotinib is approved in more than 85 countries across the world. These results also enabled us to aware that patients with ALK-positive NSCLC have a high risk of

Table 16.1 Clinical trials of ALK inhibitors

Trial	Drug	Phase	ORR (%)	Median PFS (months) HR (95% CI)	Median OS (months) HR (95% CI)
PF1011	Crizotinib	I	60.8%	9.7	–
PF1005	Crizotinib	II	60%	8.1	–
PF1007	Crizotinib vs. PEM/DTX	III	65% vs. 45% $P < 0.001$	HR; 0.49 (0.37–0.64); $P < 0.001$	HR; 1.02 (0.68–1.54); $P = 0.54$
PF1004	Crizotinib vs. platinum doublet	III	74% vs. 45% $P < 0.0001$	HR; 0.45 (0.35–0.69); $P < 0.001$	–
ASCEND-1	Ceritinib	I	72% in crizotinib naïve; 56% in crizotinib resistant	18.4 in crizotinib naïve; 6.9 in crizotinib resistant	–
ASCEND-2	Ceritinib	II	38.6%	5.7	–
ASCEND-3	Ceritinib	II	63.7%	11.1	–
ASCEND-4	Ceritinib vs. platinum doublet	III	72.5% vs. 26.7%	HR; 0.55 (0.42–0.73); $P < 0.00001$	Not reached
AF-001JP	Alectinib	I–II	93.3%	–	–
AF-002JG	Alectinib	I–II	53%	–	–
NP28673	Alectinib	II	50%	8.9	–
J-Alex	Alectinib vs. crizotinib	III		Not reached	Not reached
NCT01449461	Brigatinib	I	72%	13.2	–

developing brain metastases, as observed in approximately 30% of cases at the time of tumor diagnosis [13] and in 60% of patients during crizotinib treatment [14]. The main reason for crizotinib failure in brain disease is its poor blood-brain barrier penetration [15]. A retrospective analysis of the PROFILE 1005 and 1007 trials documented that the intracranial overall response rate (IC-ORR) was 18% in patients who did not receive radiation therapy.

16.3.2 Second- and Third-Generation ALK Inhibitors

16.3.2.1 Ceritinib

Ceritinib is a second-generation ALK TKI that is approximately 20 times more potent than crizotinib at the level of IC50 [16]. Ceritinib has been shown to strongly inhibit ALK-positive cell lines harboring mutations that cause resistance to crizotinib, especially the L1196M, G1269A, I1171T, and S1206Y. The efficacy and safety of ceritinib were evaluated in a phase I trial (ASCEND-1) that included patients with ALK-positive NSCLC [17]. The ORR was 72% in ALK inhibitor-naïve patients compared with 56% in ALK inhibitor-pretreated patients, and the median PFS was 18.4 months and 6.9 months, respectively (Table 16.1). Based on these results, ceritinib was approved by the FDA for patients with advanced or metastatic ALK-positive NSCLC progressing to crizotinib. In terms of the efficacy of ceritinib on brain metastases or leptomeningitis, the IC-ORR was 63% and 36% in ALK-inhibitor-naïve and ALK-inhibitor-pretreated patients, respectively, in the ASCEND-1 trial. ASCEND-7 trial which evaluates the efficacy of ceritinib in patients with ALK-positive NSCLC with brain metastases or leptomeningitis is currently ongoing. The phase II ASCEND-2 trial enrolled patients who had previously received cytotoxic chemotherapy and had also progressed to crizotinib. The ORR was 38.6% [18] (Table 16.1). Another phase II ASCEND-3 trial is evaluating the role of ceritinib in patients with ALK-positive crizotinib-naïve NSCLC. ASCEND-4, the phase III trial comparing the efficacy of ceritinib with first-line chemotherapy, demonstrated that the median PFS was 16.6 months in the ceritinib group and 8.1 months in the chemotherapy group (hazard ratio 0.55), respectively [19]. Another phase III trial (ASCEND-5), comparing the efficacy of ceritinib with chemotherapy in further lines in crizotinib-resistant disease progressing after previous chemotherapy, is currently ongoing.

16.3.2.2 Alectinib

Alectinib is a highly selective oral ALK TKI active in crizotinib-naïve and crizotinib-resistant ALK-positive NSCLC. Importantly, it has an activity against the mutation related to crizotinib resistance such as L1196M, G1269A, C1156Y, F1174L, L1152R, and S1206Y [20]. Two phase I/II trials have evaluated the efficacy and safety of alectinib in ALK-positive NSCLC (Table 16.1). In the AF-001JP trial, conducted in Japan, 70 patients with ALK-positive crizotinib-naïve NSCLC were enrolled [21]. In the phase I part, 300 mg of alectinib twice daily was defined as the recommended dose for the phase II. The ORR of crizotinib-naïve patients entered in the phase II part of the trial was 93.5%, with a PFS at 12 months of 83%. Based on the results of the AF-001JP trial, alectinib was firstly approved in Japan for the treatment of patients with ALK-positive NSCLC who had not previously received other ALK inhibitors. In the AF-002JG phase I/II study, conducted in the USA, 47 patients with ALK-positive NSCLC who had progressed on crizotinib were enrolled [22]. In the phase I part, 600 mg of alectinib twice daily was defined as the recommended dose for the phase II. The ORR to alectinib in the phase II part of the trial was 55% (Table 16.1).

In terms of brain metastasis, alectinib is suggested to be effective against brain metastasis. Since alectinib is not a substrate of P-glycoprotein, it seems that it may reach effective therapeutic concentrations in the brain. In the AF-002JG study, out of 47 enrolled patients, 21 had asymptomatic brain metastases, and 6 of the 21 had a complete response, 5 had a partial response, and 8 had stable disease. One patient with leptomeningeal metastases attained a partial response. Alectinib has also been tested in two phase II clinical trials in crizotinib-resistant ALK-positive NSCLC, including central nervous system (CNS) metastases (Table 16.1). In the NP28673 trial, the ORR was 50% and median PFS was 8.9 months [23]. The efficacy of alectinib in patients with brain metastasis was confirmed by IC-ORR of 57%.

The comparison of alectinib with crizotinib as the first-line treatment in patients with ALK-positive advanced NSCLC is currently on study by two randomized phase III trials, Japan J-ALEX and the worldwide ALEX trial. Both trials were also designed to investigate the potential superiority of alectinib over crizotinib for the management of brain metastases. The preliminary data of J-ALEX showed reduced risk of PFS by 66% in favor of alectinib compared with crizotinib (hazard ratio 0.34, 99% CI: 0.17–0.70, $P < 0.0001$) in 207 enrolled patients. Median PFS was not reached in the alectinib arm (95% CI: 20.3 months not estimated) vs. 10.2 months in the crizotinib arm (95% CI: 8.2–12).

The efficacy of alectinib in the further-line treatment of *ALK*-rearranged NSCLC is being studied in another ongoing phase III study (NCT02604342). This study evaluates and compares between treatment groups the efficacy of alectinib versus chemotherapy in patients with ALK-positive advanced NSCLC who were previously treated with chemotherapy and crizotinib.

16.3.2.3 Brigatinib

Brigatinib is a potent second-generation ALK TKI which showed in preclinical studies a dual inhibition of ALK (including L1196M mutation conferring resistance to crizotinib) and EGFR T790 M [7]. For this inhibitory mechanism, brigatinib could be an encouraging therapeutic option for patients who showed resistance to crizotinib by the activation of the EGFR bypass track [7]. The activity and safety of brigatinib were recently evaluated in a phase I/II trial (NCT01449461) [24]. Patients with treatment-naïve or crizotinib-resistant ALK-positive NSCLC, with or without CNS metastases, have been enrolled. In the phase I part, a dose of 180 mg once daily was chosen for the recommended dose. In the phase II part, the ORR was 72%, and median PFS was 13.2 months in patients with ALK-positive NSCLC with previous crizotinib treatment (Table 16.1). In the small group of crizotinib-naïve patients, the ORR was 100%, while median PFS have not yet been reached. For the 21 assessable patients with brain metastasis without previous brain irradiation, including 18 patients who had received previous crizotinib, 5 (56%) of 9 patients with measurable lesions had a response, and 7 (58%) of 12 patients with only non-measurable lesions had complete disappearance of brain lesions.

16.3.2.4 Lorlatinib

Lorlatinib is a third-generation ATP-competitive selective ALK inhibitor, specifically designed and optimized to penetrate the blood-brain barrier. It also inhibits ROS1. Importantly, lorlatinib is the only ALK TKI that has an activity of G1202-related mutations that show resistance to the rest of ALK TKIs [25]. However, it is not approved by any regulatory agency in the world at the time of writing this text.

Lorlatinib is approximately tenfold more potent against wild-type EML4-ALK and approximately 40-fold more potent against L1196M-mutated EML4-ALK compared with crizotinib, and it regresses brain tumors at doses much lower than the maximum tolerated dose [26]. The phase I/II trial in ALK-positive and ROS1-positive NSCLC patients with or without CNS metastases is ongoing.

16.4 Mechanisms of Resistance to ALK Inhibitors

ALK TKIs are generally effective in the patients with *ALK*-rearranged NSCLC; however, those clinical benefits with ALK TKIs are almost universally limited due to the emergence of acquired resistance. Diverse mechanisms are considered to contribute to the acquired resistance to ALK TKIs, for example, the presence of secondary *ALK* mutations (some of them are stated above), *ALK* fusion gene amplification, and activation of alternative signaling pathways are reported. Among these, the emergence of secondary *ALK* mutations is most intensively studied. The mutation profiles that related to acquired resistance of each ALK TKI are listed in Table 16.2. Notably, each ALK TKI has different mutation profiles which would be very important to consider the sequential use of ALK TKIs.

In addition to acquired resistance, intrinsic resistance can be also seen in the clinical setting. Even though ALK TKIs were proven by multiple clinical studies to represent strong effects on *ALK*-rearranged NSCLCs, there was small number of patients who did not show the initial response. Logically, any of the mechanisms of acquired resistance stated above could cause intrinsic resistance if they were preexisting in the tumor cells before the treatment with ALK TKIs; however, the mechanisms of primary resistance to ALK TKIs are currently poorly understood.

Table 16.2 ALK mutations related to acquired resistance to each TKIs

	Crizotinib	Alectinib	Ceritinib	Brigatinib	Lorlatinib
L1196M	×	○	○	○	○
G1269A	×	○	○	○	○
C1156Y	×	○	×	○	○
F1174L/C/V	×	○	×	○	○
1151Tins	×	○	×	○	○
L1252R	×	○	×	○	○
S1206Y	×	○	○	○	○
I1171N/S/T	×	×	○	-	○
V1180 L	×	×	○	-	○
G1202R	×	×	×	×	○
G1202del	×	×	×	×	○
G1123S	○	○	×	-	-
L1198F	○	×	×	×	×

Abbreviations: *ALK* Anaplastic lymphoma kinase, *TKIs* Tyrosine kinase inhibitors

16.5 Treatment Strategies for *ALK*-Rearranged NSCLC

Currently, three ALK TKIs (crizotinib, alectinib, and ceritinib) are available in clinic, and the others (brigatinib and lorlatinib) are expected to be approved in the near future. At that time, we will have five "bullets" to fight with *ALK*-rearranged NSCLCs, which would be the optimistic news for physicians and, most importantly, for lung cancer patients. However, at the same time, various issues and questions are also arisen to develop effective therapeutic strategies. The clinical questions would be summarized in twofold: (1) What is the optimal sequence of ALK TKIs for the individual patient? (2) Can ALK TKIs be combined with other treatment arms?

16.5.1 What Is the Optimal Sequence of ALK TKIs?

16.5.1.1 Importance of Repeat Biopsies

First strategy to consider the sequence of ALK TKIs is to effectively treat the refractory diseases by overcoming the dominant resistance mechanisms. Although not all the mechanisms underlying the resistance to ALK TKIs are covered, we at least know that a certain mutations in *ALK* cause resistance to ALK TKIs (Table 16.2). These recent advances to understand the mechanisms of resistance to ALK TKIs underscore the critical need for re-biopsies to guide the optimal therapeutic strategies. When feasible and safe, there is no question about pursuing repeat biopsies to be strongly recommended in patients progressing on an ALK TKI [5]. For example, when a patient showed refractory disease after crizotinib treatment, and if L1196M mutation was detected by re-biopsy of the progressing tumor, then alectinib may be expected to show the clinical response as the next drug. If no mutation was detected, conventional chemotherapy would have a priority than next ALK TKI as the following treatment line.

However, it is also true that this ideal treatment strategy cannot be fit in many ways into the "real world" of the treatment of *ALK*-rearranged NSCLCs in clinic. Because generally ALK TKIs are effective and strong shrinkage of the tumor is often obtained, the refractory disease may not be suitable for the re-biopsy (tumor may be too small, or the location is not suitable for the biopsy). Not all the patient is agreeable to the repeat biopsies (especially patients with high age), and we always need to consider the risk for pursuing biopsies (especially for patients with poor performance status). Most importantly, the detection of the mutation of *ALK* is not approved, at least in Japan to date, as the companion diagnostic tool. This means that the detection of *ALK* mutation is possible in a limited institution. The development of companion diagnostic tools along with the next-generation drug is necessary and urgent. Furthermore, if applied, a liquid biopsies using peripheral blood of the patients may become more useful tool to identify the mechanisms of resistance with minimally invasive procedures.

16.5.1.2 Enhancing the Strength of Tumor Response Up Front

Thus far, it seems that most efforts to overcome the resistance to ALK TKIs have focused on to uncover the mechanisms of resistance. Indeed, many mutations related to the resistance are reported as stated above, although there are many obstacles to fit those findings in clinic. Alternatively, strategies to prevent resistance up front are likely to have greater impact in clinic. Although general guidelines recommend crizotinib as a first-line drug for the treatment of *ALK*-rearranged NSCLCs and are emerging for determining the optimal later-line ALK TKI, which TKI to use in the first-line setting remains unclear [5]. The up-front use of a more potent and selective second-generation ALK inhibitor may substantially delay disease progression through various mechanisms. First, next-generation ALK TKIs have activity against multiple crizotinib-resistant mutations, including the most common L1196M and G1269A mutations, and may thus suppress the outgrowth of any preexisting clones that harbor these mutations and also prevent them from emerging de novo. Second, most next-generation TKIs have greater CNS activity than crizotinib and would hence delay the development of brain and leptomeningeal metastases, which are commonly experienced in crizotinib-treated patients.

From this point of view, it is worth of notice that the phase III studies comparing second-generation TKI with crizotinib as a first-line setting are currently ongoing. The first reported results comparing a second-generation ALK TKI with crizotinib in the TKI-naive setting came from the J-ALEX study, comparing alectinib with crizotinib in Japanese patients with ALK-positive NSCLC. As stated in alectinib section, preliminary results suggest that first-line alectinib may be superior to crizotinib. Based on these results, alectinib was recently granted FDA breakthrough therapy designation for first-line treatment of ALK-positive NSCLC. Although this study has reported to have some limitations, including an imbalance of patients with baseline brain metastases and a higher than expected rate of toxicities with crizotinib [5], the results of this study will likely be practice-changing. A similar global phase III trial (ALEX) comparing first-line alectinib to crizotinib in ALK-positive NSCLC is ongoing. Importantly, it remains unclear whether first-line use of alectinib can prolong OS of patients compared with crizotinib, as these trials have not allowed patient crossover at the time of progression. Therefore, more relevant comparison of first-line alectinib versus sequential crizotinib followed by alectinib needs to be elucidated.

16.5.2 Combination Use of ALK TKIs and Other Drugs

16.5.2.1 Conventional Chemotherapy

In this era of translational medicine, molecular-targeted agents such as TKIs and specific antibodies have received much attention in the treatment of lung cancer. However, one should remember that the cytotoxic chemotherapy is still one of the standard treatment regimens for lung cancer including *ALK*-rearranged NSCLCs. The results from previous clinical studies with crizotinib (PROFILE 1007 and 1014) demonstrated that, although high efficacy of crizotinib was confirmed compared to chemotherapy, pemetrexed or docetaxel appeared to be still effective in patients with *ALK*-rearranged NSCLC. In particular, multiple retrospective analyses suggested that patients with *ALK*-rearranged NSCLC benefit more from pemetrexed than those with other oncogene-driven NSCLCs. Therefore, pemetrexed-based chemotherapy needs to be considered in *ALK*-rearranged NSCLC patients, and more importantly, it is crucial to include both ALK TKIs and cytotoxic agents in total treatment setting in each patient. In this regard, the main concern in clinic would be the timing of conventional chemotherapy. As stated above, the second ALK TKI can be administered after the resistance to the first ALK TKI, ideally with determining the resistant mechanism with re-biopsy. However, it might be difficult with many reasons in the real world to perform re-biopsy and determine the acquired gene mutation. Do we still choose next ALK TKI? At present, it appears that cytotoxic chemotherapy, especially pemetrexed-based chemotherapy, is another choice to be considered in such cases. Another question is whether ALK TKIs can be continuously used beyond progression of the tumor with combined use of cytotoxic chemotherapy. There is no evidence at this point for this issue. A trial investigating crizotinib plus pemetrexed for crizotinib-failed patients (NCT02134912) is ongoing. Additionally, in-turn use of ALK TKI and conventional chemotherapy may be effective. Learning from the strategy using EGFR TKI, it is reported that the insertion of conventional chemotherapy during the first-line use of gefitinib for patients with *EGFR*-mutated NSCLC showed prolonged PFS compared to monotherapy with gefitinib, and similar result might be able to achieve with ALK TKIs and pemetrexed-based chemotherapy in patients with *ALK*-rearranged NSCLC.

16.5.2.2 Anti-angiogenic Agents

An adequate blood supply is essential for cancer cells to survive and grow; thus, the concept of inhibiting tumor angiogenesis has been applied to cancer therapy. Among the factors associated with tumor angiogenesis, vascular endothelial growth factor (VEGF) and its receptor VEGFR are reported to be the key factors to form new vessels, and inhibition of the VEGF signaling pathway exhibits an additive effect when combined with conventional chemotherapy. Currently, anti-VEGF antibody (bevacizumab) and anti-VEGFR antibody (ramucirumab) are available in clinic. The results from phase III clinical trials have demonstrated that the addition of bevacizumab to platinum-based chemotherapy improves the response rate and prolongs survival of patients with various types of cancer including NSCLC [27]. In addition, malignant pleural effusion induced by the increased permeability of the blood vessels, which is caused by tumor-secreting VEGF, can be improved with bevacizumab [28]. Furthermore, bevacizumab was shown to exhibit a preventive role in brain metastases formation [29]. In addition to bevacizumab, ramucirumab in combination with docetaxel exhibited a significantly improved survival in comparison to docetaxel monotherapy in a second-line setting for advanced NSCLC (Garo neb lancet 2014).

In addition to prevent new vessel formation in the tumor, another important mechanism of anti-VEGF therapy against tumors is considered to be the normalization of the tumor vasculature, which results in improvement of the delivery of the drug used along with anti-VEGF(R) agent. The combination use of anti-angiogenesis agents with cytotoxic drugs could therefore improve the access of cytotoxic drugs to the tumor.

One might consider that not only cytotoxic drugs but also other molecular-targeted agents could be combined to enhance the drug delivery. Indeed, in patients with *EGFR*-mutated NSCLC, the JO25567 trial demonstrated that erlotinib in combination with bevacizumab was significantly superior to erlotinib alone for advanced NSCLC harboring *EGFR*-sensitive mutations. PFS achieved by combination therapy and monotherapy were 16.0 and 9.7 months, respectively (HR; 0.54, 95% CI; 0.36–0.97, P = 0015) [30]. Thus, it seems logical to consider that the efficacy of ALK TKIs might also enhanced by addition of anti-angiogenic agents. When ALK TKIs were combined with anti-angiogenic agents, several favorable results could be expected: (1) prolonged survivals compared with monotherapy using ALK TKIs, (2) enhanced antitumor activity against brain metastasis, and (3) suppression of radiation necrosis and subsequent brain edema. In particular, radiation necrosis mimicking progression in the brain was demonstrated by several reports when alectinib was used as postradiation therapy, and anti-VEGF therapy is expected to suppress this pseudoprogression [20].

Collectively, inhibition of the angiogenic pathway in addition to the therapy with ALK TKIs appears to be promising in several ways for the management of patients with lung cancer.

16.5.2.3 Immune Checkpoint Therapy

When nonself-antigens are invaded in human body, those antigens are recognized and presented by antigen-presenting cells (APCs) to T cells. T cells are then activated and eliminate pathogens that have those antigens. At the same time, the cross talk between APCs and T cells has negative feedback systems to prevent overzealous T cell activation and inflammation, and one of the negative feedback systems is regulated by programmed cell death-1 (PD-1) which is expressed by T cells and programmed cell death ligand-1 (PD-L1) which is expressed by APCs. Notably, in the tumor microenvironment, tumor cells do express PD-L1 to downregulate the immune response of T cells that were infiltrated to attack cancer cells. Therefore, targeting the immune checkpoint factors, such as PD-1 and PD-L1, has now become one of the standards of care in the treatment of lung cancer. Inhibition of the interaction of PD-1 and PD-L1 by blocking antibodies suppresses the immune escape of cancer cells and induces immune response in T cells against cancer cells. Currently, multiple clinical trials assessing the efficacy of anti-PD-1 or anti-PD-L1 antibodies are ongoing. Recent CheckMate and KEYNOTE trials demonstrated that nivolumab and pembrolizumab, representative PD-1 inhibitors, exhibited a survival benefit in comparison to conventional chemotherapy in lung cancer [31, 32]. Nivolumab was demonstrated to exhibit a significantly prolonged survival compared with docetaxel in the second-line setting for both squamous NSCLC and non-squamous NSCLC. Furthermore, the second-line use of pembrolizumab was also shown to be significantly superior to docetaxel in patients with PD-L1-positive NSCLC previously treated with platinum-based chemotherapy [33]. Thus, immune checkpoint inhibition has emerged as a novel and promising therapeutic option in the management of lung cancer.

Regarding the combination use of ALK TKIs and immune checkpoint inhibitors, several studies are investigating the efficacy and tolerability of the combination therapy [5]. For example, studies assessing crizotinib with nivolumab or ipilimumab (NCT01998126) or pembrolizumab (NCT02511184), ceritinib with nivolumab (NCT02393625), alectinib with atezolizumab (NCT02013219), and lorlatinib with avelumab (NCT02584634) are ongoing. However, careful interpretation of the results will be needed, as many of ongoing studies are not logically biomarker driven, and there are limited preclinical data so far to support these combination strategies. One should note that PD-1/PD-L1 inhibitors have demonstrated durable activity in a subset of NSCLC; responses are limited to approximately 20% of patients, although most of the patients with durable response achieved prolonged survival, suggesting that there are a distinct subset of the patients who are expected to have strong benefit to PD-1/PD-L1 inhibitors. Although the precise biomarker of immune therapy is not yet covered, patients with *ALK*-rearrangement may not be included in the subset with good response to PD-1/PD-L1 inhibitors. So far, the efficacy of PD-1/PD-L1 inhibitors is associated with high PD-L1 expression, high tumor mutational load, and smoking history [5]. Patients with *ALK*-rearranged NSCLC tend to be never smokers with a low tumor mutational load. Moreover, a recent retrospective analysis demonstrated that *ALK*-rearranged NSCLCs tend to have low PD-L1 expression and low T cell infiltration in the tumor microenvironment [34]. Indeed, no responses were seen among six patients with *ALK*-rearranged NSCLC treated with immune checkpoint inhibitors in the study.

With the reasons stated above, the potential benefit of combining immune checkpoint inhibitors with ALK TKIs is currently unclear and questionable. However, it is reported that the PD-L1expression can be induced by translocated ALK through the activation of PI3K-AKT and MEK-ERK pathways, which was demonstrated by in vitro analyses and clinical investigation using samples (although only a small number) from *ALK*-rearranged patients [35]. A larger cohort is needed to clarify the level and mechanism of PD-L1 expression in *ALK*-rearranged tumor, and the continuous efforts are warranted to determine the biomarkers predictive of response to immune checkpoint inhibitors. Furthermore, it should be carefully investigated how we use both drugs (sequentially or in combination) and how we assess the efficacy (PFS or OS, when combined) of these therapies.

16.6 Other Genetic Alterations in Lung Cancer

As stated above, oncogenic driver gene alterations such as *ALK*-rearrangement (and also *EGFR* mutations) have successfully been targeted with corresponding TKIs. Recent development of technologies, such as introduction of next-generation sequencer, has been enabled to detect other oncogenic driver mutations in genes such as *ROS1*, *RET*, *MET*, and *BRAF* in various types of cancer including NSCLC, and several targeted drugs have already been investigated in early phase clinical trials with some success (Table 16.3).

16.6.1 ROS1 *Rearrangements*

The prevalence of aberrant fusions in *ROS1* gene is described to be 1–2% of NSCLCs. More than ten fusion partners have been reported including *CD74*, *EZR*, *TPM3*, *SDC4*, *SLC34A2*, and *LRIG3*. The clinical features of patients with *ROS1* rearrangement resemble that of patients with *ALK* rearrangement or *EGFR* mutations; they are mostly found in adenocarcinomas with never or light smokers (very rarely found in squamous cell carcinomas or smokers) and are more prevalent among the young and females. The common clinical features between patients with *ROS1* and *ALK* rearrangements could be explained by the fact that the kinase domains of *ROS1* and *ALK* are highly homologous, and thus their rearrangements in lung cancer share common carcinogenic properties. In line with this premise, crizotinib has been investigated as a therapeutic agent for *ROS1*-rearranged NSCLC patients in an expansion cohort of the PROFILE 1001 trial [36]. Crizotinib achieved an ORR of 72% and median PFS of 19.2 months, with 85% OS at 12 months in this 50 patient cohort. With this result, crizotinib has been recently approved by FDA for

Table 16.3 Rare oncogenic drivers in NSCLC

Gene alteration	Prevalence in NSCLC	Typical clinical features	Targeted drugs
ROS1 rearrangement	1–2%	Adenocarcinoma, younger age, never smoker	Crizotinib
RET rearrangement	1–2%	Adenocarcinoma, younger age, never smoker	Alectinib, sunitinib, sorafenib, lenvatinib, vandetanib, cabozantinib
MET amplification	3–4%	Older age	Crizotinib, cabozantinib
MET mutation	2–3%	Older age	Crizotinib, cabozantinib
BRAF mutation	1–2%	–	Vemurafenib, dabrafenib, trametinib
HER2 mutation	1–2%	Adenocarcinoma, younger age, never smoker	Afatinib, trastuzumab

ROS1-rearranged NSCLC patients. Phase II study of crizotinib for *ROS1*-rearranged NSCLC patients is currently ongoing in Asian countries. Moreover, clinical development of next-generation dual ALK and ROS1 inhibitors (lorlatinib, ceritinib, brigatinib, and entrectinib) and other ROS1 inhibitors (cabozantinib and foretinib) is also currently ongoing. Similarly to that described in *ALK*-rearranged cancer, the individual resistance mechanisms against above molecular-targeted agents are also needed to be elucidated.

16.6.2 RET *Rearrangements*

RET rearrangements are found in approximately 1% of NSCLC. This prevalence will increase up to 2–3% when patients are selected to have tumors without other gene aberrations. Gene alterations in *RET* was initially identified in thyroid cancer in the 1990s, followed by in NSCLC in 2012. *RET* rearrangements are known to be mutually exclusive with *EGFR*, *ALK*, *Kirsten rat sarcoma viral oncogene homolog* (*KRAS*), or *HER2* gene aberration. Several fusion partners have been identified including *KIF5B*, *CCDC6*, *NCO4*, and *TRIM33*. Among these partners, *KIF5B* is reported to be the most frequent. The clinical features of patients with *RET* rearrangement resemble that of patients with EGFR mutations (female adenocarcinomas with never or light smokers) with slight tendency to the young. These evidences suggest that *RET* rearrangements are also oncogenic driver in NSCLC, and the treatment strategies are investigating in multiple clinical studies. Many RET TKIs are multi-kinase inhibitors already in clinical use, including vandetanib, cabozantinib, lenvatinib, sunitinib, sorafenib, and alectinib. Among these, the effect of vandetanib on *RET*-rearranged NSCLS was recently evaluated in the phase II trial in Japan (LURET trial) [37]. In this trial, *RET*-rearranged patients were screened using a nationwide genomic screening network (LC-SCRUM-Japan) of about 200 participating institutions in Japan. Among 1536 patients with *EGFR* mutation-negative NSCLC screened, 34 were *RET*-positive (2%), and 19 patients were enrolled in this study. Vandetanib was orally administered with daily dose of 300 mg. Among 17 eligible patients included in primary analysis, 9 (53%, 95% CI; 28–77) achieved an objective response, which met the primary endpoint. In the intention-to-treat population of all 19 patients treated with vandetanib, 9 (47%, 95% CI; 24–71) achieved an objective response. Median PFS was 4.7 months (95% CI; 2.8–8.5). Interestingly, higher clinical activity was seen in vandetanib-treated patients harboring the *CCDC6–RET* fusion variant (response rate 83%, median PFS of 8.3 months). The most common grade 3 or 4 adverse events were hypertension (58%), diarrhea (11%), rash (16%), dry skin (5%), and QT prolongation (11%), which could be explained by the inhibition of VEGFR and EGFR. Cabozantinib and lenvatinib were also reported to have objective response rates in phase II trials including pretreated NSCLC patients. Collectively, several drugs that are already approved in other types of cancer also have antitumor activities in *RET*-rearranged NSCLC; however, further efforts are warranted to screen the rare population of lung cancer and verify the preference of RET inhibitors.

16.6.3 MET *Amplification and Mutations*

MET, also known as hepatocyte growth factor receptor, was initially identified in osteosarcoma in 1980s. Since then, much attention has been paid to MET pathway activation as a potential therapeutic target in a number of cancers including NSCLC, as MET pathway activation correlates with malignant grade of cancer and poor patient's survival. MET pathway activation is thought to occur through a diverse set of mechanisms that influence properties affecting cancer cell survival, growth, and invasiveness. Among the mechanisms, high level of *MET* amplification and exon 14 alterations have recently been described to play important role in lung cancer. *MET* amplification has been considered as a therapeutic target as it was found in approximately 10% of NSCLC patients with EGFR active mutation who acquired the resistance to EGFR TKI. Subsequently, the prevalence of *MET* amplification and *MET* mutations within exon 14 was found to be relatively common (approximately 15%) in NSCLC regardless of drug resistance, suggesting that these *MET* alterations could be oncogenic drivers. *MET* amplification strengthens the downstream signal to activate the proliferation of cancer cells; however, *MET* mutations were initially thought to be inactive since most mutations were found outside the kinase domain. Later it was found that they could lead to the decreased degradation of MET, resulting in sustained and constitutive MET signaling [38]. Importantly, *MET* amplification and exon 14 alterations could occur independently or in combination in NSCLC, and separately they represent approximately 3–4% of NSCLC. Of note, typical clinical features of patients with *MET* aberrations are different from those of *EGFR* or *ALK* alterations in NSCLC. Both *MET* alterations seem more frequent among older lung cancer patients, with no apparent major differences according to smoking status or between adenocarcinomas and squamous cell carcinomas [38].

Considering to target MET, crizotinib could be expected as a choice, since this drug was developed as a MET inhibitor in the first place. The encouraging antitumor activity of crizotinib against NSCLC patients with *MET* alterations was presented in American Society of Clinical Oncology (ASCO) 2014. The preliminary data showed that crizotinib had antitumor activity in NSCLC patients either with high *MET* amplification or *MET* exon 14 alterations within the subsequently expanded independent cohorts of the still ongoing PROFILE1001 trial. Importantly, crizotinib showed objective responses in 67% of previously treated patients with high *MET* amplification ($n = 14$), but this activity dropped to 0% and 17% in patients with low and intermediate *MET* amplification, respectively. These results suggested that the level of *MET* amplification in the tumor is important to achieve the benefit of MET TKIs. In addition, clinical case reports have shown that crizotinib was also effective in *MET* exon 14-altered tumors. Moreover, small studies have shown that other MET TKIs, such as cabozantinib and capmatinib, had also shown strong activity in patients with tumor harboring MET exon 14 alterations [39].

Collectively, *MET* amplification and alteration in exon 14 are distinctive oncogenic drivers and target of MET inhibitors. Continuous efforts are warranted to determine the importance of the status of *MET* alterations (single or overlap), to enrich the biomarker to select patients who accept the benefit of MET inhibitor, and to investigate the mechanism of resistance to MET TKIs which could be different from that determined in other population of gene aberrations. The prospective studies investigating the efficacy of MET TKIs for *MET*-amplified and/or *MET* exon 14-altered patients are ongoing.

16.6.4 **BRAF** *Mutations*

BRAF is a member of the RAF family of serine/threonine protein kinases. BRAF is located downstream of KRAS and plays a role in regulating the MAPK/ERK signaling pathway, which affects cell division, differentiation, and secretion. Mutations in *BRAF* are associated with cardiofaciocutaneous syndrome, a disease characterized by heart defects, mental retardation, and a distinctive facial appearance. Mutations in this gene have also been associated with various cancers, including NSCLC, non-Hodgkin lymphoma, colorectal cancer, malignant melanoma, and thyroid carcinoma. Among the mutations seen in *BRAF*, V600E mutation is most well known, and this mutation activates BRAF kinase activity, which results in aberrant cell proliferation and survival through sustained and constitutive downstream signaling. The representative malignancy that harbors V600E mutation is malignant melanoma, and V600E accounts for 80–90% of *BRAF* mutations detected in this disease. For patients with malignant melanoma who have V600E mutation, BRAF inhibitors (vemurafenib and dabrafenib) are reported to have encouraging activities, and, moreover, the addition of MEK inhibitor to BRAF inhibitor resulted in better clinical efficacy compared to the single treatment with BRAF inhibitor.

In NSCLC, the prevalence of *BRAF* kinase domain mutations is approximately 1–2%. Unfortunately, unlike malignant melanoma, V600E mutation was detected in only half of the cases and the other half harbor non-V600E mutations, of which the drug sensitivity and biological properties are much less well known than those of V600E. Some mutation does not activate BRAF kinase activity. There seems to be no distinct distribution according to smoking status, sex, or age [38].

As in the case in malignant melanoma, the encouraging antitumor effect of dabrafenib with or without trametinib, an allosteric MEK1/2 inhibitor, was shown in phase II trials. Planchard et al. have reported the efficacy of single treatment of dabrafenib in patients with NSCLC positive for V600E mutation. In this report, oral dabrafenib was administered 150 mg twice daily, and 26 of the 78 previously treated patients achieved an investigator-assessed overall response (33%, 95% CI; 23–45). Four of the six previously untreated patients had an objective response. Serious adverse events were reported in 42% of patients including one patient died from an intracranial hemorrhage that was judged by the investigator to be due to the study drug. The most frequent grade 3 or worse adverse events were cutaneous squamous cell carcinoma (12%), asthenia (5%), and basal-cell carcinoma (5%) [40]. Two months after the above study was published, the antitumor activity and safety of dabrafenib plus trametinib in patients with V600E-mutant NSCLC were reported by the same group of investigators [41]. In this global study, 57 patients were enrolled and received oral dabrafenib (150 mg twice daily) plus oral trametinib (2 mg once daily) in continuous 21-day cycles until disease progression. As a result, 36 patients (63.2%, 95% CI; 49·3–75·6) achieved an investigator-assessed overall response. Serious adverse events were reported in 56% of the patients and included pyrexia (16%), anemia (5%), confusional state (4%), decreased appetite (4%), hemoptysis (4%), hypercalcaemia (4%), nausea (4%), and cutaneous squamous cell carcinoma (4%). The most common grade 3–4 adverse events were neutropenia (9%), hyponatremia (7%), and anemia (5%). Four patients died during the study from fatal adverse events judged to be unrelated to treatment (one retroperitoneal hemorrhage, one subarachnoid hemorrhage, one respiratory distress, and one from disease progression that was more severe than typical progression, as assessed by the investigator). Thus, dabrafenib with or without trametinib could represent a new targeted therapy with robust antitumor activity in NSCLC patients harboring V600E *BRAF* mutation. The safety profile was overall consistent with that in patients with malignant melanoma.

16.6.5 HER2 *Aberrations*

HER2 gene amplification and mainly kinase domain mutations have been identified as oncogenic drivers in NSCLC. Among *HER2* aberration detected in NSCLC, in-frame insertion in exon 20 is most frequently seen. NSCLC patients with *HER2* aberration share common clinical and pathological features with those with EGFR mutation [38]. The prevalence of *HER2* aberrations in NSCLC is roughly 1–2%. Although *HER2* aberration in NSCLC is mutually exclusive, low frequencies of concomitant *EGFR* mutations, *ALK* translocations, and *ROS* translocations were reported [42].

In the treatment of NSCLC patients with *HER2* aberrations, several HER2-targeted therapies could be considered including trastuzumab, a monoclonal antibody against HER2, and pan-HER TKIs such as afatinib, neratinib, and dacomitinib. Combination therapies with trastuzumab and chemotherapy have shown activity in retrospective European cohorts [42], and the activities of pan-HER TKIs are also reported. However, clinical efficacies of HER2-targeted therapies seemed to be relatively low compared to that of other targeted agents. Recently, the efficacy of dacomitinib on lung cancer patients with *HER2* mutation or amplification was reported [43]. In this phase II study, oral dacomitinib was administered 30–45 mg daily in 28-day cycles to 30 patients (*HER2* mutation in 26, amplification in 4 patients). Three of 26 patients with tumors harboring HER2 exon 20 mutations (12%, 95% CI; 2–30) had partial responses, and no partial responses occurred in 4 patients with tumors with *HER2* amplifications. The median OS was 9 months from the start of dacomitinib (95% CI; 7–21 months) for patients with *HER2* mutations and ranged from 5 to 22 months with amplifications. Treatment-related toxicities included diarrhea (90%, grade 3/4: 20%/3%), dermatitis (73%, grade 3/4: 3%/0%), and fatigue (57%, grade 3/4: 3%/0%). One patient died on study likely due to an interaction of dacomitinib with mirtazapine.

Currently, the reason why the clinical efficacy of HER2-targeted therapy in NSCLC is not as good as that of other molecular-targeted therapy is not yet defined. Further efforts are needed to determine the specific molecular context that predicts responsiveness of HER2-targeted therapy and to develop the optimal treatment strategy for patients with *HER2* aberrations.

16.6.6 NTRK *Rearrangements and Other Potential Targets*

The tropomyosin receptor kinase (Trk) receptor family comprises three transmembrane proteins referred to as Trk A, B, and C receptors that are encoded by the *NTRK1*, *NTRK2*, and *NTRK3* genes, respectively [38]. These receptor tyrosine kinases are expressed in human neuronal tissue and play an essential role in the physiology of development and function of the nervous system through activation by neurotrophins. In lung cancer, rearrangements in *NTRK1* have been reported with the frequency of approximately 1% of NSCLC. Gene fusions involving *NTRK1* genes lead to transcription of chimeric Trk proteins, resulting in constitutive activation of kinase function. To target *NTRK1* rearrangement, several pan-Trk inhibitors including entrectinib are in development, and clinical studies are ongoing.

Candidates for other molecular targets such as KRAS, insulin-like growth factor 1 receptor (IGFR1), fibroblast growth factor receptor 1 (FGFR1), and discoidin domain receptors (DDR) are being studied preclinically and clinically; however, no effective therapy is available at this point.

16.7 Conclusion

Twenty years ago, lung cancer was classified only by its histological features, and even after the classification, treatment strategies using conventional cytotoxic drugs were similar among histological subtypes except small cell lung cancer. After the discovery of *EGFR* mutation, however, the concept of driver mutation in carcinogenesis has been widely recognized, and strong and durable effect of molecular-targeted agents revolutionarily changed the treatment strategy of NSCLC. Moreover, recent development of technologies has enabled us to deeply and widely investigate the genomic alteration of cancer, and as reviewed in this chapter, several minor mutations were already identified. Our final goal is personalized medicine, where individual patients are treated differently based on their molecular profiles. At this point, before reaching the final goal, we need to "fractionate" patients to rare populations based on their molecular profile using the available tools and administer the appropriate treatment strategies to obtain the maximum benefit of the treatment. This concept is important even after the resistance to the therapy as patients may be further fractionated based on the profiles of resistant mechanisms. To do this, clinicians are needed to be well versed in molecular biology in addition to their experience in clinic to understand the molecular profiles of both efficacy and safety, some of which are common in the profiles of gene aberrations, and to construct the optimal treatment strategies for the patients.

Reference

1. Siegel RL, Miller KD, Jemal A. Cancer Statistics, 2017. CA Cancer J Clin. 2017;67:7–30. https://doi.org/10.3322/caac.21387.
2. Passaro A, Lazzari C, Karachaliou N, Spitaleri G, Pochesci A, Catania C, et al. Personalized treatment in advanced ALK-positive non-small cell lung cancer: from bench to clinical practice. Onco Targets Ther. 2016;9:6361–76.
3. Ullrich A, Schlessinger J. Signal transduction by receptors with tyrosine kinase activity. Cell. 1990;61:203–12.
4. Morris SW, Kirstein MN, Valentine MB, Dittmer KG, Shapiro DN, Saltman DL, et al. Fusion of a kinase gene, ALK, to a nucleolar protein gene, NPM, in non-Hodgkin's lymphoma. Science. 1994;263:1281–4.
5. Lin JJ, Riely GJ, Shaw AT. Targeting ALK: precision medicine takes on drug resistance. Cancer Discov. 2017;7:137–55. https://doi.org/10.1158/2159-8290.CD-16-1123.
6. Soda M, Choi YL, Enomoto M, Takada S, Yamashita Y, Ishikawa S, et al. Identification of the transforming EML4-ALK fusion gene in non-small-cell lung cancer. Nature. 2007;448:561–6.
7. Caccese M, Ferrara R, Pilotto S, Carbognin L, Grizzi G, Caliò A, et al. Current and developing therapies for the treatment of non-small cell lung cancer with ALK abnormalities: update and perspectives for clinical practice. Expert Opin Pharmacother. 2016;17:2253–66.
8. Shaw AT, Yeap BY, Mino-Kenudson M, Digumarthy SR, Costa DB, Heist RS, et al. Clinical features and outcome of patients with non-small-cell lung cancer who harbor EML4-ALK. J Clin Oncol. 2009;27:4247–53. https://doi.org/10.1200/JCO.2009.22.6993.
9. Shaw AT, Engelman JA. ALK in lung cancer: past, present, and future. J Clin Oncol. 2013;31:1105–11. https://doi.org/10.1200/JCO.2012.44.5353.
10. Camidge DR, Bang YJ, Kwak EL, Iafrate AJ, Varella-Garcia M, Fox SB, et al. Activity and safety of crizotinib in patients with ALK-positive non-small-cell lung cancer: updated results from a phase 1 study. Lancet Oncol. 2012;13:1011–9. https://doi.org/10.1016/S1470-2045(12)70344-3.
11. Solomon BJ, Mok T, Kim DW, Wu YL, Nakagawa K, Mekhail T, et al. First-line crizotinib versus chemotherapy in ALK-positive lung cancer. N Engl J Med. 2014;371:2167–77. https://doi.org/10.1056/NEJMoa1408440.
12. Shaw AT, Kim DW, Nakagawa K, Seto T, Crinó L, Ahn MJ, et al. Crizotinib versus chemotherapy in advanced ALK-positive lung cancer. N Engl J Med. 2013;368:2385–94. https://doi.org/10.1056/NEJMoa1214886.
13. Rangachari D, Yamaguchi N, VanderLaan PA, Folch E, Mahadevan A, Floyd SR, et al. Brain metastases in patients with EGFR-mutated or ALK-rearranged non-small-cell lung cancers. Lung Cancer. 2015;88:108–11. https://doi.org/10.1016/j.lungcan.2015.01.020.
14. Costa DB, Shaw AT, Ou SH, Solomon BJ, Riely GJ, Ahn MJ, et al. Clinical experience with crizotinib in patients with advanced ALK-rearranged non-small-cell lung cancer and brain metastases. J Clin Oncol. 2015;33:1881–8. https://doi.org/10.1200/JCO.2014.59.0539.
15. Costa DB, Kobayashi S, Pandya SS, Yeo WL, Shen Z, Tan W, et al. CSF concentration of the anaplastic lymphoma kinase inhibitor crizotinib. J Clin Oncol. 2011;29:e443–5. https://doi.org/10.1200/JCO.2010.34.1313.
16. Marsilje TH, Pei W, Chen B, Lu W, Uno T, Jin Y, et al. Synthesis, structure-activity relationships, and in vivo efficacy of the novel potent and selective anaplastic lymphoma kinase (ALK) inhibitor 5-chloro-N2-(2-isopropoxy-5-methyl-4-(piperidin-4-yl)phenyl)-N4-(2-

(isopropylsulfonyl)phenyl)pyrimidine-2,4-diamine (LDK378) currently in phase 1 and phase 2 clinical trials. J Med Chem. 2013;56:5675–90. https://doi.org/10.1021/jm400402q.
17. Kim DW, Mehra R, Tan DS, Felip E, Chow LQ, Camidge DR, et al. Activity and safety of ceritinib in patients with ALK-rearranged non-small-cell lung cancer (ASCEND-1): updated results from the multicentre, open-label, phase 1 trial. Lancet Oncol. 2016;17:452–63. https://doi.org/10.1016/S1470-2045(15)00614-2.
18. Crinò L, Ahn MJ, De Marinis F, Groen HJ, Wakelee H, Hida T, et al. Multicenter Phase II study of whole-body and intracranial activity with ceritinib in patients with ALK-rearranged non-small-cell lung cancer previously treated with chemotherapy and crizotinib: results from ASCEND-2. J Clin Oncol. 2016;34:2866–73. https://doi.org/10.1200/JCO.2015.65.5936.
19. Soria JC, Tan DS, Chiari R, Wu YL, Paz-Ares L, Wolf J, et al. First-line ceritinib versus platinum-based chemotherapy in advanced ALK-rearranged non-small-cell lung cancer (ASCEND-4): a randomised, open-label, phase 3 study. Lancet. 2017;389:917–29. https://doi.org/10.1016/S0140-6736(17)30123-X.
20. Toyokawa G, Seto T, Takenoyama M, Ichinose Y. W'ALK' into the next stage. Clin Lung Cancer. 2017;18:122–6. https://doi.org/10.1016/j.cllc.2016.10.005.
21. Seto T, Kiura K, Nishio M, Nakagawa K, Maemondo M, Inoue A, et al. CH5424802 (RO5424802) for patients with ALK-rearranged advanced non-small-cell lung cancer (AF-001JP study): a single-arm, open-label, phase 1-2 study. Lancet Oncol. 2013;14:590–8. https://doi.org/10.1016/S1470-2045(13)70142-6.
22. Gadgeel SM, Gandhi L, Riely GJ, Chiappori AA, West HL, Azada MC, et al. Safety and activity of alectinib against systemic disease and brain metastases in patients with crizotinib-resistant ALK-rearranged non-small-cell lung cancer (AF-002JG): results from the dose-finding portion of a phase 1/2 study. Lancet Oncol. 2014;15:1119–28. https://doi.org/10.1016/S1470-2045(14)70362-6.
23. Ou SH, Ahn JS, De Petris L, Govindan R, Yang JC, Hughes B, et al. Alectinib in crizotinib-refractory ALK-rearranged non-small-cell lung cancer: a phase II global study. J Clin Oncol. 2016;34:661–8. https://doi.org/10.1200/JCO.2015.63.9443.
24. Gettinger SN, Bazhenova LA, Langer CJ, Salgia R, Gold KA, Rosell R, et al. Activity and safety of brigatinib in ALK-rearranged non-small-cell lung cancer and other malignancies: a single-arm, open-label, phase 1/2 trial. Lancet Oncol. 2016;17:1683–96. https://doi.org/10.1016/S1470-2045(16)30392-8.
25. Gainor JF, Dardaei L, Yoda S, Friboulet L, Leshchiner I, Katayama R, et al. Molecular mechanisms of resistance to first- and second-generation ALK inhibitors in ALK-rearranged lung cancer. Cancer Discov. 2016;6(10):1118–33.
26. Johnson TW, Richardson PF, Bailey S, Brooun A, Burke BJ, Collins MR, et al. Discovery of (10R)-7-amino-12-fluoro-2,10,16-trimethyl-15-oxo-10,15,16,17-tetrahydro-2H-8,4-(metheno)pyrazolo[4,3-h][2,5,11]-benzoxadiazacyclotetradecine-3-carbonitrile (PF-06463922), a macrocyclic inhibitor of anaplastic lymphoma kinase (ALK) and c-ros oncogene 1 (ROS1) with preclinical brain exposure and broad-spectrum potency against ALK-resistant mutations. J Med Chem. 2014;57:4720–44. https://doi.org/10.1021/jm500261q.
27. Sandler A, Gray R, Perry MC, Brahmer J, Schiller JH, Dowlati A, et al. Paclitaxel-carboplatin alone or with bevacizumab for non-small-cell lung cancer. N Engl J Med. 2006;355:2542–50.
28. Bradshaw M, Mansfield A, Peikert T. The role of vascular endothelial growth factor in the pathogenesis, diagnosis and treatment of malignant pleural effusion. Curr Oncol Rep. 2013;15:207–16. https://doi.org/10.1007/s11912-013-0315-7.
29. Ilhan-Mutlu A, Osswald M, Liao Y, Gömmel M, Reck M, Miles D, et al. Bevacizumab prevents brain metastases formation in lung adenocarcinoma. Mol Cancer Ther. 2016;15:702–10. https://doi.org/10.1158/1535-7163.MCT-15-0582.
30. Seto T, Kato T, Nishio M, Goto K, Atagi S, Hosomi Y, et al. Erlotinib alone or with bevacizumab as first-line therapy in patients with advanced non-squamous non-small-cell lung cancer harbouring EGFR mutations (JO25567): an open-label, randomised, multicentre, phase 2 study. Lancet Oncol. 2014;15:1236–44. https://doi.org/10.1016/S1470-2045(14)70381-X.

31. Brahmer J, Reckamp KL, Baas P, Crinò L, Eberhardt WE, Poddubskaya E, et al. Nivolumab versus docetaxel in advanced squamous-cell non-small-cell lung cancer. N Engl J Med. 2015;373:123–35. https://doi.org/10.1056/NEJMoa1504627.
32. Garon EB, Rizvi NA, Hui R, Leighl N, Balmanoukian AS, Eder JP, et al. Pembrolizumab for the treatment of non-small-cell lung cancer. N Engl J Med. 2015;372:2018–28. https://doi.org/10.1056/NEJMoa1501824.
33. Herbst RS, Baas P, Kim DW, Felip E, Pérez-Gracia JL, Han JY, et al. Pembrolizumab versus docetaxel for previously treated, PD-L1-positive, advanced non-small-cell lung cancer (KEYNOTE-010): a randomised controlled trial. Lancet. 2016;387:1540–50. https://doi.org/10.1016/S0140-6736(15)01281-7.
34. Gainor JF, Shaw AT, Sequist LV, Fu X, Azzoli CG, Piotrowska Z, et al. EGFR mutations and ALK rearrangements are associated with low response rates to PD-1 pathway blockade in non-small cell lung cancer: a retrospective analysis. Clin Cancer Res. 2016;22:4585–93. https://doi.org/10.1158/1078-0432.CCR-15-3101.
35. Ota K, Azuma K, Kawahara A, Hattori S, Iwama E, Tanizaki J, et al. Induction of PD-L1 expression by the EML4-ALK oncoprotein and downstream signaling pathways in non-small cell lung cancer. Clin Cancer Res. 2015;21:4014–21. https://doi.org/10.1158/1078-0432.CCR-15-0016.
36. Shaw AT, Ou SH, Bang YJ, Camidge DR, Solomon BJ, Salgia R, et al. Crizotinib in ROS1-rearranged non-small-cell lung cancer. N Engl J Med. 2014;371:1963–71. https://doi.org/10.1056/NEJMoa1406766.
37. Yoh K, Seto T, Satouchi M, Nishio M, Yamamoto N, Murakami H, et al. Vandetanib in patients with previously treated RET-rearranged advanced non-small-cell lung cancer (LURET): an open-label, multicentre phase 2 trial. Lancet Respir Med. 2017;5:42–50. https://doi.org/10.1016/S2213-2600(16)30322-8.
38. Zugazagoitia J, Molina-Pinelo S, Lopez-Rios F, Paz-Ares L. Biological therapies in nonsmall cell lung cancer. Eur Respir J. 2017;49. pii: 1601520. https://doi.org/10.1183/13993003.01520-2016.
39. Paik PK, Drilon A, Fan PD, Yu H, Rekhtman N, Ginsberg MS. Response to MET inhibitors in patients with stage IV lung adenocarcinomas harboring MET mutations causing exon 14 skipping. Cancer Discov. 2015;5:842–9. https://doi.org/10.1158/2159-8290.CD-14-1467.
40. Planchard D, Kim TM, Mazieres J, Quoix E, Riely G, Barlesi F, et al. Dabrafenib in patients with BRAF(V600E)-positive advanced non-small-cell lung cancer: a single-arm, multicentre, open-label, phase 2 trial. Lancet Oncol. 2016;17:642–50. https://doi.org/10.1016/S1470-2045(16)00077-2.
41. Planchard D, Besse B, Groen HJ, Souquet PJ, Quoix E, Baik CS, et al. Dabrafenib plus trametinib in patients with previously treated BRAF(V600E)-mutant metastatic non-small cell lung cancer: an open-label, multicentre phase 2 trial. Lancet Oncol. 2016;17:984–93. https://doi.org/10.1016/S1470-2045(16)30146-2.
42. Mazières J, Barlesi F, Filleron T, Besse B, Monnet I, Beau-Faller M, et al. Lung cancer patients with HER2 mutations treated with chemotherapy and HER2-targeted drugs: results from the European EUHER2 cohort. Ann Oncol. 2016;27:281–6. https://doi.org/10.1093/annonc/mdv573.
43. Kris MG, Camidge DR, Giaccone G, Hida T, Li BT, O'Connell J, et al. Targeting HER2 aberrations as actionable drivers in lung cancers: phase II trial of the pan-HER tyrosine kinase inhibitor dacomitinib in patients with HER2-mutant or amplified tumors. Ann Oncol. 2015;26(7):1421. https://doi.org/10.1093/annonc/mdv186.

Part IV
Current Topics

Chapter 17
Application of High-Throughput Technologies in Personal Genomics: How Is the Progress in Personal Genome Service?

Kaoru Mogushi, Yasuhiro Murakawa, and Hideya Kawaji

Abstract The advent of high-throughput profiling technologies, in particular next-generation sequencing, has revolutionized our genomic studies and provided unprecedented insights into the human diseases. The use of genetic testing in the clinical settings has grown substantially and has now entered medical practice around the world. Here we provide an overview of recent advances in various high-throughput methods for genomic and functional genomic analyses. Next we review recent findings in genomics, ranging from single nucleotide polymorphisms associated with respiratory diseases and genomic alterations in lung cancers to aberrant gene expressions in lung diseases. Finally, we summarize the current status of clinical sequencing efforts and further describe challenges in the clinical implementation of personal genomic medicine. We anticipate increase in the use of clinical sequencing, which require sufficient resource of computation to interpret large genomic datasets in a clinical laboratory. It is also crucial to extend existing

K. Mogushi
Intractable Disease Research Center, Juntendo University Graduate School of Medicine, Tokyo, Japan

Preventive Medicine and Applied Genomics Unit, RIKEN Center for Integrative Medical Sciences, Yokohama, Kanagawa, Japan

Y. Murakawa (✉)
RIKEN Preventive Medicine and Diagnosis Innovation Program, Yokohama, Kanagawa, Japan

RIKEN-HMC Clinical Omics Unit, Riken Baton Zone Program, Yokohama, Kanagawa, Japan
e-mail: yasuhiro.murakawa@riken.jp

H. Kawaji
Preventive Medicine and Applied Genomics Unit, RIKEN Center for Integrative Medical Sciences, Yokohama, Kanagawa, Japan

RIKEN Preventive Medicine and Diagnosis Innovation Program, Yokohama, Kanagawa, Japan

T. Kaneko (ed.), *Clinical Relevance of Genetic Factors in Pulmonary Diseases*, Respiratory Disease Series: Diagnostic Tools and Disease Managements, https://doi.org/10.1007/978-981-10-8144-6_17

electronic medical record systems so that we can interact with genomic data and make full use of personal genomic information. Furthermore, standardization of genomic data is also necessary for the efficient exchange of patients' genomes between hospitals.

Keywords Next-generation sequencing · Personal genomics · Clinical sequencing

17.1 Introduction

High-throughput profiling of the genomic landscape provides unprecedented opportunities to understand human diseases. Of particular importance, the use of genetic testing using next-generation sequencing (NGS) in the clinical settings has grown substantially over the last years around the world. This review provides an overview of the state-of-the-art technologies as well as recent genomic findings based on these technologies. We summarize the current status of clinical sequencing efforts and further describe challenges in the clinical implementation of genomic medicine.

17.2 Recent Advances in Omics Technologies

Comprehensive profiling of the genomic landscape provides unprecedented opportunities to understand the cellular mechanisms that underlie diseases. From the early to mid-1990s, DNA microarray technology was developed and has since been widely used in numerous research fields including molecular biology, medical biology, pharmacology, and agricultural science. DNA microarray is a high-throughput method for quantitation of nucleic acids by hybridization of oligonucleotides or cDNA probes spotted on a solid surface such as glass or plastic slides. One of the main uses of DNA microarray is to quantitate expressed mRNA in cells or tissues; another popular use is the detection of single nucleotide polymorphisms (SNPs) by designing probe sequences for each genotype in a target allele.

The next-generation sequencers have revolutionized genomic studies by enabling us to profile dozens of genes (panel sequencing), all exons (WXS, whole exome sequencing), or the entire genome (WGS, whole genome sequencing), and sequencing costs have decreased dramatically (by more than four orders of magnitude) over the last 10 years. Panel sequencing, that is, profiling a limited set of alternations related to diseases, is now widely employed. WXS extends the opportunity to uncover the contribution of an entire set of genes to various diseases. Of note, many alterations genetically associated with diseases are located outside of the protein-coding genes, which underlines the importance of WGS for our understanding of non-exonic regions. Furthermore, technological developments have enabled us to obtain molecular profiles that could not previously be assessed (Fig. 17.1). One

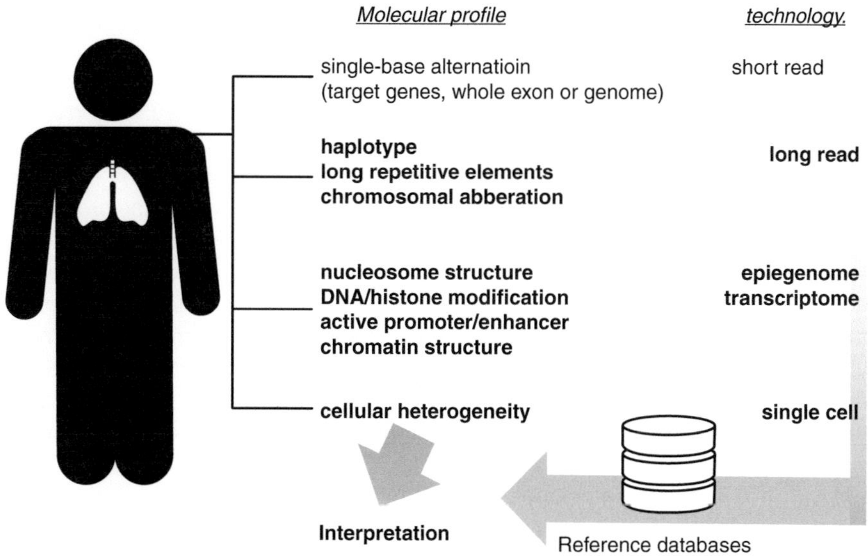

Fig. 17.1 An overview of recent technological advances

major direction of development is the extension of read length. The "short-read" next-generation sequencers currently used can determine several hundred base pairs at most, which is inadequate to capture all of our genome complexities, such as haplotype, long repetitive elements, and chromosomal aberrations, despite their impact on diseases. "Long-read" technologies have been developed to overcome this limitation. For example, single-molecule real-time sequencing (by Pacific Biosciences) and nanopore-based sequencing (by Oxford Nanopore), as well as synthetic long reading (by Illumina) and linked reading (by 10× Genomics), have increased read length by two to three orders of magnitude [1].

Another developmental direction of this technology is to obtain functional information about genomic regions, in particular non-protein-coding regions. Interpretation of genomic alterations requires assessment of their effects, and the contribution of non-coding regions to cellular functions, and subsequent traits, is still a challenging problem particularly in a clinical context. DNA methylation profiles can be obtained using bisulfite-sequencing (BS-seq) at a single-base resolution by sequencing DNAs where unmethylated cytosines are converted to uracils [2]. Chromatin accessibility and nucleosome structure, which provide the physical space for gene regulation, can be monitored with footprinting by using MNase (MNase-seq), DNaseI (DNase-seq), and transposase (ATAC-seq) [3]. Histone modification and transcription factor binding sites can be assessed with ChIP-seq, by sequencing DNAs that interact with proteins recognized by specific antibodies [4], whereas higher-resolution profiles can be obtained by digesting unbound DNAs with exonucleases. Although epigenomic profiling from formalin-fixed paraffin-embedded (FFPE) tissues has been a challenge, several protocols have been developed to assess FFPE samples (bisulfite-sequencing [5], DNaseI sequencing [6], and

ChIP-seq [7]). The gene regulatory machinery acts at the proximal region of transcription initiation sites (promoters), regulating the transcription of DNA segments into RNA molecules. These regulatory regions can be identified by examining the transcribed RNAs, particularly their 5′ ends. Interestingly, distal regulatory regions (enhancers) also produce RNAs in a bi-directional manner. CAGE (cap analysis of gene expression) monitors the frequency of transcription initiation by counting 5′-capped ends of RNA molecules. It has been effectively used to define promoters and enhancers across the human genome in broad ranges of cell types [8, 9]. Furthermore, profiling of chromatin interactions between cis- and distal-regulatory regions (promoters and enhancers) can be achieved with a technology called chromosome conformation capture by examining ligated DNA fragments that share close physical proximity [10]. Hi-C is a protocol that targets the entire genome through high-throughput sequencing; however, its resolution is not sufficiently high to focus on individual regulatory regions. Employment of a process to enrich genomic regions of interest before sequencing is effective to increase the resolution. ChIA-PET (Chromatin Interaction Analysis by Paired-End Tag Sequencing), combination of immunoprecipitation with chromosomal conformation capture, can identify interactions mediated by a specific protein of interest. Recently, a unique approach was proposed to study chromatin interaction, termed genome architecture mapping or GAM [11], which monitors the frequencies of DNA segments co-occurring in a single slice of a single cell without relying on ligation.

The last developmental direction we should mention is the effort to reduce the amount of sample required to a single cell or even single nuclei. All of the above technologies require a certain amount of "bulk" cells and assume that the samples are homogenous or predominantly contain a single cell type. They are unable to obtain accurate profiles from minor but important cells, such as tumor stem and progenitor cells that reside in a "niche." Manipulation of individual cells with manual operation, cell sorter, or specialized microfluidic devices [12] that rely on valves, droplets, and nanowells may facilitate genome [13], epigenome [14], and transcriptome [15] monitoring at the single-cell level.

The "omics" technologies have not only provided a means to examine patient specimens to obtain a precise understanding of the cellular mechanisms underlying individual diseases, but they have also produced a wealth of reference information from animal models, cultured cells, and reference samples, including cells obtained from healthy and patient donors. Extensive efforts have been made to compile these data into databases, which will facilitate their use for clinical interpretation of patient data, for example, evaluating the impact of genomic alterations in noncoding regions. In addition to compiled datasets of SNPs genetically associated with traits (GWAS catalog [16], GWASdb [17]) and a curated archive of relationships among genomic variations and phenotypes (ClinVar [18]), genomic data obtained from cancer patients (GDC [19], COSMIC [20]) and cancer cell lines (CCLE [21]) will provide direct insights into diseases. Genomic data obtained from healthy donors, in particular information on genome variation provided by population-scale genome sequencing [22, 23]; epigenetic marks provided by the international epigenome consortium (IHEC [24], BLUEPRINT [25]), including roadmap epigenomics [26];

and transcriptome profiles of individual cell types provided by the FANTOM5 project [8, 9, 27] will be of enormous value to understand genomic function underlying cells of disease state.

17.3 Impact of Genomic Analysis on Respiratory Diseases

17.3.1 SNPs Associated with Respiratory Diseases

The emergence and evolution of SNP array technology has enabled researchers to determine hundreds of thousands of SNPs in single experiments in a cost-effective manner (e.g., several hundred US dollars for an analysis of SNPs in an individual, depending on the type of assay used). A number of large studies of SNP frequencies using SNP arrays, called genome-wide association studies, have been conducted in the last decade. Furthermore, commercial genotyping services such as 23andMe and Pathway Genomics provide predicted risk reports based on individual's genotypes. NGS technology is another method to obtain personal genome information. While an SNP array can only determine genotypes at predesigned alleles, NGS directly analyzes the DNA sequence on the genome (e.g., via WXS and WGS, as discussed in the previous section). One of the largest differences between SNP array and NGS-based analysis is that NGS can capture rare variants (single nucleotide variants, SNVs) or novel mutations (e.g., non-synonymous mutations, mutations in splicing sites or promoter regions, insertions, and deletions) for both germline and somatic mutations. Furthermore, the cost of WGS has dramatically reduced in recent years: from 100 million US dollars in 2001 to 1000 US dollars in 2015 (https://www.genome.gov/sequencingcosts/). However, WGS yields a huge amount of sequence data (50–100 gigabytes) for each individual, and interpretation of a variant of uncertain significance (VUS) is still a daunting task. Recent advances in bioinformatics have provided tools to predict the pathogenicity of a VUS, which helps researchers and physicians to interpret SNVs in an individual. In the following, we overview the recent progress in genomic studies of respiratory diseases. Several GWAS projects have identified SNPs strongly associated with chronic obstructive pulmonary disease (COPD), lung cancer, asthma, idiopathic pulmonary fibrosis (IPF), and other respiratory diseases.

17.3.1.1 SNPs Associated with COPD

Emphysema and COPD are strongly associated with alpha-1 antitrypsin deficiency (AATD or A1AD). AATD is frequently caused by a germline mutation in the alpha-1 antitrypsin gene [AAT; the official gene symbol is serpin family A member 1 (SERPINA1) according to the HUGO Gene Nomenclature Committee] [28]. Genetic polymorphisms in glutathione S-transferase mu 1 (GSTM1) and epoxide hydrolase 1 (EPHX1) are also risk factors for COPD [29, 30]. Recent GWAS studies identified an association between COPD and gene variants in the 15q25 region, which includes the genes for nicotinic acetylcholine receptor subunits (CHRNA5, CHRNA3, and CHRNB4) [31]; hedgehog interacting protein (HHIP) [32]; eukaryotic elongation factor, selenocysteine-tRNA specific (EEFSEC); desmoplakin (DSP); microtubule cross-linking factor 1 (MTCL1); and surfactant protein D (SFTPD) [33].

17.3.1.2 SNPs Associated with Lung Cancer

Although hereditary lung cancer is rare, germline mutation of T790 M in epidermal growth factor receptor (EGFR) was reported in a family with non-small cell lung cancer [34]. Three novel loci (rs7086803 in 10q25.2, rs9387478 in 6q22.2, and rs2395185 in 6p21.32) were associated with lung cancer in never-smoking women in Asia, and four loci (rs2853677 in 5p15.33 and rs10937405 in 3q28, as well as rs7216064 in 17q24.3 and rs3817963 in 6p21.3) were associated with lung cancer in the Japanese population [35].

In lung cancer treatment, irinotecan (CPT-11) is often used as an antitumor agent but is known to cause adverse effects such as neutropenia and delayed diarrhea. The frequency of these adverse effects is reportedly associated with the uridine diphosphate glucuronosyltransferase 1A1 (UGT1A1) genotype of the patient. UGT1A1 has two major genotypes, *6 and *28, that are associated with decreased glucuronidation of irinotecan and a higher risk of hematologic toxicity and severe diarrhea. Dose adjustment is recommended for patients with the UGT1A1*6 or UGT1A1*28 genotype.

17.3.1.3 SNPs Associated with Asthma and Allergic Disease

Asthma and allergic disease have a strong relationship, and they have common and distinct etiologies [36]. A meta-analysis of several GWAS of asthma in the North American population identified several loci, such as 17q21 near interleukin 1 receptor-like 1 (IL1RL1), thymic stromal lymphopoietin (TSLP), and interleukin 33 (IL33), as well as pyrin and HIN domain family member 1(PYHIN1), that were associated with asthma [37]. Another GWAS analysis suggested that loci in 4q31 (USP38-GAB1), 10p14, and 12q13 as well as 5q22 (TSLP/WDR36) and 6p21 (MHC class III region) were significantly associated with asthma in the Japanese population [38]. Furthermore, 11 genes including zinc finger and BTB domain containing 10 (ZBTB10) and C-type lectin domain containing 16A (CLEC16A) are reportedly associated with the risk of having asthma with hay fever [39].

17.3.1.4 SNPs Associated with IPF

Genetic studies have revealed that germline mutations in surfactant protein A2 (SFTPA2) [40] and C (SFTPC) [41], telomerase RNA component (TERC), and telomerase reverse transcriptase (TERT) [42] may be the underlying cause of IPF

[43]. A recent GWAS study showed that variants in the TOLLIP, MUC5B, MDGA2, and SPPL2C loci were strongly associated with IPF in the United States [44]. Furthermore, an SNP in intron 2 of the TERT gene (rs2736100) has been shown to be associated with IPF in the Japanese population [45].

17.3.2 Somatic Point Mutations in Lung Cancer

Somatic point mutations in lung cancers have been studied by means of high-throughput NGS analysis. A whole genome sequencing study revealed thousands of somatic point mutations in non-small cell lung cancer, with an average mutation frequency much higher in smokers than in never-smokers. Importantly, many genes that were potentially targetable with drugs were found to be mutated [46]. More recently, a whole genome sequencing analysis was performed in small-cell lung cancer, which showed that genes involved in several key biological processes were mutated, thereby identifying candidate therapeutic targets [47].

17.3.3 Genomic Rearrangements in Lung Cancers

The advent of NGS has enabled us to detect genomic rearrangements and has thus revolutionized the field of lung cancer genomic research by revealing a number of novel drug targets. Genomic translocation can underlie lung cancer development through the expression of fusion transcripts with oncogenic properties. Importantly, identification of these fusion transcripts can provide novel therapeutic candidates. The EML4-ALK fusion gene was first reported in non-small cell lung cancer by Soda et al. in 2007 [48]. Crizotinib, which was approved by the FDA in 2011, shows promising efficacy in the treatment of EML4-ALK-positive lung cancer by inhibiting the constitutively activated ALK kinase [49]. In recent years, RNA-seq has been employed to identify fusion transcripts on a genome-wide scale and has successfully detected a number of novel gene fusions [50]. Various computational tools have been developed to detect fusion transcripts from RNA-seq data, and attempts have been made to compare the performance of available software packages [51].

17.3.4 Utility of CAGE in Lung Cancer Diagnostics

In addition to genomic rearrangements and point mutations, aberrant gene activations in disease states can also be used for clinical diagnostics and treatment. One example is aberrant promoter activities in lung cancer, as measured by CAGE. CAGE is a method that can quantify promoter activities genome-wide by using NGS to determine the 5′ ends of capped RNAs. A recent study, in which CAGE analysis was performed on 97 frozen tissues from surgically resected lung cancers [22 squamous cell carcinoma (SCC) and 75 adenocarcinoma (AD)], identified two novel marker candidates, the SPATS2 promoter for SCC and the ST6GALNAC1 promoter for AD [52]. This finding will contribute to a more accurate diagnosis of lung cancer, which is an important step toward precision medicine for this disease.

17.4 Challenges in the Clinical Implementation of Genomic Medicine

17.4.1 Clinical Use and Interpretation

As mentioned in the previous sections, recent studies in genomic research have revealed many SNPs and SNVs associated with respiratory diseases. Well-known germline mutations in combination with common risk alleles found by GWAS can be used to diagnose specific diseases. Several genetic tests are being made available for clinical use in respiratory diseases. Conventional techniques (i.e., polymerase chain reaction-restriction fragment length polymorphism (PCR-RFLP), PCR invader assay, TaqMan PCR, and capillary sequencing) can still be used for this purpose if the number of target genes is limited.

Genetic tests based on targeted gene panels using NGS are being developed. In target gene resequencing, regions in the genomic DNA are selectively amplified using specific primers designed for the genes of interest. The obtained mixture of amplicons is analyzed by NGS to examine SNPs and SNVs in the target genes. In addition, DNA from multiple patients can be analyzed in a single sequencing run by adding "index" DNA sequences for multiplexing and demultiplexing each sample. MiSeq (Illumina) and Ion Torrent Personal Genome Machine Ion PGM (Thermo Fisher Scientific) are suitable for such target gene resequencing. For example, the Laboratory for Molecular Medicine at Partners HealthCare provides "PulmoGene Panel Tests" for comprehensive genetic testing for hereditary lung disease (8 genes for cystic lung disease, 17 genes for bronchiectasis, 12 genes for basic fibrosis, 21 genes for Hermansky–Pudlak syndrome, 5 genes for pulmonary hypertension, and 6 genes for central hypoventilation syndrome) [53]. Similarly, The DNA Diagnostic Laboratory at Johns Hopkins Medicine offers a "Comprehensive Diffuse Lung Disease NGS Panel." For hereditary lung cancer, Blueprint Genetics provides the "Hereditary Lung Cancer Panel" for targeted resequencing of EGFR, breast cancer 2 (BRCA2), cyclin-dependent kinase inhibitor 2A (CDKN2, also known as p16), and tumor protein p53 (TP53).

Therefore, SNPs and SNVs that are strongly associated with hereditary lung diseases can be screened for by using target gene resequencing at relatively low cost. However, patients without candidate SNVs in the target genes may nonetheless have a novel mutation for a disease. WXS or WGS might be helpful to further screen for possible pathogenic mutations, and the knowledge obtained would help to improve the diagnosis of hereditary lung diseases.

17.4.2 Implementation of Genomic Databases for Clinical Use

Genetic tests performed by NGS typically produce a huge amount of raw and processed data (about 100 MB–100 GB, depending on the type of sequencing strategy and data used). These data are not directly interpreted by a physician, but future reanalysis of the data with improved software and a genetic database would be beneficial for patients. Therefore, sufficient storage devices to handle large genomic datasets would be needed in a clinical laboratory.

In addition, most genetic testing services provide text-based reports for candidate pathogenic SNVs as well as information on VUS so that physicians can interpret the significance of the mutations. These reports can be stored in an existing electronic medical record (EMR) system. However, it is sometimes difficult to search the contents of the reports if they are imported into the EMR as a scanned image such as a Portable Document Format (PDF) file. Therefore, an extension of existing EMR systems specifically to handle genomic data would be important to make full use of personal genomic information (Fig. 17.2).

Standardization of genomic data is also necessary for the efficient exchange of patients' genomes between hospitals. One approach is the Electronic Medical Records and Genomics (eMERGE) Network in the United States [54]. The eMERGE Network consists of the following cohorts who provided written informed consent: approximately 20,000 participants in the Marshfield Clinic Personalized Medicine Research Project biobank, 1687 cases from the Mayo biobank, about 10,000 participants in the Northwestern University biorepository, 3793 participants in the Group Health biobank, and 75,000 patients in the Vanderbilt biobank. Such large networks have the potential to improve clinical care and discover novel findings in genomic medicine, including respiratory diseases.

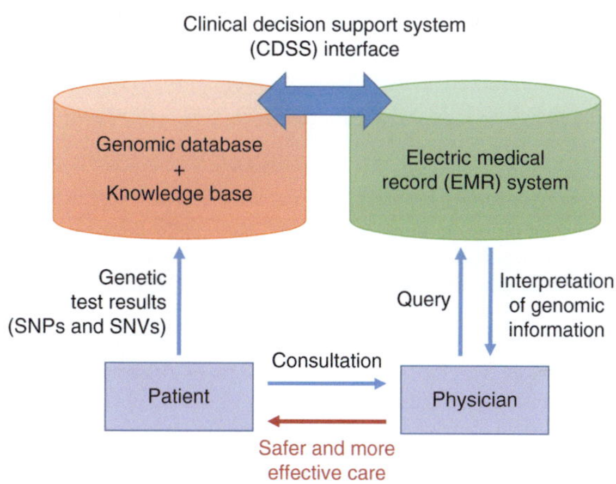

Fig. 17.2 A schematic diagram of relationship between electronic medical record (EMR) system and genomic database

17.5 Conclusion

Various technological advances in high-throughput sequencing methods have provided unprecedented insights into the genomic and functional genomic information underlying diseases. Of particular importance, genetic testing for clinical applications has now entered medical practice around the world, and we anticipate increase in the use of clinical sequencing. To further facilitate the use of genetic testing in the clinical settings, sufficient storage devices to handle large genomic datasets would be needed in a clinical laboratory. In addition, an extension of existing EMR systems specifically to handle genomic data would be crucial to make full use of personal genomic information. Furthermore, standardization of genomic data is also necessary for the efficient exchange of patients' genomes between hospitals.

References

1. Goodwin S, McPherson JD, McCombie WR. Coming of age: ten years of next-generation sequencing technologies. Nat Rev Genet. 2016;17(6):333–51. https://doi.org/10.1038/nrg.2016.49.
2. Krueger F, Kreck B, Franke A, Andrews SR. DNA methylome analysis using short bisulfite sequencing data. Nat Methods. 2012;9(2):145–51. https://doi.org/10.1038/nmeth.1828.
3. Zentner GE, Henikoff S. High-resolution digital profiling of the epigenome. Nat Rev Genet. 2014;15(12):814–27. https://doi.org/10.1038/nrg3798.
4. Furey TS. ChIP-seq and beyond: new and improved methodologies to detect and characterize protein-DNA interactions. Nat Rev Genet. 2012;13(12):840–52. https://doi.org/10.1038/nrg3306.
5. Gu H, Smith ZD, Bock C, Boyle P, Gnirke A, Meissner A. Preparation of reduced representation bisulfite sequencing libraries for genome-scale DNA methylation profiling. Nat Protoc. 2011;6(4):468–81. https://doi.org/10.1038/nprot.2010.190.
6. Jin W, Tang Q, Wan M, Cui K, Zhang Y, Ren G, et al. Genome-wide detection of DNase I hypersensitive sites in single cells and FFPE tissue samples. Nature. 2015;528(7580):142–6. https://doi.org/10.1038/nature15740.
7. Cejas P, Li L, O'Neill NK, Duarte M, Rao P, Bowden M, et al. Chromatin immunoprecipitation from fixed clinical tissues reveals tumor-specific enhancer profiles. Nat Med. 2016;22(6):685–91. https://doi.org/10.1038/nm.4085.
8. Consortium F, the RP, ClST, Forrest AR, Kawaji H, Rehli M, et al. A promoter-level mammalian expression atlas. Nature. 2014;507(7493):462–70. https://doi.org/10.1038/nature13182.
9. Andersson R, Gebhard C, Miguel-Escalada I, Hoof I, Bornholdt J, Boyd M, et al. An atlas of active enhancers across human cell types and tissues. Nature. 2014;507(7493):455–61. https://doi.org/10.1038/nature12787.
10. Schmitt AD, Hu M, Ren B. Genome-wide mapping and analysis of chromosome architecture. Nat Rev Mol Cell Biol. 2016;17(12):743–55. https://doi.org/10.1038/nrm.2016.104.
11. Beagrie RA, Scialdone A, Schueler M, Kraemer DC, Chotalia M, Xie SQ, et al. Complex multi-enhancer contacts captured by genome architecture mapping. Nature. 2017;543(7646):519–24. https://doi.org/10.1038/nature21411.
12. Prakadan SM, Shalek AK, Weitz DA. Scaling by shrinking: empowering single-cell 'omics' with microfluidic devices. Nat Rev Genet. 2017;18(6):345–61. https://doi.org/10.1038/nrg.2017.15.

13. Gawad C, Koh W, Quake SR. Single-cell genome sequencing: current state of the science. Nat Rev Genet. 2016;17(3):175–88. https://doi.org/10.1038/nrg.2015.16.
14. Clark SJ, Lee HJ, Smallwood SA, Kelsey G, Reik W. Single-cell epigenomics: powerful new methods for understanding gene regulation and cell identity. Genome Biol. 2016;17:72. https://doi.org/10.1186/s13059-016-0944-x.
15. Ziegenhain C, Vieth B, Parekh S, Reinius B, Guillaumet-Adkins A, Smets M, et al. Comparative analysis of single-cell RNA sequencing methods. Mol Cell. 2017;65(4):631–43. e4. https://doi.org/10.1016/j.molcel.2017.01.023.
16. Welter D, MacArthur J, Morales J, Burdett T, Hall P, Junkins H, et al. The NHGRI GWAS catalog, a curated resource of SNP-trait associations. Nucleic Acids Res. 2014;42(Database issue):D1001–6. https://doi.org/10.1093/nar/gkt1229.
17. Li MJ, Wang P, Liu X, Lim EL, Wang Z, Yeager M, et al. GWASdb: a database for human genetic variants identified by genome-wide association studies. Nucleic Acids Res. 2012;40(Database issue):D1047–54. https://doi.org/10.1093/nar/gkr1182.
18. Landrum MJ, Lee JM, Benson M, Brown G, Chao C, Chitipiralla S, et al. ClinVar: public archive of interpretations of clinically relevant variants. Nucleic Acids Res. 2016;44(D1):D862–8. https://doi.org/10.1093/nar/gkv1222.
19. Grossman RL, Heath AP, Ferretti V, Varmus HE, Lowy DR, Kibbe WA, et al. Toward a shared vision for cancer genomic data. N Engl J Med. 2016;375(12):1109–12. https://doi.org/10.1056/NEJMp1607591.
20. Forbes SA, Beare D, Bindal N, Bamford S, Ward S, Cole CG, et al. COSMIC: high-resolution cancer genetics using the catalogue of somatic mutations in cancer. Curr Protoc Hum Genet. 2016;91:10 1 1–1 37. https://doi.org/10.1002/cphg.21.
21. Barretina J, Caponigro G, Stransky N, Venkatesan K, Margolin AA, Kim S, et al. The cancer cell line encyclopedia enables predictive modelling of anticancer drug sensitivity. Nature. 2012;483(7391):603–7. https://doi.org/10.1038/nature11003.
22. Genomes Project C, Abecasis GR, Altshuler D, Auton A, Brooks LD, Durbin RM, et al. A map of human genome variation from population-scale sequencing. Nature. 2010;467(7319):1061–73. https://doi.org/10.1038/nature09534.
23. Gudbjartsson DF, Helgason H, Gudjonsson SA, Zink F, Oddson A, Gylfason A, et al. Large-scale whole-genome sequencing of the Icelandic population. Nat Genet. 2015;47(5):435–44. https://doi.org/10.1038/ng.3247.
24. Bujold D, Morais DA, Gauthier C, Cote C, Caron M, Kwan T, et al. The international human Epigenome consortium data portal. Cell Syst. 2016;3(5):496–9. e2. https://doi.org/10.1016/j.cels.2016.10.019.
25. Fernandez JM, de la Torre V, Richardson D, Royo R, Puiggros M, Moncunill V, et al. The BLUEPRINT data analysis portal. Cell Syst. 2016;3(5):491–5. e5. https://doi.org/10.1016/j.cels.2016.10.021.
26. Roadmap Epigenomics C, Kundaje A, Meuleman W, Ernst J, Bilenky M, Yen A, et al. Integrative analysis of 111 reference human epigenomes. Nature 2015;518(7539):317–330. doi:https://doi.org/10.1038/nature14248.
27. Hon CC, Ramilowski JA, Harshbarger J, Bertin N, Rackham OJ, Gough J, et al. An atlas of human long non-coding RNAs with accurate 5′ ends. Nature. 2017;543(7644):199–204. https://doi.org/10.1038/nature21374.
28. Stoller JK, Aboussouan LS. Alpha1-antitrypsin deficiency. Lancet. 2005;365(9478):2225–36. https://doi.org/10.1016/S0140-6736(05)66781-5.
29. Cheng SL, Yu CJ, Chen CJ, Yang PC. Genetic polymorphism of epoxide hydrolase and glutathione S-transferase in COPD. Eur Respir J. 2004;23(6):818–24.
30. Smith CA, Harrison DJ. Association between polymorphism in gene for microsomal epoxide hydrolase and susceptibility to emphysema. Lancet. 1997;350(9078):630–3. https://doi.org/10.1016/S0140-6736(96)08061-0.
31. Hung RJ, McKay JD, Gaborieau V, Boffetta P, Hashibe M, Zaridze D, et al. A susceptibility locus for lung cancer maps to nicotinic acetylcholine receptor subunit genes on 15q25. Nature. 2008;452(7187):633–7. https://doi.org/10.1038/nature06885.

32. Pillai SG, Ge D, Zhu G, Kong X, Shianna KV, Need AC, et al. A genome-wide association study in chronic obstructive pulmonary disease (COPD): identification of two major susceptibility loci. PLoS Genet. 2009;5(3):e1000421. https://doi.org/10.1371/journal.pgen.1000421.
33. Hobbs BD, de Jong K, Lamontagne M, Bosse Y, Shrine N, Artigas MS, et al. Genetic loci associated with chronic obstructive pulmonary disease overlap with loci for lung function and pulmonary fibrosis. Nat Genet. 2017;49(3):426–32. https://doi.org/10.1038/ng.3752.
34. Bell DW, Gore I, Okimoto RA, Godin-Heymann N, Sordella R, Mulloy R, et al. Inherited susceptibility to lung cancer may be associated with the T790M drug resistance mutation in EGFR. Nat Genet. 2005;37(12):1315–6. https://doi.org/10.1038/ng1671.
35. Shiraishi K, Kunitoh H, Daigo Y, Takahashi A, Goto K, Sakamoto H, et al. A genome-wide association study identifies two new susceptibility loci for lung adenocarcinoma in the Japanese population. Nat Genet. 2012;44(8):900–3. https://doi.org/10.1038/ng.2353.
36. Ober C, Yao TC. The genetics of asthma and allergic disease: a 21st century perspective. Immunol Rev. 2011;242(1):10–30. https://doi.org/10.1111/j.1600-065X.2011.01029.x.
37. Torgerson DG, Ampleford EJ, Chiu GY, Gauderman WJ, Gignoux CR, Graves PE, et al. Meta-analysis of genome-wide association studies of asthma in ethnically diverse North American populations. Nat Genet. 2011;43(9):887–92. https://doi.org/10.1038/ng.888.
38. Hirota T, Takahashi A, Kubo M, Tsunoda T, Tomita K, Doi S, et al. Genome-wide association study identifies three new susceptibility loci for adult asthma in the Japanese population. Nat Genet. 2011;43(9):893–6. https://doi.org/10.1038/ng.887.
39. Ferreira MA, Matheson MC, Tang CS, Granell R, Ang W, Hui J, et al. Genome-wide association analysis identifies 11 risk variants associated with the asthma with hay fever phenotype. J Allergy Clin Immunol. 2014;133(6):1564–71. https://doi.org/10.1016/j.jaci.2013.10.030.
40. Wang Y, Kuan PJ, Xing C, Cronkhite JT, Torres F, Rosenblatt RL, et al. Genetic defects in surfactant protein A2 are associated with pulmonary fibrosis and lung cancer. Am J Hum Genet. 2009;84(1):52–9. https://doi.org/10.1016/j.ajhg.2008.11.010.
41. Nogee LM, Dunbar AE 3rd, Wert SE, Askin F, Hamvas A, Whitsett JA. A mutation in the surfactant protein C gene associated with familial interstitial lung disease. N Engl J Med. 2001;344(8):573–9. https://doi.org/10.1056/NEJM200102223440805.
42. Armanios MY, Chen JJ, Cogan JD, Alder JK, Ingersoll RG, Markin C, et al. Telomerase mutations in families with idiopathic pulmonary fibrosis. N Engl J Med. 2007;356(13):1317–26. https://doi.org/10.1056/NEJMoa066157.
43. Kropski JA, Lawson WE, Young LR, Blackwell TS. Genetic studies provide clues on the pathogenesis of idiopathic pulmonary fibrosis. Dis Model Mech. 2013;6(1):9–17. https://doi.org/10.1242/dmm.010736.
44. Noth I, Zhang Y, Ma SF, Flores C, Barber M, Huang Y, et al. Genetic variants associated with idiopathic pulmonary fibrosis susceptibility and mortality: a genome-wide association study. Lancet Respir Med. 2013;1(4):309–17. https://doi.org/10.1016/S2213-2600(13)70045-6.
45. Mushiroda T, Wattanapokayakit S, Takahashi A, Nukiwa T, Kudoh S, Ogura T, et al. A genome-wide association study identifies an association of a common variant in TERT with susceptibility to idiopathic pulmonary fibrosis. J Med Genet. 2008;45(10):654–6. https://doi.org/10.1136/jmg.2008.057356.
46. Govindan R, Ding L, Griffith M, Subramanian J, Dees ND, Kanchi KL, et al. Genomic landscape of non-small cell lung cancer in smokers and never-smokers. Cell. 2012;150(6):1121–34. https://doi.org/10.1016/j.cell.2012.08.024.
47. George J, Lim JS, Jang SJ, Cun Y, Ozretic L, Kong G, et al. Comprehensive genomic profiles of small cell lung cancer. Nature. 2015;524(7563):47–53. https://doi.org/10.1038/nature14664.
48. Soda M, Choi YL, Enomoto M, Takada S, Yamashita Y, Ishikawa S, et al. Identification of the transforming EML4-ALK fusion gene in non-small-cell lung cancer. Nature. 2007;448(7153):561–6. https://doi.org/10.1038/nature05945.
49. Awad MM, Shaw ATALK. Inhibitors in non-small cell lung cancer: crizotinib and beyond. Clin Adv Hematol Oncol. 2014;12(7):429–39.

50. Fernandez-Cuesta L, Sun R, Menon R, George J, Lorenz S, Meza-Zepeda LA, et al. Identification of novel fusion genes in lung cancer using breakpoint assembly of transcriptome sequencing data. Genome Biol. 2015;16:7. https://doi.org/10.1186/s13059-014-0558-0.
51. Kumar S, Vo AD, Qin F, Li H. Comparative assessment of methods for the fusion transcripts detection from RNA-Seq data. Sci Rep. 2016;6:21597. https://doi.org/10.1038/srep21597.
52. Takamochi K, Ohmiya H, Itoh M, Mogushi K, Saito T, Hara K, et al. Novel biomarkers that assist in accurate discrimination of squamous cell carcinoma from adenocarcinoma of the lung. BMC Cancer. 2016;16(1):760. https://doi.org/10.1186/s12885-016-2792-1.
53. Bowser MJ, Duffy-Hynes E, Mahanta LM, Rehm HL, Raby BA, Funke BH. Integrating genetics into subspecialty care: The PulmoGene Test - comprehensive testing for hereditary causes of lung disease. Immunologic and genetic biomarkers of inflammatory lung disease American Thoracic Society International Conference, 16–21 May 2014, San Diego, CA, USA, A2175.
54. McCarty CA, Chisholm RL, Chute CG, Kullo IJ, Jarvik GP, Larson EB, et al. The eMERGE network: a consortium of biorepositories linked to electronic medical records data for conducting genomic studies. BMC Med Genet. 2011;4:13. https://doi.org/10.1186/1755-8794-4-13.

Chapter 18
Nucleic Acid Amplification-Based Diagnostics for Pulmonary Diseases: What Is the Current State and Perspectives of Nucleic Acid Amplification Technologies Used in Diagnostics Associated with Pulmonary Diseases?

Oleg Gusev, Yoshihide Hayashizaki, and Kengo Usui

Abstract Rapid advances of genomic technologies in medical sciences resulted in growth of identified molecular biomarkers, including those required for proper drug administration and therapy selection in pulmonary diseases. While high-throughput technologies are powerful tool for wide screening, targeted real-time monitoring using nucleic acid amplification is still the most important method for DNA and RNA detection widely employed in clinical diagnostics. In this chapter, we overview the key nucleic acid amplification platforms successfully used in the clinical diagnostics, including that associated with pulmonary diseases, and briefly outline their advantages and pitfalls. We further focus on the specific isothermal amplification technology SmartAmp and Eprobes developed by RIKEN outlining its implementation in quick and robust detection of several clinically important SNP and cancer-associated somatic mutations. Finally, we describe the further potential of expansion of utilization of Eprobes platform for direct protein detection for clinical diagnostic needs.

O. Gusev
RIKEN Preventive Medicine and Diagnosis Innovation Program, Kanagawa, Japan

KFU-RIKEN Translational Genomics Unit, RIKEN Innovation Center, Kanagawa, Japan

Institute of Fundamental Medicine and Biology, Kazan Federal University, Kazan, Russia

Y. Hayashizaki
RIKEN Preventive Medicine and Diagnosis Innovation Program, Kanagawa, Japan

K. Usui (✉)
Genetic Diagnosis Technology Unit, RIKEN Center for Integrative Medical Sciences, Kanagawa, Japan
e-mail: kengo.usui@riken.jp

T. Kaneko (ed.), *Clinical Relevance of Genetic Factors in Pulmonary Diseases*, Respiratory Disease Series: Diagnostic Tools and Disease Managements,
https://doi.org/10.1007/978-981-10-8144-6_18

Keywords Nucleic acid amplification · Clinical diagnostics
Companion diagnostics

18.1 Introduction

Variety of biological molecules of metabolized products in the body is used for evaluation of our health by mean of analysis of blood and other derivatives. These molecules called "biomarkers" are measured quantitatively from the human specimens, allowing to assess or predict health conditions or pathogenesis of diseases by comparing with reference value. Along with classical biochemical and metabolic biomarkers, genomic sequence-based human-inherited factors have been dramatically investigated to become novel biomarkers, after the completion of Human Genome Project [1, 2]. The genomic variations such as single-nucleotide polymorphisms (SNPs) associated with several diseases were identified by the clinical cohort assays of genome-wide association study (GWAS) with SNP tilling array. Recently, rise of next-generation sequencing technologies (NGS) paves for speedy comprehensive analysis of genomic data. Current registered in 1000 Genomes Project number of SNPs exceeds 150 million records [1]. NGS contributes to identify not only hereditary variants but also novel cancer-specific somatic mutation (cancer driver mutation) from the cancer cell or tissue-derived genomic DNA. In fact, over four million mutations were described in the Catalogue of Somatic Mutations in Cancer (COSMIC), release v78 [3].

While we observe drastic accumulation of information on genomic variations associated with human diseases (reviewed in Chap. 17 of this book), one should note that analyzing of whole genome information for routine diagnosis of each patient may not be unrealistic due to time and money cost issues. Additionally, overload of complicated genomic information has a risk causing delay in making decision for personalized medical strategy. Therefore, target genetic technologies for time and cost-effective analyzing well-evaluated and annotated in relation to certain disease, individual SNP, mutation, or pathogen RNA/DNA are essential for routine medical use. Notably, the Food and Drug Administration (FDA) requires or recommends gene diagnosis for constantly increasing list of drugs (186 titles as of April, 2017) before actual medication to prevent individual adverse effects and to optimize effective dose volume.

18.2 Nucleic Acid Amplification Technologies

In approaches focused on a single nucleotide variation (SNV), or limited genome re-arrangements as biomarkers, nucleic acid amplification methods are the optimal solution, due to the highest specificity targeted on the unique sequence from a tiny amount of sample volume, such as a drop of blood. The key and the most adapted technique for amplification of nucleic acids for its further visualization has long been and still is the polymerase chain reaction (PCR), based on the thermal cycling equipment and some mechanism of amplification detection, either through post-reaction electrophoresis or real-time monitoring (e.g., fluorometry discussed further in this chapter).

Remarkably, utilization of diagnostic nucleic acid amplification has already expanded out of specialized diagnostics laboratories, driven by improvements in cost and evolving new amplification techniques for wider access [4]. Among the directions, the active employment of sequence-specific isothermal nucleic acid amplification is a promising alternative to classical PCR allowing, in principle, to eliminate the need for even basic laboratory equipment in favor of stand-alone diagnostic devices. Examples of the methods using this approach include strand-displacement amplification (SDA) [5], nucleic acid sequence-based amplification (NASBA) [6], helicase-dependent amplification (HDA) [7], loop-mediated isothermal amplification (LAMP) [8], recombinase polymerase amplification (RPA) [9], and Smart Amplification Process (SmartAmp) [10, 11].

Here, we introduce detailed mechanism of an isothermal amplification taking SmartAmp as an example. SmartAmp employs a combination of two primers designed asymmetrically with different motifs on the tails, which primers are called as turn-back primer (TP) and folding primer (FP). The TP tail has a complementary sequence of downstream of TP annealing region (Fig. 18.1). At the same time, FP has an artificial hairpin sequence as the tail sequence. While the TP tail hybridizes newly synthesized DNA from TP and forms step-loop at the end of amplicon, FP tail forms a hairpin structure by itself. DNA amplification process in SmartAmp system includes two steps: the first step push the aiming sequence to be flanked on

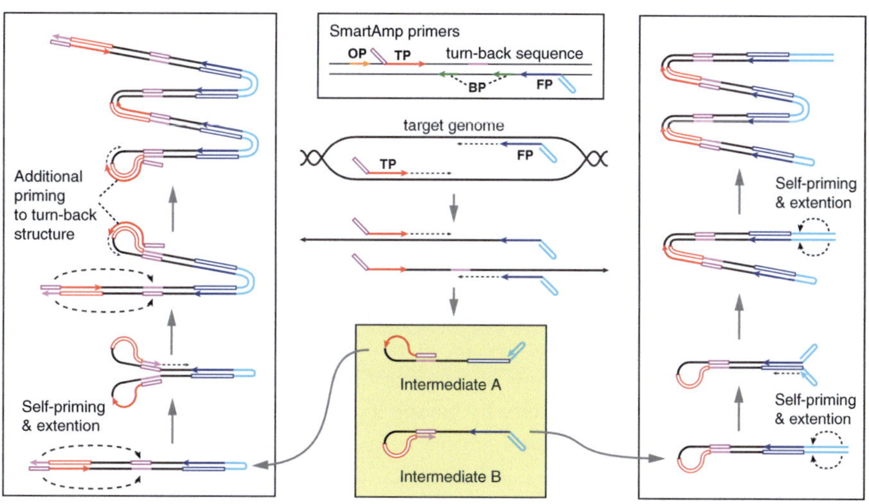

Fig. 18.1 Main reaction pathway of SmartAmp. TP, turn-back primer; FP, folding primer; BP, boost primer; OP, outer primer

3′ and 5′ ends with fold-back domains providing self-priming ability; and then the key intermediate products undergo repeated self-priming and target amplification with strand-displacement DNA polymerase (*Aac* DNA polymerase I) producing concatenated, primer inclusive amplification products. In addition, SmartAmp employs background suppression technology to increase specificity with boost primer (BP) and its hybridization-mediated fluorescence primer (see Sect. 18.3) and, thus, allowing an "amplification is detection" assay use. Among other amplification technologies, SmartAmp has one of the highest specificities, high sensitivity (as low as 10 copies), and strong amplification (100-fold larger than PCR), allowing detection of target DNA even in crude cell lysate such as a drop of the blood. This combination of features make SmartAmp technology a promising platform for utilization in point-of-care (POC) and over-the-counter (OTC) diagnostic devices, as one can expect less than an hour turnover time from taking biopsy to DNA/RNA analysis result.

18.3 Fluorogenic Oligonucleotide Probe-Based Solutions

Double-stranded DNA (dsDNA)-specific intercalating dyes, such as *SYBR Green I*, are widely used to evaluate the result of DNA amplification [12]. Designed for sensitive diagnostics, the main components of real-time PCR instruments are the thermal controlling system, excitation light source, photodetector, and excitation/detection filters. In the process of real-time PCR, intensity of DNA amplification is reflected by alteration of fluorescence intensity, resulting in amplification curve of sigmoid shape. The timing of uprising amplification curve in the studied sample depends on initiate copy numbers of template DNA. Using this dynamic, quantitative PCR (qPCR) allows quantitative analyses of DNA in the studied sample by comparing the curve with that derived from control DNA.

Furthermore, a real-time PCR instrument can perform DNA melting analysis after the amplification reaction. This assay allows assessing amplified product size based on Tm value from fluorescence melting curve [13]. At the same time, SYBR green-based real-time PCR has some remarkable technical disadvantages. The most important issue here is the association of the dye with any amplified dsDNA including false-positive amplified products such as primer dimer. Therefore, in this case, preparing highly specific PCR primers is critical.

Alternatively, highly specific results in real-time PCR or other amplification method can be achieved by using fluorogenic oligonucleotide probes (Fig. 18.1). The probes allow higher specificity by having a part of internal sequence of amplified region (amplicon) [14]. Each fluorophore in such probes is designed so that the alteration of florescence signal is taking place only after the hybridization of the probe to the amplicon. *TaqMan probes (Thermo Fisher Scientific)*, for example, utilize 5′-end conjugated reporter fluorophore and 3′-end quenching dye for the targeting oligonucleotide (Fig. 18.2a) [15]. The probes produce the fluorescence

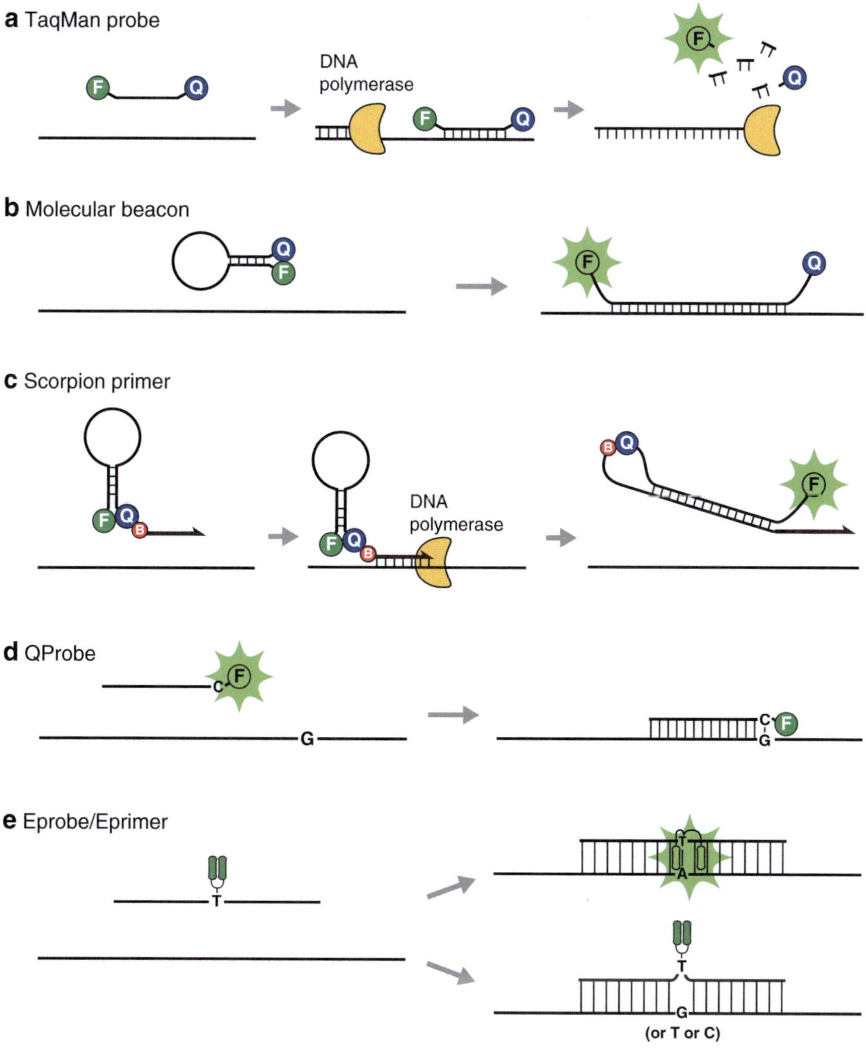

Fig. 18.2 Schematic model of the fluorogenic oligonucleotide probes. F, fluorophore; Q, quenching dye; B, PCR-blocking linker (**a**) TaqMap probe; (**b**) Molecular beacon; (**c**) Scorpion primer; (**d**) QProbe; (**e**) Eprobe/Eprimer

signal from the hydrolysis of the probe by 5′- to 3′-exonuclease activity of DNA polymerase. Hydrolysis of hybridized probe releases the fluorophore from the quenching dye; thus, the fluorescence signal increases with a progression of the amplification.

Molecular Beacon probes, an alternative solution, also contain 5′-end conjugated reporter fluorophore and 3′-end quenching dye [16]. At the same time, the probe has longer, compared to that of TaqMan one, oligonucleotide sequence and forms stem-loop structure by itself [17]. Two dyes are kept in close proximity and the fluorescence is quenched by energy transfer. In a process of hybridization of Molecular Beacon with the target sequence, the fluorophore separates enough from quenching dye by formation of loop sequence/target-dsDNA, and target-specific fluorescence signal is derived (Fig. 18.2b).

Scorpion primer is a fluorescent primer conjugating Molecular Beacon-like stem-loop fluorogenic probe to the 5′ end of the primer [18]. Difference of such primer from Molecular Beacon is that the loop-sequence self-hybridizes to newly synthesized DNA strand from 3′ end of primer by DNA polymerase and the fluorescence signal is appeared. Scorpion primer contains hexamethylene glycol linker between stem-loop probe and primer segments, where the linker prevents synthesis of complementary DNA strand for the stem-loop segment. Therefore, the fluorescence signal causes only self-hybridization after DNA synthesis of the amplicon, and the blocking linker plays a role of preventing primer-dimer-based false-positive signal generation (Fig. 18.2c).

QProbe employs the opposite approach to obtaining upraised by amplification fluorescent signal. The probe design is simple: the fluorophore is conjugated at either 5′ or 3′ end of an oligonucleotide. The fluorophore used for QProbe is BODIPY® FL (4,4-difluoro-5,7-dimethyl-4-bora-3a,4a-diaza-s-indacene-3-propionic acid). The fluorophore is diminished by the interaction with a guanine (G) base on the hybridized targeted DNA. Therefore, quenching rate of the fluorescence increase along with DNA amplification (Fig. 18.2d).

Eprobe/Eprimer is an exciton-controlled hybridization-sensitive fluorescent oligonucleotide (ECHO) containing two DNA-intercalating dye moieties (e.g., thiazole orange) conjugated to single nucleotide (thymidine base) in an oligonucleotide (Fig. 18.2e) [19, 20]. When in the single-stranded form, its fluorescent signal is strongly suppressed by an excitonic interaction between the dyes. Upon hybridization of the Eprobe to a complementary target DNA strand, the dyes are separated and intercalate into the double-strand leading to strong fluorescence signal. Intercalation of dyes can further stabilize the DNA/DNA hybrid and increase the melting temperature compared to standard DNA oligonucleotides [21]. This feature of Eprobe opens opportunities to use this type of probes in clamping oligonucleotide-based applications such as peptide nucleic acids (PNA) or locked nucleic acids (LNA) (see Sect. 18.4.1).

18.4 Clinical Applications by the Nucleic Acid Amplification with Fluorogenic Oligonucleotide Probe and Eprimer/Eprobe

As described above, several nucleic acid amplification methods and fluorogenic oligonucleotide probes were developed for genomic biomarker detection. In this section, examples of diagnostic applications by the nucleic acid amplification combined with Eprimer or Eprobe as a fluorophore oligonucleotide probe are introduced for each kinds of the biomarker.

18.4.1 Somatic Point Mutation Detection in Cancer

Cancer driver mutations often affect effectiveness of the anticancer drugs, and its detection assists the appropriate dosing decision of the drug or preventing adverse effect for individual cancer patients. However, the tumor or blood specimens used for isolation of genomic DNA include not only cancer cell but also healthy one; therefore, highly sensitive and specific detection method for the target mutation is required. To achieve specific detection, suppression technologies of PCR amplification from wild-type genomic DNA by using "clamping oligonucleotide" such as LNA and PNA were developed [22, 23].

Recently, Atsumi et al. developed novel highly sensitive detection method for somatic mutations: "Eprobe-clamping PCR" (Fig. 18.3) [24]. In the method, Eprobe is designed to be a full-match sequence for reference wild-type genome. Additionally, the probe has competitive sequence against 3′ terminal sequence either forward or reverse primers (reverse primer in Fig. 18.3). In case of wild-type genome, Eprobe strongly hybridizes to the genome and inhibits annealing of reverse primer. On the other hand, since the probe against mutated genome makes mismatch at the target SNP, the hybridization is unstable and allows the DNA synthesis from reverse primer. In this condition, amplified products from mutated genome are accumulated in the reaction. After the amplification, Eprobe also plays a role of fluorogenic oligonucleotide, and following results of melting curve analysis can identify existence of the mutation with high sensitivity.

In fact, Atsumi et al. applied the method to detection of *KRAS* codon 12 and 13 mutations [24]. By combining Eprobe-clamping PCR method and high-resolution melting curve analysis based on Rotor-Gene Q system (QIAGEN), they achieved high sensitivity for detecting at least 0.05% mutation ratio. In the results of clinical

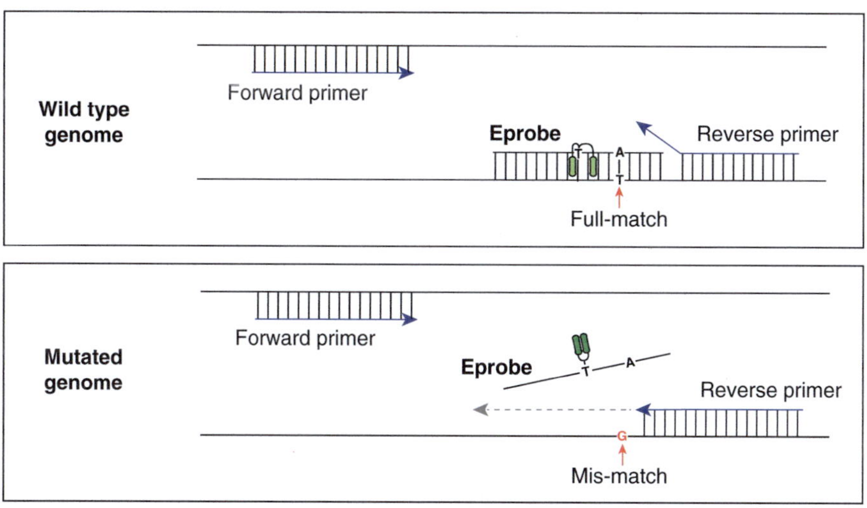

Fig. 18.3 Mechanism of Eprobe-clamping PCR

study with 92 genomic DNA derived from frozen tumor specimens, the method could dramatically improve the mutation detection level, which detected 33/92 mutated samples (36%), whereas Sanger sequencing identified mutation in 20 samples (22%).

18.4.2 HER2 12-bp Duplicated Insertion Detection in Lung Cancer

Somatic mutations in the cancer cells or tissues are represented not only by point mutation but also by insertion/deletion (indel) mutations. The frameshift or in-frame patterns are caused by indel mutations at the protein-coding region, and the cancer-signaling pathway often activates by lose of function or gain of function of the expressed proteins from such the mutated genes.

Human epidermal growth factor 2 (HER2) is one of typical biomarker proteins in breast cancer. The HER2 protein is overexpressed on the cell membrane and triggers progression of the breast cancer [25]. On the other hand, lung cancer-specific insertion mutation in *HER2* gene is also reported [26]. The mutation causing 12 base pair insertion at exon 20 of the gene results in four amino acid residue duplication, Tyr-Val-Met-Ala, in the sequence of expressed protein. A previous study demonstrated that anti-HER2 drug used for treatment of breast cancer, trastuzumab, had highly disease control rate of 93% with *HER2* 12-bp duplicated insertion mutation [27]. Therefore, detection of the insertion mutation in the biopsy of lung cancer patients is promising to suggest about efficacy of trastuzumab for lung cancer treatment.

As a diagnosis tool for *HER2* 12-bp duplicated insertion, Takese et al. developed highly sensitive mutation analysis by Eprobe-mediated PCR method (Eprobe-PCR) [28]. The method avoided wild-type-dependent amplification result by combining insertion-specific PCR primers and *HER2*-exon 20-specific Eprobe, and then at least 0.1% mutation detection was achieved. In clinical study for 446 of the lung adenocarcinoma, Eprobe-PCR could detect the *HER2* mutation in 2.02% (9/446), while Sanger sequencing detected it in 1.57% (7/446) only. Additionally, the authors revealed via detection of Eprobe-PCR that the insertion mutation was not found in any other lung cancer type tested (squamous cell carcinoma, adenosquamous carcinoma, small-cell lung cancer, and large-cell neuroendocrine carcinoma).

18.4.3 Detection of SNPs in the MDM2 Gene by Using the Duplex SmartAmp Method

For SNP genotyping, the PCR technology with fluorogenic probe such as TaqMan has been generally developed. On the other hand, several isothermal nucleic acid amplification technologies have been mainly applied for infectious diseases identification because of its performance of rapid amplification. In our study, there was a following example of development of the rapid SNP genotyping by using one of isothermal amplification method "SmartAmp" with Eprimer.

One of genetic polymorphisms in the human *MDM2* gene is a tumor susceptibility marker and a prognostic factor for cancer. Enokida et al. have investigated an c.309T>G SNP in the *MDM2* gene, which attenuates the tumor suppressor activity of p53 and accelerates tumor formation in humans. To detect this SNP, the authors have developed a new SNP detection method with two different colored exciton dye-labeled primers (Eprimers) for each variant (309T and 309G, respectively). The method, named Duplex SmartAmp, enables us to simultaneously detect both alleles in one tube and to detect them directly in a small amount of genomic DNA or blood sample [29]. The authors, then, confirmed effectiveness of Duplex SmartAmp by comparing the results derived from 96 genomic DNA and 24 blood samples to those obtained by using the conventional PCR-restriction fragment length polymorphism (RFLP) method; the results of both methods were in a full agreement. In the clinical setting, Duplex SmartAmp can be used to detect c.309T>G in the *MDM2* gene to assess a patient's cancer susceptibility and that the method enables rapid clinical diagnosis with larger number of samples.

18.4.4 Other Types of Molecular Biomarkers Analysis by Nucleic Amplification Method: Protein Detection Via PLA Assay

Remarkably, the methods originally developed for nucleic acid detection can be successfully employed for detection other types of biomolecules, including proteins.

Heme oxygenase 1 (HO-1) is one of the oxidative stress-responsive enzymes. The enzyme catalyzes the initial rate-limiting step in the oxidative degradation of heme to bilirubin. The reaction of HO-1 with heme releases iron and carbon monoxide, which can be measured in exhaled breath and has been shown to be elevated in patients with COPD; therefore, quantitative analyses of the protein are useful for suggesting COPD as protein biomarker.

ELISA is generally used for measurement of the protein level. However, limit of detection is often lower than clinical needs [30]. Söderberg et al. have recently developed a new approach for highly sensitive protein detection method called proximity ligation assay (PLA), which is combined antibody-based target protein detection with DNA amplification [31] (Fig. 18.4a). The assay uses three antibodies recognizing one target protein. One antibody (3rd antibody in Fig. 18.4a) is conjugated to magnetic beads, and the other two antibodies (1st and 2nd antibodies in Fig. 18.4a) each carry a single-stranded DNA probe. First, when the DNA probe-conjugated antibodies bind to the target protein, their terminal ends come into close proximity. Second, a splint oligo hybridizes both ends, the two DNA probes are ligated by T4 ligase and a linear single-stranded DNA template consisted of the two

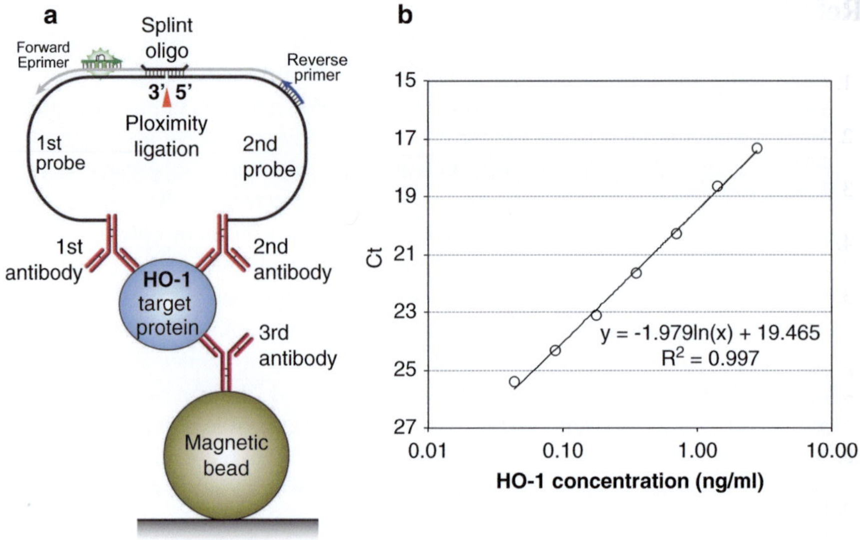

Fig. 18.4 PCR-mediated proximity ligation assay (PCR-PLA) for HO-1 detection. (**a**) Schematic model of PLA. After proximity ligation reaction by T4 ligase at splint oligo-hybridized 5′ or 3′ end of the probes (indicated a red arrow head), PCR is performed with Forward-Eprimer and reverse primer. Since Forward-Eprimer anneals synthetic DNA strand (gray line) from reverse primer only, there is no fluorescent signal before the PCR amplification. (**b**) Result of in vitro quantitative detection for HO-1 by PCR-PLA. In the graph, Y axis indicates crossing point (Cp) of real-time PCR analysis

probes is produced. Third, captured target-protein complexes are accumulated and isolated by the 3rd antibody conjugated to magnetic beads. Finally, positive fluorescence signal after Eprobe-mediated PCR indicates the existence of the target protein. In the in vitro feasibility study for HO-1 protein quantitative detection, the assay achieved high sensitivity (>50 pg/ml, i.e., >0.9 pM) and good linearity of quantification (0.5–5.0 ng/ml, $r^2 > 0.99$) (Fig. 18.4b, our unpublished data).

18.5 Conclusion

Despite the development of effective next-generation sequencing methods, allowing high-throughput genomic analysis of clinical samples and targeted gene diagnostics, based on nucleic acid amplification, remains to be a key tool in laboratory diagnostics. There is obvious decrease of running cost and turnover (from biological sample to the result of analysis) time, as well as promising improvement in sensitivity and robustness of amplification methods and probes. In the next decade, we expect to observe further active development of POCT- and OTC-based gene diagnostic solutions, to cope with rapid progress in genetic aspects of personalized medicine.

References

1. Genomes Project C, Auton A, Brooks LD, Durbin RM, Garrison EP, Kang HM, et al. A global reference for human genetic variation. Nature. 2015;526(7571):68–74.
2. Lele RD. The human genome project: its implications in clinical medicine. J Assoc Physicians India. 2003;51:373–80.
3. Forbes SA, Beare D, Boutselakis H, Bamford S, Bindal N, Tate J, et al. COSMIC: somatic cancer genetics at high-resolution. Nucleic Acids Res. 2017;45(D1):D777–D83.
4. Craw P, Balachandran W. Isothermal nucleic acid amplification technologies for point-of-care diagnostics: a critical review. Lab Chip. 2012;12(14):2469–86.
5. Spargo CA, Fraiser MS, VanCleve M, Wright DJ, Nycz CM, Spears PA, et al. Detection of M-tuberculosis DNA using thermophilic strand displacement amplification. Mol Cell Probes. 1996;10(4):247–56.
6. Compton J. Nucleic acid sequence-based amplification. Nature. 1991;350(6313):91–2.
7. Vincent M, Xu Y, Kong H. Helicase-dependent isothermal DNA amplification. EMBO Rep. 2004;5(8):795–800.
8. Notomi T, Okayama H, Masubuchi H, Yonekawa T, Watanabe K, Amino N, et al. Loop-mediated isothermal amplification of DNA. Nucleic Acids Res. 2000;28(12)
9. Piepenburg O, Williams CH, Stemple DL, Armes NADNA. Detection using recombination proteins. PLoS Biol. 2006;4(7):1115–21.
10. Mitani Y, Lezhava A, Kawai Y, Kikuchi T, Oguchi-Katayama A, Kogo Y, et al. Rapid SNP diagnostics using asymmetric isothermal amplification and a new mismatch-suppression technology. Nat Methods. 2007;4(3):257–62.
11. Mitani Y, Lezhava A, Sakurai A, Horikawa A, Nagakura M, Hayashizaki Y, et al. Rapid and cost-effective SNP detection method: application of SmartAmp2 to pharmacogenomics research. Pharmacogenomics. 2009;10(7):1187–97.
12. Chang HS, Mizukami K, Yabuki A, Hossain MA, Rahman MM, Uddin MM, et al. A novel rapid genotyping technique for collie eye anomaly: SYBR green-based real-time polymerase chain reaction method applicable to blood and saliva specimens on flinders technology associates filter paper. J Vet Diagn Investig. 2010;22(5):708–15.
13. Elenitoba-Johnson KSJ, Bohling SD, Wittwer CT, King TC. Multiplex PCR by multicolor fluorimetry and fluorescence melting curve analysis. Nat Med. 2001;7(2):249–53.
14. Juskowiak B. Nucleic acid-based fluorescent probes and their analytical potential. Anal Bioanal Chem. 2011;399(9):3157–76.
15. Arikawa E, Sun Y, Wang J, Zhou Q, Ning B, Dial SL, et al. Cross-platform comparison of SYBR green real-time PCR with TaqMan PCR, microarrays and other gene expression measurement technologies evaluated in the MicroArray quality control (MAQC) study. BMC Genomics. 2008;9:328.
16. Tyagi S, Kramer FR. Molecular beacons: probes that fluoresce upon hybridization. Nat Biotechnol. 1996;14(3):303–8.
17. Tapp I, Malmberg L, Rennel E, Wik M, Syvanen AC. Homogeneous scoring of single-nucleotide polymorphisms: comparison of the 5 '-nuclease TaqMan (R) assay and molecular beacon probes (vol 28, pg 732, 2000). BioTechniques. 2000;29(3):546.
18. Whitcombe D, Kelly S, Mann J, Theaker J, Jones C, Little S. Scorpions (TM) primers - a novel method for use in single-tube genotyping. Am J Hum Genet. 1999;65(4):A412.
19. Okamoto A. ECHO probes: a concept of fluorescence control for practical nucleic acid sensing. Chem Soc Rev. 2011;40(12):5815–28.
20. Hanami T, Delobel D, Kanamori H, Tanaka Y, Kimura Y, Nakasone A, et al. Eprobe mediated real-time PCR monitoring and melting curve analysis. PLoS One. 2013;8(8)
21. Kimura Y, Hanami T, Tanaka Y, de Hoon MJL, Soma T, Harbers M, et al. Effect of thiazole orange doubly labeled thymidine on DNA duplex formation. Biochemistry. 2012;51(31):6056–67.
22. Murdock DG, Wallace DC. PNA-mediated PCR clamping. Applications and methods. Methods Mol Biol. 2002;208:145–64.

23. Efrati E, Elkin H, Peerless Y, Sabo E, Ben-Izhak O, Hershkovitz D, LNA-based PCR. Clamping enrichment assay for the identification of KRAS mutations. Cancer Biomark. 2010;8(2):89–94.
24. Atsumi J, Hanami T, Enokida Y, Ogawa H, Delobel D, Mitani Y, et al. Eprobe-mediated screening system for somatic mutations in the KRAS locus. Oncol Rep. 2015;33(6):2719–27.
25. Mitri Z, Constantine T, O'Regan R. The HER2 receptor in breast cancer: pathophysiology, clinical use, and new advances in therapy. Chemother Res Pract. 2012;2012:743193.
26. Arcila ME, Chaft JE, Nafa K, Roy-Chowdhuri S, Lau C, Zaidinski M, et al. Prevalence, clinicopathologic associations, and molecular spectrum of ERBB2 (HER2) tyrosine kinase mutations in lung adenocarcinomas. Clin Cancer Res. 2012;18(18):4910–8.
27. Mazieres J, Peters S, Lepage B, Cortot AB, Barlesi F, Beau-Faller M, et al. Lung cancer that harbors an HER2 mutation: epidemiologic characteristics and therapeutic perspectives. J Clin Oncol. 2013;31(16):1997–U307.
28. Takase Y, Usui K, Shimizu K, Kimura Y, Ichihara T, Ohkawa T, et al. Highly sensitive detection of a HER2 12-base pair duplicated insertion mutation in lung cancer using the Eprobe-PCR method. PLoS One. 2017;12(2):e0171225.
29. Enokida Y, Shimizu K, Atsumi J, Lezhava A, Tanaka Y, Kimura Y, et al. Rapid detection of SNP (c.309T > G) in the MDM2 gene by the duplex SmartAmp method. PLoS One. 2013;8(4)
30. Bayer PM, Fabian B, Hubl W. Immunofluorescence assays (IFA) and enzyme-linked immunosorbent assays (ELISA) in autoimmune disease diagnostics - technique, benefits, limitations and applications. Scand J Clin Lab Invest Suppl. 2001;61:68–76.
31. Soderberg O. Detection of proteins and their interactions by proximity-ligation. Chromosom Res. 2007;15:2–3.